In Praise of *Nutraerobics*:

"*Nutraerobics* could be the nutritional Bible of the 80s."
—*Your Good Health*

"Loaded with charts, tables, and simple self tests, *Nutraerobics*, in a clear and enjoyable style, is a complete guide to healthy eating."
—*East West Journal*

"*Nutraerobics* is a good general discussion and guide to the benefits of an improved lifestyle . . . . Recommended."
—*Library Journal*

"*Nutraerobics* cannot be read passively, as Bland constantly challenges the reader with hard facts, probing inquiries, common situations one can identify with (from stress, low energy, muscle weakness and fatigue to proper weight management) . . . . He gives practical solutions on how to overcome these conditions. This is the book to read when you have decided your life requires a change and you're ready to face an honest health appraisal."
—*Total Health*

"*Nutraerobics* is a comprehensive preventative health plan. Bland's commonsense approach is thorough and well documented."
—*Publishers Weekly*

"Just the book for those of us who . . . can stand up, look down and no longer see our shoes . . . . *Nutraerobics* is a personalized system of diet and exercise designed for the prevention of the diseases that ail modern people. The plan recognizes that we are all different, both in body type and the condition in which we begin a health program . . . . Dr. Bland's book is as much a workbook as it is an introduction to the latest studies of nutrition and fitness . . . . it tells what you can (must) do in order to achieve optimum health through a balanced program of nutrition, exercise and vitamin supplements."
—Tom Carter, *The Washington Times*

NUTRA

EROBICS

**The
Complete
Individualized
Nutrition and Fitness Program**

Jeffrey Bland, Ph.D.

1817

Harper & Row, Publishers, San Francisco

Cambridge, Hagerstown, New York, Philadelphia
London, Mexico City, São Paulo, Sydney

Designed by Paul Quin
Illustrations by Barry Geller

Library of Congress Cataloging in Publication Data
Bland, Jeffrey, 1946–
    Nutraerobics : the complete nutrition and fitness program for life after thirty.
    Includes index.
    1. Nutrition.   2. Nutritionally induced diseases.
3. Middle age—Health and hygiene.   I. Title.
RA784.B56   1983   613.2   83–47716
ISBN 0–06–250053–8
ISBN 0–06–250054–6 (pbk.)

88 89 10 9 8 7 6 5 4 3 2

To all the B's who sacrificed—
thanks to P, K, K, and the newest, JB

Contents

List of Figures and Tables   x

Preface   xi

Acknowledgments   xiii

1 Another Health Book?   1
What Is Vertical Disease? · What Is the **Aerobics** in Nutraerobics? · Benefits of the Nutraerobics Program · Specializing in Health Care · Risk Factor Intervention · Notes

2 Assessing Your Biotype   11
Genetotype Questionnaire · Interpretation of the Genetotype Questionnaire · Stress Indicator Questionnaire · Interpretation of the Stress Indicator Questionnaire · Physical Evaluation Questionnaire · Interpretation of the Physical Evaluation Questionnaire · Dietary Evaluation Questionnaire · Interpretation of the Dietary Evaluation Questionnaire · Symptoms Evaluation Questionnaire · Interpretation of the Symptoms Evaluation Questionnaire · Summarizing Your Biotype · Biotype Summary Worksheet · Notes

3 Assigning Your Unique Nutritional Needs   53
Optimal Versus Adequate Nutrition · The Changing U.S. Diet · Vitamins and Minerals as Supplements · The Empty-Calorie Diet · Food Fortification · Historical Diet Habits · Marginal Undernutrition · Recognizing Your Nutritional Status · Toxicity of Vitamins · Nutrients as Therapeutic Agents · The Test of Success · Notes

4 The Aging Process: Life After 30   77
Testing Your Lifestyle · Does Function Decline with Age? · Determining Your Own Biological Age · Your View of Yourself and Your Health · The Medical Profession and Prevention · Nutraerobics and Aging · Vitamins and Minerals and the Aging Process · Memory Loss and Nutraerobics · Aging Pigments and Nutraerobics · The B Vitamins and Aging · Immunity and Aging · Toxic Minerals and Aging · Blood Pressure and Aging · Notes

5 Emotions, Fatigue, or Lack of Sleep Got the Best of You?   103
Neurotransmitters and Diet · Personality Disorders and Diet · Orthomolecular Psychiatry · Strengths and Weaknesses of the Orthomolecular Model · A Case Study of Orthomolecular Control · Your Biotype and Personality Disorders · Learning Ability and Nervous System Disorders · Cerebral Allergy · Depression Management · Hormones and Behavior · Blood Sugar and Mood · The Use of Dietary Gums and Fibers · Chromium and Its Effect on Blood Sugar · Long-Term Effects of Poor Blood Sugar Control · Toxic Elements and Brain Chemistry · Seizure Disorders and Taurine · Conclusions of Your Biotype · Notes

6 Overweight or Underweight?   133

Genetics and Weight Problems · Designing a Weight Control Program · Some Causes
and Effects of Obesity · Approaches to Weight Loss · Thermodynamics of Weight Loss
· Lean Body Mass · Keeping the Weight Off · Brown Fat · Thyroid and Weight Gain
· Diet, Exercise, and Brown Fat · Appetite and Appetite Problems · The Use of Fiber
to Supplement Appetite · Nutrients and Appetite · The "Diet" · The Protein-Sparing
Modified Fast · The Safe Approach to Dieting · Exercise and Dieting · The Plateau ·
Vitamins and Minerals · Underweight Problems · Notes

7 Heart Disease and Nutraerobics   165

Determining Heart Disease Risk Factors · Lifestyle Changes and Heart Disease · The
MRFIT Study · Target of the Nutraerobics Program · Diet and HDL Cholesterol ·
Other Risk Factors · Treatment of Existing Heart Problems · Exercise as Therapy ·
Diet as Therapy · Eggs and Heart Disease · Meat Consumption and Cholesterol · Fiber
and Cholesterol · What Type of Cooking Oil? · Eskimos and Heart Disease · Minerals
and Heart Disease · Trace Elements and Heart Disease · Vitamins, Accessory
Nutrients, and Heart Disease · Summary Review · Notes

8 Cancer and Your Biotype   195

Cancers of Affluence · Cancer and the Environment · Recommendations to Reduce
Cancer · Treatment of Cancer · Alternative Cancer Therapies · Evaluating the
Treatment Options · Cause of Cancer · Lung Cancer Prevention · Nutrients and Cancer
Defense · Trace Elements and Cancer · Vitamin and Mineral Therapy · Vitamins and
Cancer · Breast Cancer and Nutraerobics · Digestive Cancers · Skin Cancer · Cancer
and Your Drinking Water · Summary of the Program · Notes

9 Male and Female Problems   225

Stress and Hormone Levels · Nutrients and Hormones · Women and Iron Deficiency
· Hypothyroidism and Women · Anorexia Nervosa and Bulimia · Premenstrual Tension
· Oral Contraceptives · Folic Acid and Cervical Dysplasia · Dysmenorrhea · Exercise
and Menstruation · Smoking and the Menses · Fibrocystic Disease · Other Nutrients
and the Female · Nutrition for Men · Infertility in Males · Wernicke-Korsakoff
Syndrome and Osteoarthritis · Prostate Problems · Light and Health · Notes

10 Bone Loss and Calcium Where It Shouldn't Be   249

Control of Calcium · Bone Loss and Aging · Calcium and Your Teeth · Vitamin D and
Your Bones · Calcium and Phosphorus Relationship · Protein and Bone Status ·
Calcium Allowance · Oral Health Effects of Calcium–Phosphorus Imbalance ·
Prevention of Tooth Loss · Osteoarthritis and Calcium · Other Nutrients in Bone
Formation · Zinc and Cavity Prevention · Osteoporosis and Calcium Therapy · Milk
Intolerance and Toxic Minerals · Fluoride and Bone Integrity · An Integrated
Approach to Bone Integrity · Exercise for Bone Integrity · Dr. Weston Price and Bone
Status · Notes

11 The Link Between Arthritis, Headache, and Intestinal Problems
269

Your Immune System · Problems with the Immune System · Water-Soluble Vitamins
and Immunity · Fat-Soluble Vitamins and Immunity · Minerals and Immunity · Protein
and Fats in Immunity · Immunity and Allergy · Migraine Headache and Allergy ·
Arthritis and Allergy · Immunity and Arthritis · Acquired Immunodeficiency
Syndrome (AIDS) · Stress and Immunity · Notes

12 Protecting the Unborn 287

Suboptimal Nutrition and Pregnancy · Factors Affecting Fetal Development · Diet and
Problem Pregnancy · Vitamin Supplementation During Pregnancy · Blood Sugar and
Fetal Development · Problems of Excessive Nutrients in Pregnancy · Calcium and
Toxemia of Pregnancy · Trace Elements and Pregnancy · Essential Fats and Pregnancy
· Protein and Pregnancy · Starting the Living Life Insurance Program · Notes

13 Children and Their Behaviors 307

The "Junk Food Syndrome" · Behavior and Biochemical Individuality · Vitamins and
Brain Function · Conditional Lethal Mutations · Intelligence and Vitamins · Nutrient
Excesses · Sugar and Its Influence on Behavior · Toxic Elements and Behavior ·
Preventing Lead Absorption · The "Feingold Diet" · Children as Indicators of Health
· Notes

14 Implementing Your Nutraerobics Program 327

The Health-Care Consumer · When to Implement the Program · The Environment and
Nutraerobics · Natural or New Is Not Always Healthy · The Importance of Exercise in
Nutraerobics · Balancing the Midline · How to Use Your Nutraerobics Program
Summary Checksheet · Nutraerobics Program Summary Checksheet · Going On to the
Next Step · Vision, Hair, and Skin · I-Centered Versus We-Centered · Putting It into
Perspective · A Case Study for Nutraerobics · Taking Responsibility for Your Health
· Notes

Index   353

List of Figures and Tables

Table 1: Drug–Nutrient Antagonism   31

Figure 1: Suggested Revisions of the Standard American Diet   56

Table 2: Ranges of Safe Daily Intakes of the Essential Vitamins and Minerals   72

Figure 2: Declining Lung Capacity with Age   84

Table 3: Assessing Your Biological Age After 30   86

Figure 3: Brown and White Rice Bread Enriched with Vegetable Gum   122

Figure 4: The Metabolic Weight Equation   140

Figure 5: Nomogram for Calculating Body Mass Index   142

Figure 6: Incidence of Heart Disease by State   168

Table 4: Summary of Aspects of Nutraerobics Heart Disease Management Program   190

Table 5: Highest Risk Factors to Cancer   199

Table 6: Summary of the Nutraerobics Program for Cancer Risk Reduction   219

Table 7: Range of Nutrients Required by Pregnant Women   302

Table 8: Daily Doses of Supplemental Vitamins and Minerals Used in Mental Retardation Study   314

Table 9: Additives and Foods to Be Eliminated in the Feingold Diet   324

Preface

Good health throughout our lives should be a reality, not a possibility. However, securing health is often obscured by our individual uniqueness. We are all individuals who have *no* duplicates. Each person's need to maximize his or her potential on this planet is different from everyone else's.

Charting a path to health through optimizing your strengths and minimizing your weaknesses is the objective of this book. You will design your own "living life insurance program," as you read through the book and learn of your biotype characteristics.

The Nutraerobics Program has been built upon the recent work of hundreds of scientific studies and clinical success in thousands of patients. The time you spend with this book will remove some of the mystery and confusion surrounding good health and give you tools for construction of your own health-promoting Nutraerobics Plan.

Acknowledgments

This book represents the collected feedback and thought-provoking discussions I have had with hundreds of scientists, researchers, and doctors at meetings, colloquies, and seminars, in print, and via the phone during the past three years. I deeply appreciate the stimulation provided by my colleagues and the many doctors who attended my meetings and seminars; the collected benefit of their experiences in health promotion made this book possible. I also thank the University of Puget Sound, and particularly the members of the Chemistry Department, for their understanding and support of my efforts in putting this book together.

The penetrating and constructively critical review of the manuscript by my agent, Susan Wray, was very important in the book's evolution and completion. The editorial expertise of Roy M. Carlisle, Kathy Reigstad, Ann Moru, and their associates at Harper & Row San Francisco was important in every phase of the development of the manuscript from the inception of the idea to its completion.

Lastly, two individuals deserve the most significant notes of commendation for their work "above and beyond." Mary Ludlow and Phyllis Hamilton (the hands behind the words) contributed more as my creative and organizational force than as secretaries. To them I am deeply indebted for their commitment to the completion of the manuscript in spite of the overwhelming whirl of the day to day.

Writing this book has made me keenly aware of the excitement of learning and our need to explore the frontier of knowledge. I thank my students for their contribution in not allowing me to get intellectually lazy and in reminding me that the horizon is always in front of us.

Jeffrey Bland
Tacoma, WA

Note

Before starting any fitness and nutrition program, check with your doctor to make sure it is appropriate for you to embark on the program you have in mind. Follow the instructions in this book carefully. Because this book is not intended as a source of medical advice, if you experience any distressing or unexpected reactions, however mild, while following this program, consult your doctor.

1

Another Health Book?

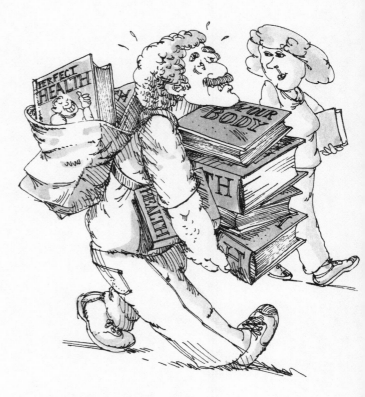

I JUST DON'T UNDERSTAND WHY I'M ALWAYS SO TIRED.

Do you:

1. Have frequent headaches or vision problems?

2. Feel overly tired or weak?

3. Have recurrent insomnia, bad dreams, or depression?

4. Find it difficult to concentrate or keep fully alert?

5. Fight to control your weight?

6. Have sore or swollen joints or muscles?

7. Feel that you are at high risk to heart attack?

8. Have high blood pressure?

9. Worry about a family history of cancer?

10. Wonder what optimal nutrition during pregnancy is?

11. Wish you could make some sense of all the nutrition information available today?

12. Wonder how to stay healthy after 30?

If so, then you may have what we call vertical disease, and this book is for you. It asks you to participate in the exercise of assessing your own health from which you will be able to identify specific ways of keeping yourself in good health or finding better health. The approach detailed in this book has proven successful for thousands of individuals who have committed themselves to the Nutraerobics Program.

What's different about this book from the hundreds of other health books on the market? By completing the questionnaires in this book, you will learn how to analyze your own needs and design your own personalized lifestyle-nutrition-exercise program. It will introduce you to the no-nonsense Nutraerobics Health Enhancement Program, which has helped reduce the biological age of thousands who have tried it. The information in this book is a result of hundreds of published clinical studies reported by researchers the past few years, as well as ten years of clinical experience with the program in many medical facilities. Life may not be prolonged by applying the information in this book, but the quality of life as measured by improved health will be increased.

Health is not a mystery; it's our most precious gift and needs to be nurtured and worked for. This book gives you the tools to get it and keep it. To be successful with this program you must be willing to honestly assess yourself by using the questionnaires provided. You will learn how to interpret your responses to the questionnaires, so you can formulate your own specific biotype—that set of biological characteristics that determines how your individual body works—from which the specific program to maximize your own good health will be developed.

What Is Vertical Disease?

Your responses to the questionnaires represent the first step in implementation of the Nutraerobics Program. This program represents a reasonably inexpensive, easily applied program for health improvement that shouldn't take much of your time. The basic premise of this program is that the absence of disease does not necessarily mean the presence of wellness. The Nutraerobics Program is designed to help improve wellness, even in people not yet diagnosed as sick. More people are suffering from undiagnosed vertical disease in this country than from diagnosed horizontal disease.

Vertical disease is the state in which an individual is living with fatigue, headaches, muscle weakness, a feeling of low energy, increased susceptibility to every new cold bug that comes around, digestive disorders, skin problems, insomnia, depression, or a variety of other symptoms that are traditionally treated as psychosomatic problems but may truly be early warning signs to later, more significant diseases. It is called vertical disease because persons with it are still standing upright, even though they are walking with stooped shoulders and shuffling feet, muttering, "When am I going to get sick enough that someone can do something for me?"

Vertical disease may be contrasted to horizontal disease. In horizontal disease you are lying flat on your back and someone looks down at you and says, "How do you feel?" You groan and say, "Not so good." This is the state in which you are symptomatically diagnosed as having a disease, and this is the time the medical community generally springs into action to help you to recover from the disease. The absence of horizontal disease does not necessarily mean the absence of vertical disease. The Nutraerobics Program is designed to identify contributors to vertical diseases and specify what components of an individual's lifestyle may be contributing to those early warning symptoms of something that, if unmanaged, may later become a diagnosed horizontal disease.

Most horizontal illnesses we are afflicted with today are members of what is called the **chronic degenerative disease family.** They include such conditions as heart disease, cancer, diabetes, emphysema, arthritis, and colitis. There are no known single causes of these diseases. They are characterized by several stages: an initiation phase, then a subclinical stage evincing a symptomatic health problem, and finally a diagnosed severe health difficulty. Most of modern medicine has focused on managing disease once diagnosed, while the Nutraerobics Program concentrates on arresting the course of the disease at its early stages. Loss of function precedes the diagnosed disease state. Conditions such as memory loss, accelerated aging, lowered sense of vitality, tiredness, and decreased immune defense are all associated with this preclinical state. Some people just call this aging, but it's really **accelerated** biological aging.

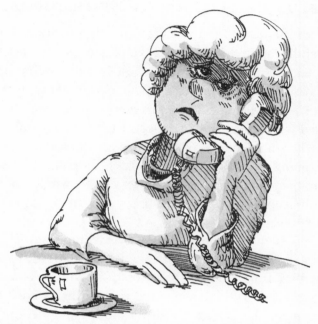

WHAT DO YOU MEAN, VERTICAL DISEASE? I'M PERFECTLY HEALTHY. I JUST DON'T FEEL WELL.

Biological age is a measure of your vital capacity and may not be equal to your actual chronological age. In fact, it is possible for you to be twenty or more years older or younger biologically than you are chronologically. (You will learn how to evaluate your biological age in Chapter 4.) We can each control our biological age to a great extent. As we reduce our biological age by implementing the Nutraerobics Program, we reduce our risk of contracting the major killer diseases. We can get better, rather than just older.

How can this happen? You must practice the Nutraerobics Program regularly; you must use self-discipline in making personal decisions. Just as you cannot become an expert tennis player without practice, neither can you succeed at the Nutraerobics approach to better health and younger biological age without commitment.

What Is the *Aerobics* in Nutraerobics?

The Nutraerobics Program uses specific nutrition, lifestyle, and exercise modification to maximize your aerobic potential. What is aerobic potential? Your body works best in maintaining health when your food, or "fuel," is converted efficiently to energy in the presence of adequate oxygen being delivered to every cell of your body. **Aerobics** is concerned with seeing that every cell has the opportunity to flourish in the presence of adequate oxygen. This is achieved not only through the conditioning effect of a proper exercise program, **but more importantly from the complete tune-up of every cell**—which the Nutraerobics Program accomplishes by adjusting your nutrition and lifestyle to your specific needs.

Aerobics is more than exercise. Everything you do to yourself, from eating to relaxing to being in stressful situations, has an impact on your aerobic functioning. The aerobics in Nutraerobics is there to remind you that everything suggested to you in this book is designed to help improve the efficiency with which you function, which increases with improved utilization of oxygen and your nutrition. You will note as you read the book that the concept of Nutraerobics takes you well beyond exercise or diet alone, and the program truly works, because of the synergy among its many components. If this program is applied in its entirety, the results will be much greater than those achieved by the individual components of exercise, diet, or lifestyle modification alone.

If you are ready to get started toward implementing your Nutraerobics Plan, the first step is to assess your general health. The questionnaires in Chapter 2 will help you to identify what areas in this book you most need to concentrate on, the areas in which you may uncover early warning signs of previously unknown health problems. Chapter by chapter you will be aided in identifying your own biotype and then designing and finally learning how to implement a specific Nutraerobics Program tailored for your need.

Benefits of the Nutraerobics Program

What type of improvements in health and function might result from implementation of the Nutraerobics Program? For one thing, even intelligence, which is thought to decline with aging, can be improved by implementation of the Nutraerobics Program. In one experiment a group with an average age of 70 was put through a program similar to the Nutraerobics Program and compared to a group of similar average age who did not implement the program. It was found that the trained group had a significant increase in intelligence as contrasted with the untrained group.[1]

Just by reading this book, you are stimulating patterns of thought, provoking intellectual activity. This concept underlies the success of the Nutraerobics Program—it is an action-oriented program that aggressively pursues good physical and intellectual health. Positive improvement from the program comes from doing. Just telling yourself each day, "It's my life and I'm going to make it healthy," is the best affirmation on the road to success with the Nutraerobics program.

Feelings of helplessness can rob you of your health. You need a program with objectives to stimulate your body's natural health-maintaining circuits. It has been found in experiments that animals suffer sudden death when forced to swim when there appears no escape, but provided with a hope for rescue, they can swim for prolonged periods of time.[2] Premature illness and early death can be related to a life with no positive options. The Nutraerobics Program provides a positive option for health. Many of us think aging is an inevitable process; we feel caught in an intractable battle with an incurable disease called aging which will rob from us the vitality and excitement of life.

Many of the aspects of aging are modifiable. When we see people who have aged chronologically without showing most of the "aging symptoms," it indicates how many of the characteristics we normally associate with aging can be postponed or eliminated by personal decisions. Most people accept the fact that aging brings loss of function and

—lo and behold—loss of function does occur because there is no positive approach to the other option. It is a self-fulfilling prophecy. What is the other option? Good health and vitality in mid to late life.

Specializing in Health Care

Now, given that there may be options available through the Nutraerobics Program for improving health and reducing the rate of biological aging, will these options necessitate strange behavior patterns and make us socially unacceptable in our community? Most of us don't want to become "health nuts" or full-time specialists in health care. Rather, what we would like is the time, energy, and health to do the things that we really enjoy doing—whether that's playing golf, learning computer programming, skiing, pursuing a second career, being a better parent, or just enjoying life in general. If we spend **all** our time becoming healthy, then we have no time left to do the things that we want to be healthy **for.**

The Nutraerobics Program is designed to reinforce subconscious patterns of behavior that will provide healthy options without taking up large amounts of time or requiring "strange" behaviors. Health improvement won from the implementation of the program by practice each day will more than pay dividends for the time spent on its mastery as you age with greater health.

Risk Factor Intervention

The underlying concept of the program is the new branch of health improvement called **early warning risk factor intervention.** What this means in simple language is that the Nutraerobics Program will help you to identify your own unique needs in managing your life to promote high-level health and then provide you options to integrate these needs into your lifestyle so as to reduce your risks to later, crisis-stage disease. Most doctors have been trained traditionally to treat disease when it is diagnosed, not to recognize the early warning signs and symptoms associated with increased risk to later-stage disease. The focus in the Nutraerobics Program is on the early warning assessment and recognition of later-stage health problems and then on providing a method of intervention using nutrition, exercise, and lifestyle modification to reduce these risks.

This approach does not focus exclusively on such well-known risk factors as smoking, high cholesterol and fat in the diet, and obesity but rather attempts to identify which features in your genetic makeup are strengths and which are weak spots in need of reinforcing. We all carry genetic weaknesses or "biochemical Achilles' heels." Among any random hundred presumably healthy people you will find a great diversity in basic states of functioning, for which differing nutrients, exercise programs, and possibly even lifestyles are required to promote individual optimal states of health.

The following chapters will help you, first, to identify your own biochemical uniquenesses, second, to introduce you to alternative concepts of health improvement based upon those uniquenesses, and then last, to reinforce those concepts through methods of positive behavior change. The chapter order in this book is designed to address the more general health concerns first, such as aging, heart disease, cancer, and digestive problems, and then the more specific problems, such as male and female difficulties, bone loss, child behavior, and problems of pregnancy and infancy.

From your responses to the questionnaires and their interpretations in the next chapter, you will know which chapters to concentrate on. You can either read this book from cover to cover or you can skip around in it, focusing on specific chapters that you feel are of more concern to you. This book is a workbook to help you improve your health and it should be used as a service manual in inspecting and improving the function of your body's machine, both physically and psychologically. To be successful with this program you must get involved in the assessment process.

It is ironic that in our culture we spend billions of dollars each year on life insurance policies, which are really "death insurance policies" in that they pay the beneficiaries for our death, yet we spend very little on true life insurance policies that promote our health while we are alive. The Nutraerobics Program puts the emphasis on your health promotion and redirects your energies toward securing your most vital and precious possession, your health.

With these concerns in mind, let's introduce you to the Nutraerobics Health Enhancement Program and get you started on the road toward preventing those symptoms of vertical disease.

Notes

1. For a discussion of Dr. James Plemons's work and other interesting information concerning lifestyle and aging, see the excellent book by James Fries, *Vitality and Aging* (San Francisco: W. H. Freeman, 1981).

2. For a discussion of the psychology of aging and its relationship to health see James Birren and K. Warren Schaie, *Handbook of the Psychology of Aging* (New York: Van Nostrand Reinhold, 1977).

2

Assessing Your Biotype

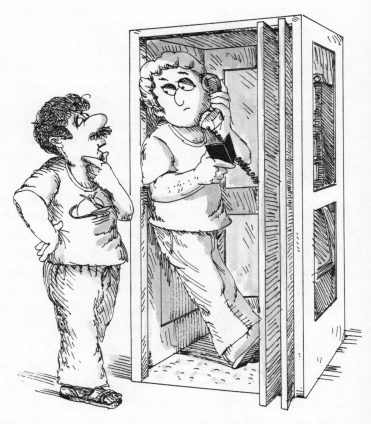

WELL, I DON'T KNOW, WHAT'S HER BIOTYPE ?

This is one of the most important chapters in this book. From the answers you provide to the questionnaires in this chapter you will identify your own specific biological needs, or **biotype.** It will take you some time to complete this chapter but, remember, the information gained in assessing your biotype will be used throughout the remainder of the book in designing and implementing your Nutraerobics Program. In Chapter 14 you will need this information to summarize your Nutraerobics Program Summary Checklist.

A little over thirty years ago Dr. Roger Williams, a pioneering biochemist and discoverer of a number of the B-complex vitamins, first proposed his novel model of disease, which he called the **genetotrophic theory of disease.** In this model he postulates that people often become ill because their unique genetic constitutions and needs for specific nutrients are not being met by their diet or lifestyle. A genetotrophic disease he defines as a disease that results from the absence of an optimal level of one or more nutrients based upon a person's own genetic need.[1] Diseases he categorizes under this heading may include many of the diseases that medical science today views as being caused by factors of unknown origin—coronary heart disease or atherosclerosis, stroke, cancer, diabetes, essential hypertension (or high blood pressure), rheumatoid or osteoarthritis, colitis, other digestive disorders, and possibly even certain psychiatric abnormalities.

Since Dr. Williams first proposed this theory, extensive research has been undertaken in laboratories and clinical settings around the world to try to uncover areas of human biochemical uniqueness and their relationship to dietary and lifestyle habits. All these studies use three categories of factors in a comprehensive assessment of an individual's unique genetic requirements. These three categories include: (1) a good physical assessment, which includes such things as family health history, personal health history, symptoms, drug and medication use, and a physical examination; (2) dietary data, in which the diet is evaluated for its quality and quantity; and (3) biochemical information from sophisticated tests including blood, urine, and other tissue analysis. The purpose of taking all of this information into account and evaluating the biochemical uniqueness of an individual is to establish an optimal program to meet his or her needs, thereby preventing later-stage health problems.

The analogy to this is, of course, preventive maintenance of a car, for which a good program must be tailored to meet that model's specific requirements. Such things as the timing, the air-to-fuel ratio in the carburetor, the gap of the spark plugs, the manifold pressure—even the oil in the crankcase and the type of gas—are all specific to an individual make and model of car. Some people are genetically tuned like racing machines and need to be managed as such. Other people have basic biochemistries more like heavy equipment or trucks, and they need a very different set of supports for their optimal function.

In this chapter we will be assessing your own biochemical uniqueness—that specific genetic profile we will call your *biotype*. Because you are not able to do biochemical tests on your body, we will have to rely primarily on those factors that relate to your symptoms, your personal health history, your genetic background, your diet, and your relationship to the environment. If after completing this book, you wish to include sophisticated biochemical tests in your evaluation, a visit to a health practitioner in your community specializing in preventive medicine is suggested.

Nutraerobics differs from other programs in that it assumes that you are not optimally healthy until proven otherwise—exactly the opposite of the assumption in a standard medical practitioner's office that you are healthy until proven diseased. With that in mind, let's start evaluating your own biochemical uniqueness. As you go through the questionnaires, remember two things.

First, be honest with yourself. This survey is for no one but you, so cheating fools no one except yourself. The value of the Nutraerobics Program will to a great extent depend upon how successful you are in looking at yourself critically and answering the questionnaires accurately and honestly. If you are confused about a question or have not really thought about it before, spend some time thinking about it or talking with someone before you provide a response. Sometimes just bringing some of these topics from the subconscious to the conscious can initiate a positive behavior modification program; therefore, the time you spend thinking about the questions and reviewing them may affect your success with the implementation of the Nutraerobics Program.

Second, be aware of any "redundancy" that appears in the course of the questionnaires. Single bits of information are in themselves of limited usefulness; however, when two or three questions elicit similar responses, the urgency to treat these items seriously becomes more profound. This is what is termed redundancy in an evaluation, and what we will be attempting to do is to define those redundant areas where your responses to various questions lead us ultimately to the same conclusion. The greater redundancy, or multiple bits of information saying the same thing, the stronger your associations and the more likely that this is an area that warrants your attention. You might want to keep notes on areas of particular concern.

Remember, also, that the explanations of the separate questionnaire items are, of necessity, brief. If you do not understand the mechanisms involved or would like a fuller explanation, be assured that we go into most of the topics in much greater detail in subsequent chapters. In many cases cross-references are provided.

Now spend some time filling out the questionnaires. An interpretation follows each one. If you feel you don't have time to do them justice now, skip on to Chapter 4 and keep reading. You do not have to use this book as a self-study book if you do not care to. By reading Chapters 4 through 14 you will learn of some of the newest concepts in how to keep healthy.

1. Do you have a low tolerance to alcohol, drugs, or medications (are you easily affected at low dose)?

2. Do you have digestive problems when consuming milk or milk products?

3. Are you sensitive to monosodium glutamate (MSG), producing "Chinese restaurant syndrome" (cramping of stomach or intestinal complaints)?

4. Do you have difficulty handling stress?

5. Are you overly sensitive to hot and cold?

6. Did either or both of your parents have an overweight or underweight problem?

7. Do you sunburn readily?

8. Do you have a crease in your earlobe?

9. Have your parents had high blood pressure, diabetes, or cancer?

10. Do you tend to get seborrheic dermatitis (a scaly skin rash commonly found on the scalp)?

11. Do you gain weight easily or have difficulty putting weight on?

12. Are you subject to recurring constipation and/or diarrhea?

13. Has there been a history of kidney stones or of calcium loss from the bones of members of your family?

14. Did you grow very rapidly as a teenager, so as to experience "growing pains"?

15. Do you tend to get disoriented or weak and shaky if you do not eat a meal on time?

16. Did either of your parents have a weak constitution or tend to get every common illness that came along?

17. Are mental illnesses or accelerated aging common in your family?

18. Do you have red or blond hair?

19. Do you tend to have an uncontrollable "sweet tooth"?

20. Do you feel you need more than eight hours sleep per night or do you get along well on less than six hours sleep?

21. Do fatty foods give you indigestion?

Interpretation of
the Genetotype Questionnaire

1. It has been found that individuals who have high alcohol sensitivity (low tolerance), associated with easy facial flushing, may have a genetic lowered ability to metabolize alcohol and other drugs due to alterations in liver function; that is, their livers cannot quickly process and eliminate these substances from their systems. People who show this symptom may be insufficient in a specific liver enzyme and should refrain from excessive drinking to avoid adverse reactions caused by raised blood levels of a chemical called acetaldehyde.[2] This condition may also indicate the genetic need for higher levels of the B vitamins, as well as zinc and magnesium, which are important in the liver for the metabolism of alcohol.

2. A large percentage of the adult population, particularly those of Hispanic, black, or Oriental ethnic background, have lactose (milk sugar) intolerance or milk sensitivity. Continued consumption of milk products in the face of this genetic uniqueness can lead to intestinal irritations, producing not only diarrhea and stomach pain but also long-term increased risk to such diseases as colitis or irritable bowel syndrome.

Using cultured milk such as yogurt or buttermilk will reduce the lactose problem but there may still be an allergic reaction to milk proteins such as casein. If such is the case, a significant mucous problem or flatulence may develop.

3. It has recently been found that a reaction to monosodium glutamate may be the result of a vitamin B-6 deficiency. Orientals are known not to be susceptible to MSG syndrome, whereas Scandinavians are. Higher levels of vitamin B-6 in those sensitive to MSG helps promote the proper metabolism of not only monosodium glutamate, but of other amino acids in dietary protein as well.[3] People susceptible to MSG problems may require two to three times the normal amount of vitamin B-6 to promote optimal protein metabolism.

4. Individuals vary considerably in their ability to translate environmental or social stress into distress. We all have a different number of "antennae" out into the environment and the sensitivities to sensory overload can vary considerably from person to person. What may be a nondistressful situation for one person may be an extremely distressful situation for another. The translation of stress to distress puts considerable load on your physiological system, which in turn creates greater nutrient need, so that it is important to regulate both dietary intake and lifestyle to minimize stress-induced disease. Increased needs for vitamin C, magnesium, and the B-complex vitamins, including pantothenic acid, are suggested for the "high-stress" individual.

5. A high sensitivity to temperature change can indicate chronic thyroid gland problems. The thyroid gland is the master gland controlling the metabolic activity of every cell in your body. Some individuals are born with either an under- or overactive thyroid gland. A number of nutrients such as iodine, copper, zinc, and the amino acid tyrosine are important for activating the thyroid gland in individuals who may be susceptible to hypothyroidism (low thyroid activity).

Other symptoms accompanying this condition include constipation, poor wound healing, a sense of mental confusion, and heart irregularities, as well as easy weight gain. A routine low body temperature upon waking (below 97.8 degrees F) may indicate borderline hypothyroidism.

6. It is now well recognized that genetics plays a role in determining one's weight throughout life. If one of your parents was obese, you have a 40 percent chance of obesity, and if both parents were obese, you have an 80 percent statistical probability. If your parents had weight problems, it is very important for you to implement proper eating habits, nutritional intake, and exercise early in life so as to beat the odds. In Chapter 6, we will be discussing in some length the whole area of weight management for those of you who may have a tendency to be either underweight or overweight.

7. Easy sunburning may indicate the poor conversion in your skin of substances to the tanning pigment melanin. This not only makes you more sensitive to the harmful effects of the sun rays but also has a relationship to the potentially increased need for the B-complex substance para-aminobenzoic acid (PABA), copper, vitamin B-6, vitamin B-3 (niacin), and the pigment in orange-red vegetables called beta-carotene.

8. A crease at the bottom portion of the earlobe has been found associated with a much increased risk to coronary heart disease and heart attack.

Individuals with this increased risk should implement rigorous control over their diet, exercise, and stress, so as to minimize their genetic tendency toward heart disease. If you answered yes to this question, you should spend considerable time studying the material in Chapter 7 on Nutraerobics and heart disease.

9. It is now well known that high blood pressure (essential hypertension), maturity-onset diabetes (diabetes beginning in adult life rather than at birth), and cancer all have familiar relationships and seem to be in part genetically related. If you have a high incidence in your blood family of one or more of these conditions, then you should be very cautious in designing your particular program to minimize the biochemical risk to these diseases. Spend some time on the chapters on brain chemistry, heart disease, and cancer (5, 7, and 8) for specific information in these areas.

10. A recurrent seborrheic dermatitis condition may indicate deficiencies in the B-complex vitamins, zinc, or essential fatty acids, or food or environmental allergy problems. Essential fatty acids are found in oil-rich grains or in oils such as peanut, soy, safflower, or sunflower-seed oil. Individuals who consume diets excessively high in saturated animal fats and who are not eating enough foods rich in the B-vitamins or zinc may have nutrient deficiency symptoms such as scaly seborrheic or eczemic dermatitis.

11. Weight gain or loss or difficulty in maintaining what would be considered ideal body mass for your height may indicate that you have either a very slow or a very fast metabolism, and that you convert foods either very poorly or very rapidly into energy. Much of this control over energy manufacture is by a tissue called brown fat, which produces heat as its by-product. There is a lengthy discussion of the control of brown fat metabolism in the chapter on weight control (6).

12. Alternating constipation and diarrhea or chronic constipation may indicate a food allergy, lack of proper levels of dietary fiber, inappropriate fluid intake, or need for more exercise. Some individuals require a considerable amount of dietary fiber for proper bowel function, whereas others may have food allergic symptoms that present themselves only as constipation and/or diarrhea with no other side effects. Remember, adequate fluid intake and regular exercise will help maintain bowel function. What for one individual may be an adequate level of exercise, fluid, or fiber, may not be for another individual. If you have a problem in this area, you should be concentrating on Chapter 4 (aging).

13. Conditions such as kidney stones, osteoporosis (decrease in bone density due to calcium loss), or periodontal disease (loss of bone from the jaw, causing teeth to become loose and ultimately to need extraction) may indicate a specific need for balancing calcium and phosphorus, decreasing dietary protein and increasing vitamin C intake. In general, diets higher in calcium and lower in phosphorus than the average American diet will help improve bone status; however, this may differ widely from individual to individual. If you have a problem in this area, concentrate on the chapter on bone loss (10).

14. A rapid growth spurt, which makes tremendous demands upon the body's reserves, can produce nutrient deficiency states. If this is the case, it may indicate a lifelong need for increased levels of zinc, iron, copper, and manganese, as well as calcium and magnesium. The discussion of the important role that these essential minerals play in promotion of proper health is discussed in Chapter 3 on nutritional needs.

15. Changes in your energy level or your ability to concentrate may be related to a tendency toward blood sugar problems. Hypoglycemia is the term applied to low blood sugar. If the sugar in your blood is low, your brain and other organs do not get enough to manufacture energy and you therefore can experience a whole range of behavioral effects, including depression, anxiety, inability to concentrate, or confusion. These conditions are discussed in the chapter on emotions (5).

16. Certain families seem to have poorer immune system protection than others. Your immune system is the system of your body that fights potentially infectious agents, such as bacteria and viruses. If your immune system is constitutionally low, it may suggest you have a higher need for immune-activating nutrients such as vitamin C, zinc, iron, and copper. A discussion of nutrition and immune status will be found in Chapter 11.

17. People with certain kinds of mental illness may respond to increasing levels of nutrition far and above what one would normally get in an average diet. This proposition, as propounded by psychiatrists Abram Hoffer and Humphrey Osmond, has been evaluated by considerable experimental testing and the indication is that in some cases the biochemically unique need for certain nutrients to normalize brain function is well above that which an individual would get in a normal diet.[4] This field is known as orthomolecular psychiatry and is discussed in Chapter 5.

18. Individuals with lighter-colored hair who are of northern European or Scandinavian background may require slightly higher levels of dietary protein than individuals of Middle Eastern or Eastern descent. They may need between 60 and 100 grams of protein per day, while 50 grams a day may be adequate for others.

19. The very high need for sugar intake in some individuals may indicate a greater need for the B-complex vitamins and/or zinc. Recent studies have indicated the important effect that B vitamins and zinc have on reducing the urge to consume sweet foods.[5]

20. The need for sleep is an indication of the length of the body's recharging time. Individuals who tend to need more sleep may not metabolize as well as people who require less sleep. The amount of sleep time needed may also depend on psychosocial variables like anxiety, worry, or depression, but there are a number of biochemical indications that individuals who require considerable sleep throughout most of their lives may be less efficient energy metabolizers than those who can thrive on lower amounts of sleep. People who sleep less are by definition active more of the day; they require a greater number of calories and vitamins and minerals in their diets to compensate for the increased activity.

Your calorie intake should be adjusted to your energy expenditure; if you sleep less you may require more daily calories. If, however, you sleep longer but are very active while awake, your calorie need will also be higher. Discussion of how to balance your calorie need to meet your metabolism is discussed in Chapter 6. Regular insomnia or recurring bad dreams may indicate you have a greater need for the B-complex vitamins, and you should concentrate on Chapter 5.

21. Those who get indigestion from fatty foods may be poor fat metabolizers and cannot break down and absorb fats properly. This produces a feeling of fullness in the stomach or indigestion or "heartburn." A light-colored, "fatty" stool confirms this problem. If you are susceptible to these conditions, the fat in your diet should be regulated carefully so as not to put too much load on the pancreas or the gall bladder, the organs responsible for fat metabolism. This sensitivity to fatty foods may produce increased risk to gall bladder or pancreatic disease in later life if the diet is not designed appropriately.

Now that you've had a chance to evaluate your responses to this part of the questionnaire, you've established whether you are likely to be a high or low energy-processor; to be a better protein, fat, or sugar metabolizer; or whether you have a higher genetic predisposition to certain health problems. Make note of these uniquenesses for later review.

Stress Indicator Questionnaire

If one of the following has been true for you in the past year, or you know it will occur in the near future, copy the score from the left column in the space provided in the right column.

Event	Score	
Death of spouse	100	_____
Divorce	75	_____
Separation or end of love relationship	65	_____
Jail term	65	_____
Personal injury or illness	53	_____
Marriage	50	_____
Fired from job	47	_____
Love reconciliation	45	_____
Retirement	45	_____
Change in health of family member	44	_____
Pregnancy	40	_____
Sexual problems	39	_____
Gain of new family member	39	_____
Business readjustment	39	_____
Death of close friend	37	_____
Arguments with spouse (change in frequency or intensity)	35	_____
New high mortgage	31	_____
Trouble with in-laws	29	_____
Son or daughter leaving home	28	_____
Trouble with boss	23	_____
Change in living conditions	20	_____
Total		

Additional Questions:
1. Do you feel distressed?
2. Does the world seem to be moving too fast?
3. Are you unable to complete what you want, because you never have enough time?
4. Is there an urgency about life?
5. Are your aspirations for success running your life?

Source: Adapted from Thomas H. Holmes and Richard H. Rahe, "Social Readjustment Rating Scale."

Interpretation of the Stress Indicator Questionnaire

The "scores" for the life changes on the Stress Indicator Questionnaire have been quantitatively correlated with the appearance of illness.[6] Total up your score on the questionnaire and you will have a number between 0 and 600. If your total score is 300 or above, it indicates that you are under very heavy stress as it relates to recent life changes, and statistically you have more than a 50 percent probability of being hospitalized during the next year due to a stress-related health condition. If your score is between 150 and 300, you are under moderate stress due to life changes and have a 30 percent probability of being ill enough to miss work over the next year. If your total is less than 100, you have no indication that recent life changes are increasing your risk to disease because of stress-related factors.

Research indicates that these types of stressors can depress the immune system and lead to increased risk to disease processes, including cancer.[7] We also know that the psychological state of individuals can directly impact upon their ability to prevent the major killer diseases or lead to increased risk to those diseases if they are under considerable emotional burden. We will come back to discuss this in greater detail in Chapter 11.

If you answered yes to **Question 1** it's important to recall that stress in life does not necessarily produce distress. Stress can actually be an energy-giving part of life that stimulates us to do work and to be productive beyond what we would normally do and be in a stressless environment. Such is the model discussed by Dr. Robert Anderson in his excellent book entitled **Stress Power.**[8]

When stress is translated from a positive force to a destructive force, it's called distress and leads to the general adaptation syndrome.[9] The **general adaptation syndrome** is a condition in which the stress has become distressful and produces a general arousal in the person, which ultimately leads to a depletion of reserves in the body and later an adaptation that may be that of compromised immunity or poor defense against disease. If you **feel** you are distressed, then you **are** distressed. Each person handles stress differently and translates it to distress under different conditions. What for one person may be a perfectly positive stress condition may be a health-eroding, distressful situation for another.

Questions 2, 3, 4, and 5 all relate to time urgency. These are questions that are commonly asked when determining if a person has a type A or type B personality.[10] The type A personality is a person with an unrealistic sense of time urgency, an overly high set of expectations or goals, and a sense that the world is moving too fast for him or her. This type of personality has an increased risk to heart attack and stroke, and again is a measure of a person's translation of stress in his or her life into health or disease risk. The type B personality, on the other hand, has the tendency not to worry about time, be a procrastinator, and be less upwardly motivated. This individual has greater problems with intestinal disorders and low blood pressure.

The long-standing philosophical debate between mind and body is truly one for historical interest only, since we now know that mind and body are inextricably tied together. What the mind perceives the body feels, and what the body feels the mind adjusts to. When we feel we are under stress, the body mirrors that stress through change in its own health status.

Have you established that you are a person whose health may be controlled by your distress level? If so, this may be the overriding feature of your biotype and you need to concentrate heavily on the material in Chapter 14.

Physical Evaluation Questionnaire

What is your:

1. Resting pulse rate (beats per minute)?
2. Blood pressure standing; sitting?
3. Weight in pounds; height in inches?
4. Waist size (inches) divided by hip size (inches)?

Do you have:

5. Lack of hair luster or recurrent bad dandruff?
6. Poor clarity of eyes, redness in whites of eyes?
7. Cracks or redness at corners of mouth and nose, or chronically chapped lips?
8. Sandpaper-like skin at back of arms?
9. A reddish-colored tongue, heavily fissured or smooth?
10. Red or infected gums, or heavily cavity-laden teeth?
11. Neck or throat tenderness?
12. Labored breathing, sinus drip, or recurrent cough?
13. Swelling of ankles or fluid retention?
14. Lower stomach swelling or pain, or excessive gas?
15. Stools that are not brown, well formed, or don't float?
16. The inability to bend fingers flat to palm of hand at the second joint?
17. Habitually foul-smelling or stale breath?
18. Recurrent eczema or dermatitis?
19. Abnormally thick ear wax or no wax at all?
20. Pain on urination or cloudiness of urine?
21. Are you now taking medications routinely? If so, what?
22. Have you been hospitalized for more than a week during the past two or three months?

Interpretation of the Physical Evaluation Questionnaire

1. Your resting pulse rate should not exceed 70 beats per minute when you are in reasonably good physical condition. A resting pulse between 70 and 85 beats per minute is considered marginal, and above 85 beats per minute there may be indication of circulatory, lung, or blood problems. If you have an elevated resting pulse and poor exercise tolerance, it would be wise to look carefully at the material on weight control and heart disease (Chapters 6 and 7).

2. Blood pressure is a good measure of risk to stroke, kidney problems, or certain forms of heart disease, as well as an indicator of the functioning of your adrenal glands. These glands are located on top of your kidneys and play an important part in your immune defense, management of blood pressure, and your reaction to stress (the stress hormone adrenaline is secreted by these glands).

Your blood pressure standing should not be above 140 over 85. The second number, called the diastolic pressure, is the most important. It is a measure of the continual strain that is being placed on the small blood vessels and arteries of your body. Diastolic values in excess of 90 are considered evidence of risk to stroke and are generally treated medically with a class of drugs called diuretics. (We'll be discussing a number of nondrug approaches toward the reduction of blood pressure, as specified by the Nutraerobics Program, in Chapters 6 and 7 on weight control and heart disease.)

The difference between standing and sitting blood pressure measures the ability of your adrenal glands to compensate for changes under stress. You should see at least a rise of 5 in the first number (systolic pressure) on going from the sitting to the standing position. If you do not see an elevation in blood pressure, you may be susceptible to what's known as postural hypotension, or dizziness that comes on when you stand up quickly because the reserves of your adrenal glands are depleted. Again, in the chapters on bone loss (10) and child behavior (13) there will be a discussion of approaches to management of this condition.

3. Your height and weight give information about your body mass index. The body mass index has been found very closely correlated to your lean body mass, which is the percent of your total weight made up of muscle and bone. These values will be used in the chapter on weight control (6) to determine your body fat percentage.

4.   Your waist size divided by your hip size gives a number somewhere between .5 and 1.5. If your waist-to-hip ratio is greater than 1.2, it suggests that you are upper-body heavy and have seven times the risk of developing diabetes in mid to late life than the person who is of an ideal body weight. If your waist-to-hip ratio is less than .8, it suggests you may be lower-body heavy. Chapter 6 deals with how to manage this problem and reduce the risk to contracting diabetes or other health problems related to body weight.

5.   Lack of hair luster or recurring bad dandruff indicate poor protein digestion or absorption, poor circulation caused by blockage of the small capillaries, or deficiencies of certain nutrients discussed in the chapter on immunity (11).

6.   Lack of clarity of the eyes or persistent redness of the whites of the eyes may be indicative of increased fragility of the small capillaries of your body, leading to what's known as microhemorrhages (small blood vessel ruptures). It's not serious if the capillaries in your eyes are fragile, producing redness, but it may be a very significant problem if this happens in your brain or other critical areas. This may be an indication of a number of nutritional imbalances, including insufficient vitamin C, zinc, vitamin K, vitamin E, or members of the B-complex vitamin family.

7.   Cracks or redness at the corners of the mouth or nose or chronically chapped lips generally indicate problems with vitamins B-1, B-2, and B-3 and may be present even when a person is getting what would normally be considered adequate levels of these vitamins in the diet. There have been a number of cases of people who were malabsorbing certain nutrients from the diet, the effect of which was to produce the deficiency-like symptoms. If you have these symptoms, you should correlate the level of B vitamins you are getting in your average daily diet with the presence of symptoms. If you are apparently getting adequate levels of vitamins in the diet, but still showing the symptoms of deficiency, then malabsorption or improper utilization of the vitamins should be reviewed. Chapter 3 on nutritional needs discusses this in some detail.

8. If you have sandpaper-like skin at the back of your arms, then a vitamin A deficiency is quite commonly implicated. Vitamin A is a fat-soluble vitamin and may be malabsorbed even when found in what would be considered adequate amounts in the diet.

9. If your tongue color is reddish, or your tongue is heavily fissured, or has no small bumps called papillae (so that it resembles a bald tire), you may have a classic example of B-complex vitamin deficiencies.[11] It has been found that when the tongue is reddish in color and is very smooth, there is an 80 percent likelihood of a vitamin B-2 or B-3 deficiency.

10. If your gums are very red and appear infected and your teeth are heavily laden with calculus (plaque), or you have a large number of filled or unfilled cavities, this is a very good indication of the reduced effectiveness of your immune system, deficiencies of folic acid, vitamin B-12, and vitamin C, and possibly an excessive amount of refined carbohydrates, especially sugars, in the diet. (These indications will be evaluated in greater detail in Chapter 7 on heart disease.) It has been found that people who have dental appliances such as false teeth or braces and subsequently develop bone loss and/or infected gums may have this problem in part due to an imbalance of dietary calcium, magnesium, and phosphorus levels and need more vitamin C, folic acid, and vitamin B-6.

11. Neck or throat tenderness may indicate the presence of an ongoing thyroid condition with deficiencies of iodine, copper, zinc, or tyrosine (one of the amino acids). Thyroid problems are discussed in greater detail in Chapter 9 on male and female problems.

12. If you have difficulty breathing or have a persistent sinus drip or recurring cough, it may indicate a low-grade infection or allergy condition, leading to reduced lung and heart efficiency. Individuals who have had a long-standing cough and a runny nose or a sinus drip have been helped by removing the food allergic substance that had been triggering this response for years. This problem is discussed in greater detail in the chapter on immunity and allergy (11).

13.   If you have swelling of the ankles or fluid retention, it again may be an indication of adrenal gland problems. The adrenal glands secrete hormones that regulate the level of salt retention in your blood. Excessive salt retention can lead to fluid retention as well as increased blood pressure. It has also been found that allergenic substances can also produce fluid retention and water weight gain. (See Chapter 6 on weight control.) Many people who feel they are too fat are really retaining too much fluid, which contributes to their excess weight.

14.   Extensive stomach swelling, pain, or gas after eating indicate a maldigestion problem, which if untreated for many years could contribute to digestive disorders such as colitis or an inflamed bowel. Long-term maldigestion may also be a cause of certain food allergic symptoms that occur when partially digested proteins are absorbed across the intestinal barrier and cause an allergic reaction once they enter the blood. This problem will be discussed in the chapter on immunity and allergy (11).

15.   Stools that are not brown, well formed, and do not float may indicate poor digestive compatibility and the buildup of toxins in the bowel, some of which may actually be cancer-producing substances. In general, one can correlate poorly formed, very dense stools with low fiber in the diet, but there may be other contributing problems as well. If the stool is very light in color, it may indicate a bile-acid deficiency. Bile is produced by the liver, stored in the gall bladder, and secreted into the intestines after you have eaten. If not enough bile is present, fats may pass through undigested, and this may be associated with gallstones and elevated blood cholesterol, which is a risk factor to heart disease. Brown-colored stools indicate the presence of adequate bile salts.

16.   The inability to bend your fingers at the second joint flat to the palm of your hand may indicate a tendency toward carpal tunnel syndrome, a condition commonly necessitating orthopedic surgery. Carpal tunnel syndrome has been found in a number of cases to be indicative of a high vitamin B-6 need, and uses of the vitamin far in excess of what one would get in the diet (levels of 125 mg or more) may be required to properly manage this condition.[12]

17. If your breath is habitually foul smelling or stale, it may indicate poor digestion and a long transit time of material in the intestines before elimination. Increased fluid intake as well as increased dietary fiber are helpful in promoting proper intestinal regularity. It may also help to remove from the diet foods that are difficult to digest. Remember, not everybody has the same digestive ability, and what may be an adequate diet for some may be a diet too difficult to digest for others, leading to longer food residence time in the intestines and putrefaction. Regular exercise can increase the tone of the abdominal muscles, aiding the intestines in moving food through them.

18. Recurrent eczema or dermatitis may indicate the lack of proper zinc, vitamin B-6, or essential fatty acids in the diet. These will be discussed in greater detail in Chapter 14.

19. No ear wax or hard, dark-colored ear wax may also indicate an essential fatty acid deficiency with increased risk to elevated blood cholesterol and potential heart disease. Use of lighter oils in the diet, staying away from animal fats, and applying the principles found in the chapter on heart disease (7) will be helpful in this area.

20. Pain on urination or cloudiness of the urine may be indications of oxalate stone formation or uric acid problems, particularly if they are also associated with swelling of certain joints or a bacterial or yeast infection of the urinary tract. In these cases, it may indicate the need for greater amounts of vitamin C, increased fluid intake, avoidance of oxalate-containing foods like spinach and rhubarb, and larger quantities of folic acid.

21, 22. Lastly, medications—whether taken yourself or administered during hospitalization—may lead to depletion of essential nutrients from your body and require supplementation. Hospital-induced malnutrition is now considered a natural problem and necessitates nutritional therapy after discharge.[13] The amounts of certain nutrients necessary to compensate for various drugs is shown in Table 1.

Table 1

Drug–Nutrient Antagonism

Nutrient	Drug	Amount of nutrient to compensate for drug
Vitamin A	mineral oil (laxative)	2000 IU
	neomycin (antibiotic)	5000 IU
Vitamin B-6	hydralazine (antipsychotic)	20–100 mg
	isoniazin (antipsychotic)	20–100 mg
	L-dopa (Parkinson's disease)	20–50 mg
	oral contraceptives	5–20 mg
	penicillamine or EDTA (chelator)	5–50 mg
Vitamin C	oral contraceptives	50–500 mg
	aspirin	50–500 mg
	tetracycline (antibiotic)	50–200 mg
Vitamin D	anticonvulsants	200–400 IU
	cholesterol-lowering drugs	200–400 IU
	mineral oil	100–400 IU
Vitamin B-12	antibiotics	10–50 mcg
	nitrous oxide	10–100 mcg
	oral contraceptives	10–20 mcg
	potassium chloride	10–50 mcg
Folic acid (folacin)	anticonvulsants	400–800 mcg
	oral contraceptives	100–400 mcg
	aspirin	100–800 mcg
	antibiotics	100–400 mcg
	pancreatic enzymes	100–800 mcg
Vitamin B-3 (niacin)	isoniazid	20–100 mg
Vitamin B-2 (riboflavin)	oral contraceptives	2–5 mg
	antipsychotics	5–30 mg
Vitamin B-1 (thiamin)	oral contraceptives	2–5 mg
	alcohol	2–20 mg
Magnesium	diuretics (antihypertensives)	100–400 mg
	alcohol	100–300 mg
Zinc	oral contraceptives	10–30 mg
	diuretics	10–20 mg
Vitamin E	Adriamycin (anticancer)	100–800 IU
	laxatives	100–400 IU

Dietary Evaluation Questionnaire

1. How many times a week do you have the following for breakfast in average portions:

   a. Citrus fruits (oranges, grapefruit, whole or juice)? ____

   b. Whole grains (hot or cold)? ____

   c. Eggs (plain or in foods)? ____

   d. Pancakes, waffles? ____

   e. Milk? ____

   f. Meats (ham, bacon, sausage)? ____

2. Of the fourteen lunches and dinners you may eat a week, how many are:

   a. Beef, lamb, pork, or organ meats? ____

   b. Poultry (chicken, turkey, duck)? ____

   c. Fish, shellfish? ____

3. How many times a week do you consume:

   a. Bread, rolls? ____

   b. Vegetables (not canned)? ____

   c. Cheese, yogurt? ____

   d. Legumes (peas, beans)? ____

   e. Pasta? ____

   f. Fruit (not canned)? ____

   g. Butter? ____

   h. Margarine? ____

   i. Vegetable oil or salad dressings? ____

   j. Ice cream? ____

   k. Alcoholic beverages? ____

   l. Snacks (potato chips, pretzels, etc.)? ____

   m. Cookies, cakes, candies? ____

   n. Nuts? ____

   o. Raisins, figs, dates? ____

   p. Soft drinks? ____

   q. Potatoes? ____

   r. Meat products? ____

4. How much water do you drink daily? ____

5. How heavily do you salt your food? ____

6. Are you a vegetarian? ____

7. Are you on a sugar- or salt-free diet? ____

8. How often do you eat out per week? ____

9. How do you prepare your vegetables and meats? ____

10. Do you use sauces and gravies often? ____

11. Do you deep-fat fry your foods frequently? ____

12. Do you often eat prepared foods, boxed or frozen? ____

13. Do you take vitamin supplements? If so, what type? ____

14. Are you on a weight loss diet?

Source: Adapted from G. Christakis, in *Nutrition and Medical Practice*, ed. L.A. Barness (Westport, CT: AVI Publishing, 1981).

Interpretation of the Dietary Evaluation Questionnaire

The Dietary Evaluation Questionnaire you've just filled out is based upon a concept called the "nutrition scan." It's not as accurate as a complete record of your diet on a food-by-food basis, but it does give us good qualitative information about what you consume in your average daily intake.

1. If you responded negatively to all parts of question 1 because you are not a breakfast eater, you are missing one of the health habits associated with long and healthy lives, according to one study.[14] In this study it was found that people who had longer, healthier lives possessed the following lifestyle characteristics:

They ate a regular breakfast.

They slept six to eight hours per night.

They had a proper weight-to-height ratio.

They did not smoke.

They drank moderately.

They got regular exercise.

They ate food from the basic seven food groups each day (meat, grains, dairy products, starchy vegetables, nonstarchy vegetables, citrus fruits, noncitrus fruits)—all reasonably fresh.

They took regular vacations.

Breakfast starts you off on your day with adequate levels of calories, vitamins, and minerals to help promote proper blood sugar levels and energy production. Citrus fruits are important as a source of vitamin C and folic acid as well as potassium. Whole grains in a breakfast provide B-complex vitamins as well as desirable fiber. Eggs are an excellent source of protein and essential fatty acids. (A discussion of the egg and heart disease controversy appears in Chapter 7.) Pancake and waffle consumption frequently indicates an excessive amount of refined carbohydrate or sugar. Milk is an excellent source of calcium, and if milk is avoided in the diet, there may be a need for calcium.

2. Your answers tell us something about the level of dietary protein and fat intake that you are achieving. If you eat a great number of your lunches and dinners with beef, lamb, pork, or organ meats in them, then you are getting very high cholesterol and fat intake. Meats such as bacon, ham, or sausage are very high in fats. Either chicken or turkey without the skin is much lower in fat, and fish is often high in certain oils that actually may help prevent heart attack, as is discussed in Chapter 7.

In general, it is probable that if you eat meat, fish, dairy products, or eggs at each meal you are getting excessive dietary protein, which can contribute to bone loss and increase the risk to osteoporosis, as discussed in Chapter 10.

3. Your answers allow you to see how you distribute protein, carbohydrate, and fat in your diet on an average daily basis. If you are eating frequent servings of bread, rolls, legumes, snacks, and potatoes, you are getting a high level of carbohydrate in your diet, primarily as starch. The more unrefined the starch, the more health-promoting the diet is. A recent study indicates that the most health-promoting diets are those that are high in complex, unrefined starches.[15] This will be discussed in greater detail in the chapter on nutritional needs (3).

If the diet is high in cheese, butter, margarine, vegetable oil or dressings, and nuts, it indicates that you are consuming a very high-fat diet, which is related to increased blood cholesterol and risk to a number of the major degenerative diseases.

If your diet is high in cheese, legumes, nuts, and meat products you may be getting excessive dietary protein; this can have an adverse effect on your bones and digestive function, as discussed in Chapters 10 and 11.

Next, inspection of the number of portions of vegetables, fruit, beans and other legumes, potatoes, and meat products you consume is an indication of your general level of vitamin and mineral intake. These are the foods known to be highest in vitamins and minerals, which are used in the metabolism of calories that come from all of your various foods. If you are low in these food groups, then you are probably marginal in your vitamin and mineral intake.

Next, we can determine relatively how much sugar you are getting in the diet by looking at your intake of ice cream, snacks, cookies, soft drinks, and raisins, figs, and dates. All of these are very high in sugar and contribute to an excessively high simple sugar dietary intake. The average American diet contains about 20 percent of its calories as sugar, which many investigators consider too high for sugar-sensitive individuals, as it contributes to a variety of health problems.[16] (See the material in Chapter 5 on blood sugar.)

Next, from the amount of vegetables, pasta, legumes, and potatoes you consume, as well as bread and rolls, you can estimate your dietary fiber intake. If the consumption of these food families is low, or if they are highly processed, then you can assume low dietary fiber intake, with increased problems of digestion and/or elimination. If, however, your intake of these food groups is higher, then you are probably getting the 15 to 20 grams of dietary fiber a day considered adequate, as is discussed in Chapter 11.

Also, from the way you answered question 3, you can know how many empty-calorie foods you are consuming. Foods such as butter, margarine, vegetable oil, ice cream, alcohol, snacks, cookies, cakes, candies, and soft drinks are all known as empty-calorie foods because they have lots of calories but very few of the vitamins and minerals necessary for their metabolism. These foods promote a whole host of problems, some of which are behavioral in nature and others of which may be related to increased risk to many of the diseases of Western society. Empty-calorie foods are discussed in greater detail in the chapter on child behavior (13).

Inspection of the number of times cheese, yogurt, or other dairy products are consumed helps establish your level of dietary calcium intake. Calcium is extremely important for bone formation and nervous system function and may be low if milk and other dairy products are not included in the diet. (See Chapter 10 on calcium and bone loss.)

4. Fluids should be consumed at the level of 3 to 4 pints per day, minimum, and should be unsugared. Drinking water is the best way of achieving proper fluid balance without adding extra calories or additives to the diet.

5. Salting of food can be a real problem. We know that salt is hidden in many processed foods and that the average American is getting an excessive amount of salt, which may contribute to blood pressure problems in the salt-sensitive individual. Modest to no salting of foods is considered desirable.

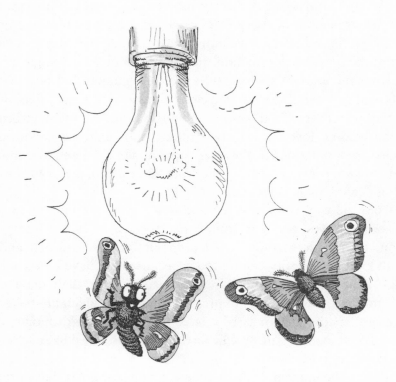

THE DOC SAID I SUFFERED FROM LOW DIETARY FIBER INTAKE.
I ASKED HIM WHAT I SHOULD EAT.
HE SAID, "SUIT YOURSELF."

6. If you are a strict vegetarian, you are highly likely to have one or more nutrient deficiencies—zinc, vitamin B-12, and possibly others.[17] If you do not have the time to closely formulate and monitor your vegetarian diet, it would be best to add a limited number of animal products such as eggs or milk products to guarantee nutrient adequacy.

7. If you are on a sugar- or salt-free diet, you are obviously limited in the amount of processed or convenience foods you can consume each day, and you are therefore by definition on a healthier diet. But where you are getting your calories and what foods do you normally consume in large quantities? A review of question 3 should allow you to answer this to see how your diet is distributed.

8. The number of times you eat out per week should be taken into account—it has now been found by national surveys that the average person in the United States eats between a quarter and a third of his or her meals in institutional settings outside of the home. Many people eat more meals away from home than they do at home, and the food they are consuming is of unknown origin. Many of these institutional foods may have been prepared hours before and warmed on a steam table, which results in loss of nutrients. It has generally been found that institutional foods have lower nutrient quality than do home-prepared entrees. Given that, if you are a frequent institutional food consumer, you should be more concerned about the level of vitamins and minerals in your diet than people who are more knowledgeable about the source of the food they are consuming.

9. High-temperature preparation or overcooking of your vegetables and meats can lead to significant nutrient depletion. Steaming your vegetables and eating your meats medium rare helps retain nutrients. The nutrient values given in food tables generally assume proper preparation of foods, so as to maintain nutrient quantities.

10. The frequent use of sauces and gravies increases the calorie content of the food considerably. In many dishes, the calorie count of the sauce or gravy is equal to that of the food it is covering. These sauces and gravies are essentially fats or oils and are usually empty calories; therefore, they increase the relative problem of nutrient depletion.

11. Deep-fat frying increases the calorie content of a food, but adds little in the way of vitamins and minerals, so, in effect, nutrients are depleted. Baked potatoes, for instance, are high in complex carbohydrates, low in fat, adequate in vitamins and minerals, and high in fiber if you eat the skin. French-fried potatoes, however, are higher in fat and lower in nutrient content due to the destruction of vitamin C in the potato during the high-temperature cooking process. The same is true of many other foods that have been deep-fat fried.

12. The consumption of prepared food from boxes or from the frozen food locker in your supermarket will lead to a much different nutrient intake than if the same entrees were made from scratch at home. Such convenience foods have suffered several steps of nutrient depletion in their manufacture, and their final nutrient quantity when put on the table is far less than what it would have been if you had prepared them yourself.

These preparation methods and processed food consumption habits are all things that may lead you to modify your confidence that you are getting an adequate level of vitamins and minerals in your basic diet and may account for some of the symptoms of chronic nutritional inadequacy that you are experiencing.

13. If you take vitamin supplements, you should be aware that excessive quantities of vitamins A and D lead to adverse side effects. A total intake of vitamin A greater than 25,000 to 30,000 units a day can be of concern in some people. Vitamin D above 1000 units per day for a long period of time in the adult may be considered hazardous. Nutrient toxicity symptoms are discussed in Chapter 3 on nutritional needs.

14. Lastly, if you are on a weight loss diet, you are by definition taking in fewer calories. If you are taking fewer calories, you are also taking in lower levels of vitamins and minerals. But your body may still require your pre-diet level of vitamins and minerals to generate the energy you require for your day's activity, and if you are marginally deprived of vitamin and mineral reserves, you may experience deficiency symptoms during the weight loss diet. Discussion of how to avoid this problem and what to do about it is covered in great detail in the chapter on weight control (6).

Summarizing the information that you have accrued from the analysis of your diet will suggest that if you're eating the average American diet, you have identified one or more nutritional problems. Recent surveys of the average American population revealed that 42 percent had intakes below 70 percent of the Recommended Dietary Allowance (RDA) for calcium, 32 percent had intakes below 70 percent for iron, 39 percent had intakes below 70 percent for magnesium, 51 percent had intakes below 70 percent for vitamin B-6, 26 percent had intakes below 70 percent for vitamin C, and 31 percent had intakes below 70 percent for vitamin A.[18] Given these sobering national statistics, it becomes very important for us to evaluate our own dietary intake and compare it to symptoms and early warning signs of underlying nutritional inadequacy that increases our risk to certain degenerative diseases.

Symptoms Evaluation Questionnaire

1. Does your hair tend to fall out or break easily?
2. Do you have poor night vision?
3. Do your gums bleed easily upon brushing your teeth?
4. Is your tongue sore or sensitive to hot beverages?
5. Do your lips or tongue burn?
6. Do you have a feeling of burning in your hands and/or feet?
7. Are you hyperexcitable?
8. Do you suffer from recurrent low back pain of unknown origin?
9. Do you have bone pain?
10. Are your fingernails ridged or spoon-shaped? Are there white spots under the nails?
11. Do you have muscle weakness or tenderness?
12. Can you not remember your dreams?
13. Do you have a racing heartbeat or missed or extra beats?
14. Do you have red areas on your skin or excessively oily skin with enlarged pores?
15. Do you have small yellowish growths under the skin, around your eyes, arms, or hands that resemble fat deposits?
16. Do you have frequent nosebleeds, prolonged bleeding, or easy bruising?
17. Do you have bluish or reddish discoloration of your legs?
18. Do you tend to heal slowly?
19. Do you have shortness of breath?
20. Do you have a poor sense of taste or smell?
21. Do you have a sensation like an electric shock when you bend your neck?
22. Do you tend to be anemic?
23. Do you have nocturnal leg cramps or muscle cramping?
24. Is your urine pink to red in color after you eat beets, or do you crave eating ice?

Interpretation of the Symptoms Evaluation Questionnaire

1. Hair loss or breakage may be an indication of protein insufficiency in the diet or maldigestion of protein or problems with regard to the sulfur-containing essential amino acids methionine, cystine, and cysteine found in dietary protein. Vegetarians and people trying to lose weight who are consuming diets that are low in the quality protein that contains these amino acids may have hair loss. These amino acids work along with the B-complex vitamin biotin as well as zinc and selenium in stimulating proper hair growth and density. Discussion of this problem will be found in Chapter 14.

2. Poor night vision may suggest a zinc and/or vitamin A deficiency. Zinc is found in higher-quality diets and may be deficient in poor-quality diets that consist of many convenience, snack, or empty-calorie foods. Vitamin A is a fat-soluble vitamin found in animal products; it is antagonized (counteracted) by excessive alcohol consumption but can be manufactured in the body by consuming adequate amounts of yellow-orange vegetables and fruits. Fat-soluble vitamins such as vitamin A are often not well absorbed; therefore, if the inspection of the diet evaluation indicates adequate vitamin A intake and there is still poor night vision, there may be a problem with the absorption of the vitamin. (For further discussion of this problem, see the chapter on nutritional needs, Chapter 3.)

3. If your gums bleed easily upon brushing your teeth, it may be an indication of vitamin C, bioflavonoid, or folic acid deficiencies. The need for vitamin C can vary dramatically from individual to individual and, therefore, what may be considered to be an adequate level of vitamin C for the average person may be suboptimal for a specific individual. A level of vitamin C between 100 and 1000 milligrams a day, along with bioflavonoids, which are found in citrus fruits in the soft white parts between the skin and the fruit, may be required to prevent increased capillary fragility and easy bruising and bleeding.

4. A tongue sore or sensitive to hot beverages may indicate a deficiency of iron, folic acid, vitamin B-2 or B-3. If this tongue sensitivity comes along with impaired taste and poor appetite, a zinc deficiency may also be involved. Increasing the nutritional quality to more B-complex-rich foods such as liver, whole grains, lean meats, and brewer's yeast may be helpful.

5. A burning tongue or lips may suggest a thiamin (vitamin B-1) deficiency. Levels of thiamin required by some individuals may be far greater, due to metabolic uniquenesses, than the 1.5 milligrams that is the Recommended Dietary Allowance. Intake levels of thiamin between 5 and 25 milligrams a day may be required for some individuals to treat this condition.

6. If you have a feeling of burning in your hands and feet, it may indicate not only a thiamin (B-1) but also a riboflavin (vitamin B-2) deficiency. Again, levels of these two B vitamins may be required at 20 to 50 milligrams along with one of the B-complex nutrients called inositol at a level of 1000 milligrams to successfully manage the tingling numbness or burning of hands or feet that is associated with certain polyneuritis (nerve) conditions.

7. Hyperexcitability may indicate a clinical deficiency of niacin (vitamin B-3) as well as magnesium deficiency. Niacin is found in high quantities in lean meats and brewer's yeast; magnesium is found in green leafy vegetables and lean muscle meats. Many individuals who are on limited incomes are unable to purchase the quality foods higher in niacin and cannot eat or do not like magnesium-rich green leafy vegetables and so may be simultaneously niacin and magnesium depleted, resulting in a hyperexcitable personality state. Levels of niacin between 10 and 15 milligrams and magnesium between 200 and 300 milligrams per day may be required.

8. Recurrent low back pain of unknown origin may indicate a folic acid, vitamin B-12, or calcium deficiency. If you also answered yes to question 21 and you have a sensation like an electric shock when you bend your neck, this is highly indicative of a vitamin B-12 deficiency. Remember, vitamin B-12 is difficult to absorb; many older people lose the ability to properly absorb this vitamin and start to exhibit deficiency state evidenced by low back pain and joint pain of unknown origin. Levels of vitamin B-12 at 5 to 10 micrograms a day along with 400 to 800 micrograms of folic acid and 500 milligrams of calcium and 5 milligrams of manganese may be helpful in managing these problems.

9. Bone pain may indicate a vitamin D deficiency, lack of exposure to sunlight, or calcium and magnesium deficiency states and may be accompanied by nocturnal leg cramps. Levels of calcium at 500 to 800 milligrams a day as a supplement, along with 200 to 300 milligrams of magnesium and 400 units of vitamin D are helpful in these conditions.

10. If your fingernails are ridged, spoon-shaped, or have white spots under them, this may indicate an iron, calcium, or zinc deficiency. Extensive white spots under the fingernails have been correlated with a zinc deficiency state, whereas ridging of the nails so that they become washboard in texture indicates an iron, zinc, or calcium deficiency. Levels of zinc between 20 and 30 milligrams a day and iron at levels between 20 and 30 milligrams a day may be required to manage these problems. These are early warning signs of later-stage, more acute problems related to the deficiency of these nutrients.

11. Muscle weakness or tenderness may indicate the presence of certain food or environmental allergies, particularly if it is accompanied by headaches. A more extensive discussion of allergies is to be found in Chapter 11.

Another source of muscle weakness and muscle tenderness is vitamin B-1 deficiency. If the sore muscles are accompanied by burning lips or tingling or numbness of the hands or feet, this is highly confirmatory of the need for increased vitamin B-1 intake.

12. If you cannot remember your dreams, it may be an indication of a vitamin B-6 deficiency. Even in the face of what appears adequate vitamin B-6 intake, lack of dream recall may signal an insufficient amount of this important nutrient. Vitamin B-6 has the function of helping aid in the proper control of substances of the brain that contribute to mood, mind, memory, and behavior and is discussed in greater detail in the chapters on aging and emotions (4 and 5). Levels of vitamin B-6 between 50 and 100 milligrams or more may be required to promote proper dream recall.

13. A racing heartbeat or missed or extra beats may be an indication of a vitamin B-1, copper, calcium, magnesium, or potassium deficiency. Vitamin B-1 at the level of 10 to 25 milligrams a day along with copper (3 to 5 mg), calcium (500 mg), magnesium (300 mg), and adequate potassium from a diet plentiful in green vegetables may be helpful in alleviating these symptoms.

14. Red areas on the skin or excessively oily skin with enlarged pores may indicate a vitamin B-2 need. Requirements for B-2 and also vitamin B-6 to manage these conditions may be from 10 to 50 milligrams per day for both of these B-vitamins. The classic picture of the red-nosed alcoholic may be related to the B-vitamin deficiency state that alcoholism produces, and not the alcohol itself, and may be corrected in part by increased B-vitamin nutriture, particularly vitamins B-2 and B-6.

15. Small yellowish growths under the skin, around the eyes, arms, or hands that resemble fat deposits are called xanthomas; they are cholesterol-rich deposits that occur when your body is trying to get rid of excessive cholesterol. This condition has been found to be related in part to your genetic background and this may indicate a very considerable risk to heart disease and other vascular complications; you should go quickly to Chapter 7 and look at the aggressive way of approaching the reduction of blood cholesterol by life-style and dietary measures. Vitamin C and chromium may be very helpful in this condition.

16. Frequent nosebleeds, prolonged bleeding, or easy bruising may indicate increased capillary fragility with deficiencies of vitamin K, vitamin C, copper, or bioflavonoids. Vitamin K is normally synthesized in your own intestines by bacteria and, therefore, is not considered to be needed in the diet as such; however, individuals who have intestinal problems or who have been on antibiotic therapy may have inadequate vitamin K synthesis and increased bleeding tendencies. Vitamin K can be gotten from green leafy vegetables. Problems with blood clotting may also produce these symptoms; if they persist they should be evaluated by your physician.

17. Bluish or reddish discoloration of the legs may indicate problems with regard to blood supply to your extremities and arteriosclerosis and require an aggressive approach toward improved circulation. (This may also come along with pain in the legs of unknown origin, and the treatment requires medical supervision.) Review the material discussed in Chapters 6 and 7 to see how exercise and diet can be used together to improve blood flow to the extremities.

18. If you tend to heal slowly, it may indicate protein insufficiencies, zinc or chromium insufficiency, or iron and copper problems, particularly if it is accompanied by a tendency toward anemia. Vitamin C has also been found to be very important in facilitating the healing process; therefore, levels of nutrients at 1000 milligrams of vitamin C, 20 milligrams of zinc, 100 micrograms of selenium, 3 milligrams of copper, 15 milligrams of iron, with adequate vitamin B-12 at 10 micrograms and folic acid at 400 micrograms should help improve wound healing in those individuals who have this biochemical need.

19. Shortness of breath may indicate lung and blood circulation problems and require exercise therapy as well as dietary improvement. (See Chapters 6 and 7 on weight control and heart disease.) It has also been found that certain toxic minerals such as lead and cadmium may also contribute to blood and lung problems (see Chapter 13).

20. A poor sense of taste or smell may indicate a zinc deficiency. This is particularly a problem in older individuals or children consuming low-quality diets. Zinc at the level of 15 to 30 milligrams per day may be required to correct this problem.

21. A sensation like an electric shock when you bend your neck is called Lhermitte's syndrome and may be related to a vitamin B-12 insufficiency. Recall that vitamin B-12 is difficult to absorb from the intestines into the bloodstream; therefore, some individuals may require a much greater amount in order to raise the level in the blood to an adequate quantity.

22. A tendency toward anemia may indicate a biochemical need for high levels of iron, copper, folic acid, or vitamin B-12. Remember that there are many other types of nutritionally related anemias other than that of iron-deficiency anemia. Some people who are anemic and do not get response from iron may be copper deficient. Levels of iron at 15 milligrams a day, copper at 3 milligrams, folic acid at 400 micrograms, and vitamin B-12 at 10 micrograms may be beneficial for people who tend to be anemic.

23. Nocturnal leg cramps or muscle cramping may indicate a calcium and/or magnesium deficiency, particularly if it is accompanied by elevated blood pressure. A calcium deficiency has been found associated with essential hypertension and nocturnal leg cramps. Levels of calcium at 800 milligrams per day and magnesium at 400 milligrams per day may be helpful in alleviating this problem, along with vitamin E at 400 units.

24. If your urine is pink to red in color after eating beets, or you crave eating ice, you may have an iron deficiency. Iron deficiency is very common in young women and older-aged individuals and can result in low-grade anemia and tiredness. Iron supplements from 14 to 50 milligrams per day may be needed to correct this problem.

Summarizing Your Biotype

You've now completed all the questionnaires and their interpretations and should have a reasonably good idea of the way you eat, your biochemical sensitivities, some of your nutritional requirements, and you are starting to establish what types of foods and lifestyle would be most appropriate for insuring your health after the age of 30, based upon your own biotype. To help you summarize your biotype, the following summary sheet is provided. Fill it out, and then continue on to learn how to tailor your Nutraerobics Program to your biotype.

Remember, we are trying to find out if you're a better protein, carbohydrate, or fat metabolizer. Do you require higher levels of the B-complex vitamins, vitamin C, or the fat-soluble vitamins? Do you properly digest and assimilate certain nutrients such as vitamin B-12? Do you require more or less exercise and what type of exercise is optimal for you? Do you have certain genetic sensitivites to health problems such as hypothyroidism, coronary heart disease, or cancer? What can you do to help compensate for those unique sensitivities? How can environmental stress and allergens modify your function?

Circle the appropriate response

Metabolic Type. *Do you have:*

Slow turnover (cold hands and feet, gain weight easily)	Normal	Rapid turnover (warmer hands and feet, can't gain weight)

Digestive Type. *Rate your ability to digest the following:*

Protein	Good	Poor
Carbohydrates: Starches from grains	Good	Poor
Cooked beans (legumes)	Good	Poor
Sugars	Good	Poor
Fats or oils	Good	Poor
Dairy products	Good	Poor

Intestinal Type. *Do you show a tendency toward:*

Constipation	Regularity	Diarrhea

Vitamin needs. *Take your response from questionnaires:*

A	Lower	Normal	Higher
B-1	Lower	Normal	Higher
B-2	Lower	Normal	Higher
B-3	Lower	Normal	Higher
B-6	Lower	Normal	Higher
B-12	Lower	Normal	Higher
B-complex	Lower	Normal	Higher
C	Lower	Normal	Higher
D	Lower	Normal	Higher
E	Lower	Normal	Higher

Mineral needs. *Take your response from questionnaires:*

Calcium	Lower	Normal	Higher
Magnesium	Lower	Normal	Higher
Iron	Lower	Normal	Higher
Copper	Lower	Normal	Higher
Zinc	Lower	Normal	Higher
Chromium	Lower	Normal	Higher
Manganese	Lower	Normal	Higher
Selenium	Lower	Normal	Higher
Potassium	Lower	Normal	Higher
Sodium	Lower	Normal	Higher
Phosphorus	Lower	Normal	Higher

Exercise Type. *Are you:*

Sedentary	Moderate	Active

Fitness Level. *Is your fitness:*

Poor	Moderate	Good

Body Weight. *Are you:*

Overweight	Normal weight	Underweight

Distress Level. *Is your response to tension, or new social situations:*

Calm	Moderately distressed	Highly distressed

Personality Type. *Do you normally function with:*

Low stress	Moderate stress	High stress

Write in problems from your present diet evaluation:

Write in any medication use:

Allergy Type. *Are you:*

Very allergic to many things	Moderately or selectively allergic	Without known allergies

Family or Personal Health Problems. *Circle if present:*

Heart	Cancer	Headaches or "nerves"
Blood pressure	Low immunity	Poor energy
Diabetes	Arthritis or muscle pain	Dental or bone problems
Obesity	Digestive disorders	

Smoker?

No   Yes

Alcohol Consumer?

No   Low   High

From this summary can you now define your Nutraerobics biotype? If not, then go back and review your responses to the questionnaires in Chapter 2 and try again. You will use this biotype throughout the remainder of the book.

If there are a few of the nutrients you are still not able to specify, don't worry, you will learn more about your needs as you go on in the book. Keep a pencil handy and make notes and modifications on your requirements for optimal health as you go through each chapter. We will put your whole program together in Chapter 14.

In the future chapters we are now going to be dealing with your biotype and applying improved lifestyle and nutrition in a Nutraerobics fashion to optimize the dividends from your Living Life Insurance Policy. Let's get going now and assign your unique nutrition and exercise needs.

Notes

1. R. Williams, *Nutrition Against Disease* (New York: Bantam, 1971).

2. S. Harada and H. W. Goedde, "Aldehyde Dehydrogenase Deficiency in Alcohol Induced Facial Flushing," *Lancet* (31 October 1981):982.

3. "Possible Vitamin B-6 Deficiency in the Chinese Restaurant Syndrome," *Nutrition Reviews, 40,* 15(1982).

4. D. Hawkins and L. Pauling, *Orthomolecular Psychiatry* (San Francisco: Freeman, 1973).

5. M. K. Hambidge and J. D. Baum, "Low Levels of Zinc in Hair of Children with Poor Growth and Appetites," *Pediatric Research, 6,* 868(1972).

6. J. Rabkin and E. L. Struening, "Life Events, Stress, and Illness," *Science, 191,* 1013(1976).

7. V. Riley, "Mouse Mammary Tumors: Alteration of Incidence as Apparent Function of Stress," *Science, 189,* 465(1975).

8. R. Anderson, *Stress Power* (San Francisco: New Age Press, 1979).

9. H. Selye, *The General Adaptation Syndrome* (New York: Bantam, 1972).

10. M. Friedman, "Modification of Type A Behavior in Postinfarction Patients," *American Heart Journal, 97,* 114(1979).

11. A. Meyer, "Tongue Color and Vitamin B Deficiency," *Lancet* (16 June 1975):116.

12. J. Ellis, Y. Watanabe, and K. Folkers, "Carpal Tunnel Syndrome and Vitamin B-6 Deficiency," *Proceedings of the National Academy of Sciences, 92,* 1141(1979).

13. D. Roe, *Drug-Induced Nutritional Deficiencies* (Westport, CT: AVI Publishing, 1976).

14. J. S. Bland, "The Improvement of Health by Risk Factor Intervention: A Tool of Preventive Medicine," *Journal of Holistic Medicine, 4,* 34(1982).

15. H. Guthrie and G. Guthrie, "Factor Analysis of Nutritional Status Data from the Ten State Nutrition Surveys," *American Journal of Clinical Nutrition, 29,* 1238(1976).

16. S. Reiser and J. Hallfrisch, "Isocalorie Exchange of Dietary Starch and Sucrose in Humans," *American Journal of Clinical Nutrition, 32,* 2206(1979).

17. J. T. Dwyer and R. M. Suskind, "Nutritional Status of Vegetarian Children," *American Journal of Clinical Nutrition, 35,* 204(1982).

18. L. Page and B. Friend, "The Changing U.S. Diet," *BioScience, 28,* 192(1978).

3

Assigning Your Unique Nutritional Needs

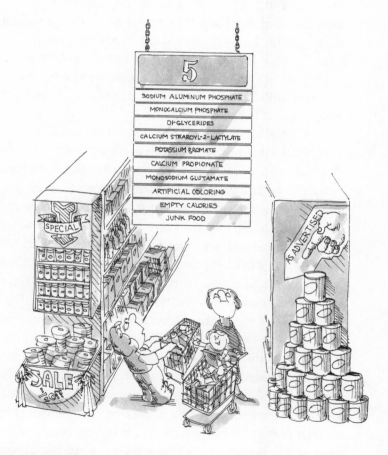

IT MUST BE BECAUSE OF THE NEW TRUTH-IN-STORE-DIRECTORIES ACT PASSED BY THE FDA.

We are now ready to design a specific Nutraerobics Program for you for the promotion of your optimal health. In designing your nutrition program and vitamin and mineral needs, many books now advocate turning to the Recommended Dietary Allowances (RDAs) to assign your level of required nutritional intake. What are the RDAs? The Recommended Dietary Allowances are "the levels of intake of essential nutrients considered, in the judgment of the Food and Nutrition Board on the basis of available scientific knowledge, to be adequate to meet the known nutritional needs of practically all healthy persons."[1] The RDAs promote adequate nutritional status; however, many people are asking not about adequate, but optimal states of nutrition, and who are the "practically all healthy persons" that the RDAs cover?

First of all, RDAs do not cover therapeutic nutritional needs. They do not take into account special needs arising from infections, metabolic disorders, chronic diseases, or any other abnormalities that require special dietary treatment, nor do they deal with specific individual requirements. They are the levels of nutrient intake suggested to promote **adequate** health. But we do know there are a number of conditions that require adjustments in the RDAs—body-size and sex, heavy physical activity or work, exposure to extreme climates, both hot and cold, changes due to illness or rehabilitation, intestinal parasites, or unique metabolic considerations based upon biochemical individuality.

Also, of the some 44 nutrients known to be essential for human function, for only about one-third of them have known Recommended Dietary Allowances been established. This does not mean that the other two-thirds are unimportant, simply that we do not know what level to establish as adequate because no acute deficiency symptom exists. The adverse health effects resulting from the absence of these nutrients may be chronic, long term, and progressive rather than producing an acute deficiency syndrome, as the absence of vitamin C produces scurvy, or the absence of vitamin B-3 produces pellagra. Such is certainly the case with vitamin E, which is considered to be an essential nutrient, but no deficiency symptom of an acute nature has been identified in the human. In establishing the RDA of vitamin E, routine food surveys of presumably healthy people were done. Inspection of their average vitamin E intake, which was considered to be adequate by definition because these people were "healthy," was found to be between 15 and 30 units per day and this was established as the RDA. So this is not necessarily an optimal level of vitamin E; it is only a crude approximation of what may be considered a desirable dietary level of vitamin E.

Many of the other essential nutrients have no Recommended Dietary Allowances because of the difficulty in assigning **any** level of adequate intake based upon existing studies. Given this, the Recommended Dietary Allowances are guidelines for general adequate nutritional intake and are not designed to be used as guidelines to promote optimal nutrition for the individual. They are helpful in providing information for nutritional surveys and the steering of governmental policy with regard to food programs, but they are only general standards to be used as goals for good nutrition.

Optimal Versus Adequate Nutrition

How then do we better establish optimal nutritional needs for you if not from the Recommended Dietary Allowances? You have already made a big step forward in answering this question by the completion of the questionnaires in Chapter 2. You have now found out about your biochemical individuality and unique specific needs. Given the kind of picture you have painted of yourself by the responses to the questionnaires in Chapter 2, you are now better able to define what may constitute optimal levels of various nutrients for your need. Let us now address the armamentarium of nutritional substances you need for the promotion of optimal health.

The body needs adequate calories in the form of protein, carbohydrate, and fat. You cannot live on vitamin or mineral pills alone; you must have the proper amount of these **macronutrients** (protein, carbohydrates, and fats) to supply your dietary calories. The Senate Select

Figure 1
Suggested Revisions of the Standard American Diet

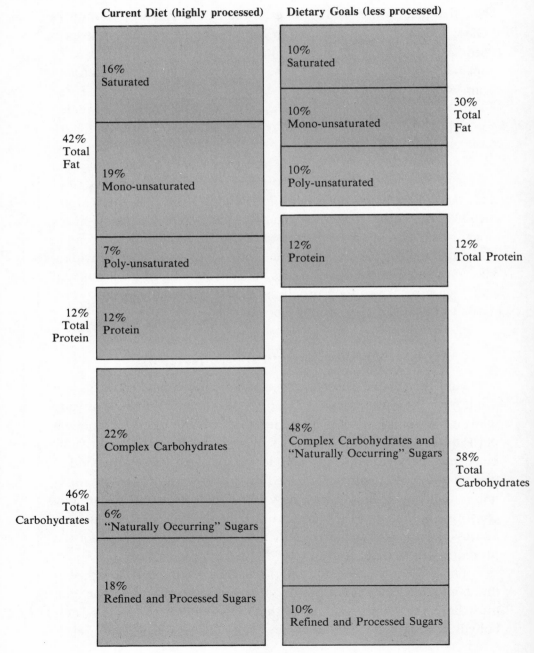

Current Diet (highly processed)

Dietary Goals (less processed)

42% Total Fat
- 16% Saturated
- 19% Mono-unsaturated
- 7% Poly-unsaturated

30% Total Fat
- 10% Saturated
- 10% Mono-unsaturated
- 10% Poly-unsaturated

12% Total Protein
- 12% Protein

12% Total Protein
- 12% Protein

46% Total Carbohydrates
- 22% Complex Carbohydrates
- 6% "Naturally Occurring" Sugars
- 18% Refined and Processed Sugars

58% Total Carbohydrates
- 48% Complex Carbohydrates and "Naturally Occurring" Sugars
- 10% Refined and Processed Sugars

Committee on Nutrition and Human Needs has promoted a set of Dietary Goals for the United States. These goals are designed to help people achieve higher levels of health through the consumption of optimal levels of protein, carbohydrate, and fat.[2] These goals can be summarized as follows:

1. Decrease calorie intake so as to promote proper body weight-to-height ratio.

2. Increase the consumption of whole grains and starchy vegetables rich in complex carbohydrates.

3. Reduce the consumption of refined and processed sugars.

4. Reduce overall fat consumption.

5. Of the fats you do eat, reduce saturated animal fat, which is a solid at room temperature, and balance it with liquid polyunsaturated vegetable oils.

6. Reduce cholesterol consumption.

7. Limit the intake of sodium from salt and other sources.

In order to achieve the dietary goals suggested above, people who are consuming a diet equivalent to the average American diet as shown in Figure 1 must make the following changes:

1. They should increase consumption of fruits and vegetables, whole-grain bread and pasta products.

2. They should decrease consumption of refined and other processed sugars by avoiding foods whose ingredients list sugars first, second, or third.

3. They should decrease consumption of foods that are known to be high in total fat, including fatty cuts of meat, deep-fried foods, fat-rich dips, spreads, butters, margarine, and high-fat

cheeses, and increase consumption of lower-fat animal products, including poultry without the skin, fish, and lean cuts
of muscle meat. There should be a substitution of low-fat or
nonfat milk for whole milk and low-fat dairy products for
high-fat dairy products. There should be a decrease in the
consumption of butterfat, eggs, and fatty cuts of meat which
are high in cholesterol.

4.   They should decrease consumption of foods with a lot of
hidden salt, which include smoked and cured meats, snack
foods, canned vegetables, and other processed foods where
salt is high on the list of ingredients or where salt is added
directly to the food. Any source of sodium, whether in salt or
other food additives, should be reduced.

Improvement in dietary intake can be achieved if a person will
consume more meals made from raw foods in the home and depend
less on institutional foods whose ingredients are of unknown origin.
The rule of thumb is when you go into the supermarket, do not get lost
in the labyrinth of highly processed foods in the market's center section, but rather take your shopping cart and quickly proceed to the
perimeter of the store where your nutritional friends are located. In
these areas you will generally find the dairy products, poultry, fish, lean
meats, fresh produce, whole-grain products, and the starchy vegetables
such as potatoes, beans, and other legumes. The central portion of the
store contains products whose lists of ingredients read more like something from an organic chemistry textbook and are found to have sugar,
salt, white flour, and fats such as mono- and diglycerides, corn oil,
partially hydrogenated palm oil, and other chemically modified fats as
the major ingredients.

The Changing U.S. Diet

Has the American diet really changed markedly in this century?
According to studies done by the U.S. Department of Agriculture

(USDA), in the past fifty years our culture has been involved in one of the most remarkable food experiments ever undertaken by humans. During this period we have altered the American food supply system away from fresh fruits, vegetables, meats, and dairy products to the highly processed, "fortified," synthetically manufactured food substitutes and convenience foods that fill the shelves of our supermarkets from coast to coast. As a result, major changes have occurred in our use of basic foods.

First, we are using more fat-rich cuts of meat and poultry than before. Second, sugars and other sweeteners, fats and oils, and processed fruits and vegetables have all increased remarkably in the standard diet. Third, we are using fewer whole-grain products, potatoes and sweet potatoes, fresh fruits and vegetables, and eggs, all of which are known to have excellent nutritive value.

Consumption of sugars and other sweeteners is up one-third since 1909–1913, largely due to the use of greater amounts of sugar hidden in highly processed foods. Use of refined sugar was high in the late 1920s, when some of it may have been diverted into illegal alcoholic beverages during Prohibition, and again in the early 1970s, when cyclamate was withdrawn. Sugar consumption declined during World War II, when sugar was one of the foods rationed. Another decline occurred in the 1970s in response to high sugar prices, although recently sugar consumption has increased as a result of the large amounts of fructose and corn syrup sweetners being used in soft drinks.

Use of sugar in processed foods and beverages now accounts for more than two-thirds of the total sugar consumed, compared to one-fourth of the total during 1910. The largest increase in the use of refined sugars is in beverages and accounts for about one-fourth of the total 125 pounds per person per year of sugar consumption.

Use of fats and oils was 50 percent greater in 1980 than it was during 1910. Use of butter and lard has declined but has more than been made up for by increasing levels of unsaturated vegetable oils, partially hydrogenated vegetable spreads, and margarines. Use of salad and cooking oils tripled between 1950 and 1976. This sharp upturn reflects the growing use of liquid oils by food processors and fast food outlets as well as by home consumers and contributes greatly to the increased fat in the average American diet.

Shifts in the kinds and amounts of foods making up the U.S. diet have altered the levels of micronutrients available for consumption. **Micronutrients** are defined as the vitamins, minerals, and other substances that help facilitate proper metabolism and energy production from the macronutrients. The vitamins can be broken down into two families: the fat-soluble family which includes vitamins A, D, E, and K; and the water-soluble family which includes the B-complex vitamins and vitamin C. The minerals can also be broken down into two families: the macroelements, which are those required in levels greater than 100 milligrams a day (such as magnesium, calcium, potassium, sodium, chlorine, and phosphorus); and the micro, or trace, elements, which are those found in the body in very small quantities and in foods sometimes at only the one-part-per-million level, such as iron, copper, zinc, manganese, chromium, selenium, vanadium, molybdenum, silicon, iodine, and fluorine.[3]

Vitamins and Minerals as Supplements

Everywhere you turn these days some advertisement is extolling the virtue of a vitamin or a mineral supplement. Vitamin and mineral supplements are a big and fast-growing business, up from about $500 million in sales in 1972 to more than $1.5 billion in 1982, with a $3.5 billion in sales projected by 1988. Today, one hundred million Americans, or 44 percent of the population, swallow one or more vitamin or mineral pills each day. Are these really necessary? Are these people taking the right supplements for their individual needs? What are the right ones for you?

We have often heard that vitamin supplements may at best produce only expensive urine and at worst produce toxicity and, therefore, should be avoided by most people who are eating a well-balanced diet. But what is the well-balanced diet?

In the past we have heard that "well-balanced" means eating

foods from the seven foods groups each day: the starchy vegetables, the nonstarchy vegetables, the meat group, the dairy and milk group, the citrus fruits, the noncitrus fruits, and the grain group. This way of designating dietary intake was very useful in the 1930s, 1940s, and 1950s, but it has lost some of its applicability in the 1980s. In what group do you put the following foods?

Count Chocula	Meat substitutes
Space food sticks	Turkey loaf
Breakfast bars	Instant mashed potatoes
Cremora	Corn or potato chips
Tang	Weight loss protein powders
Desserta	Soft drinks or sweetened fruit
Jello	drinks

This is but a partial list of the many hundreds of foods now filling our supermarket shelves that have no clear designation as to what food family they fall into. Many people have called these "empty-calorie" foods, which means they provide a large number of calories without the levels of the supporting vitamins and minerals necessary for their proper metabolism. These foods encourage obesity and lead to a new type of malnutrition commonly called "the malnutrition of too much of too little," or "overconsumptive undernutrition." This type of malnutrition does not show the classic signs of a vitamin or mineral deficiency such as scurvy, caused by vitamin C deficiency, or beriberi, from a B-1 deficiency; instead we see an increased risk to the major degenerative diseases such as heart disease, cancer, diabetes, obesity, oral health problems, and reduced effectiveness of the immune system.

Whether it is necessary for you to take vitamin or mineral supplements depends very much on what you determined was the quality of your diet from the nutrition scan you completed in Chapter 2 and the relationship of your diet to your symptoms and genetic background. However, it is very difficult these days for an individual applying the American way of eating that depends upon processed foods, restaurant and take-out meals, and nutritionally empty snacks to meet the body's need for the forty-four essential nutrients. When you consider that this basic need may also be modified by specific biochemical uniquenesses that vary from individual to individual and require higher than average levels of specific nutrients, the problem of nutrient depletion becomes even more severe.

If you consider that almost two-thirds of the daily calories in the average American diet come from fats and sugar, which are virtually devoid of vitamins and minerals, it is clear that the remaining one-third of the calories in the diet must provide all of the vitamins and minerals needed for metabolism. This is very hard to accomplish unless the remaining one-third of the diet is extremely nutrient rich.

The Empty-Calorie Diet

Starting with a very poor quality diet that depends primarily on empty-calorie foods and taking a vitamin or mineral supplement to guarantee nutritional adequacy, however, is total foolishness. The quality of the total diet starts with the food that we put in our mouths. You cannot make a high-performance automobile run well by putting low-octane gasoline in the tank but still using premium oil. Both premium oil and high-quality fuel are necessary for the car to run optimally. Likewise, you should begin designing your Nutraerobics diet with quality food items based on your specific needs as identified through your biotype; if as you continue reading, you note a need for selective nutritional supplementation, it should be just that—supplementation—based on your genetic requirements and lifestyle.

You might say at this point, "Well, I don't see people falling dead from nutritional deficiency, so why should I worry? After all, it's all food, isn't it?" From the perspective of vitamin and mineral intake, all is clearly not well today with the American diet. In fact, the most recent nationwide food consumption surveys of 1977–1978, involving a three-day dietary analysis for 37,785 individuals, show that large percentages of Americans are consuming significantly less than the recommended levels of at least six nutrients, including vitamins A, C, B-6, calcium, iron, and magnesium. Intakes of vitamins D and E, folic acid, zinc, and iodine were not measured in the study, but judging from the known deficiencies, several of these are also likely to be problem nutrients. The irony is that even though people may be eating more today than they were in 1910, they may actually be getting less in the way of the vitamins and minerals necessary for the metabolism of these calories due to the higher dependency on processed and nutrient-poor foods.

The survey showed that vitamin and mineral intake was particularly poor for adolescent girls and adult women, many of whom were on low-calorie diets that, even with the best of planning, could not fully meet their nutrient requirements. Much of the population is on certain medications, such as birth control pills or a high blood pressure or anti-ulcer medication, all of which are known to have impact upon nutritional status. Women on birth control pills are urged to increase their level of intake of vitamin B-6, zinc, and folic acid; individuals who smoke or consume alcohol may need higher levels of vitamin C, vitamin E, and the B-complex vitamins.

Food Fortification

And do we think our foods must be adequate because they are "vitamin fortified"? A number of foods are now fortified with nutrients: iodine has been added to salt since 1923 to prevent thyroid goiter; milk was first fortified with vitamin D in the 1930s. Skim milk is also fortified with vitamin A, because the naturally occurring vitamin is removed from the milk along with the milk fat. In the 1940s, millers and bakers began restoring to white flour several of the many nutrients lost in the refining process.

In the past ten years the impetus to fortify foods has shifted from the public health community to the food industry. The big push toward a fortified food supply may have begun around 1970 in the breakfast cereal market when it was found from a study that rats fed commercial breakfast foods seemed to grow and survive no better than the rats fed the boxes that the breakfast cereals came in. From that time, there was a great push to fortify with several vitamins breakfast cereals and many other convenience or snack foods or beverages commonly consumed by children.

Everything from Kool Aid to candy bars and tomato juice to baby foods is seen as an appropriate carrier for extra vitamins. As one consumer affairs spokesperson points out, "Candy dressed up in nutritional claims, even supportable claims, can play a decidedly destructive role by replacing necessary dietary elements." Of course, the food industry will not admit publicly that it uses vitamins as a promotional gimmick, but it seems quite clear that capitalizing on the public's awareness that vitamins are important does not, in fact, hurt sales.

For example, contrast the General Mills cereals Total and Wheaties. Total is a vitamin- and mineral-fortified form of Wheaties. Total provides 100 percent of the RDA for nine vitamins and one mineral, (iron), while Wheaties is fortified with only 10 to 25 percent of the RDA for eight vitamins and one mineral. It costs General Mills about one to two cents more per 12-ounce box to manufacture Total than Wheaties; however, at the supermarket a 12-ounce box of Total sells at a price 37 percent higher than that of Wheaties, or approximately 35 to 40 cents more. It is clear, then, that profits are closely correlated to fortification.

The wary consumer must be aware of the fact that fortified products do not carry the full spectrum of all the essential nutrients necessary to metabolize them. This is selected fortification and does not address the complete question of proper nutrition. Many of these products are still deficient in dietary fiber, ultratrace elements, and may be excessively high in sugars which have their own adverse effects upon human function, as will be discussed later in Chapter 7.

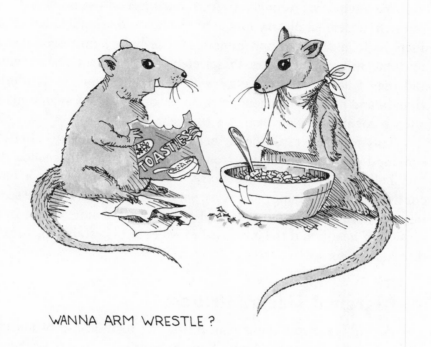

WANNA ARM WRESTLE ?

Historical Diet Habits

The study of dietary habits of people who lived some ten thousand years ago seems to indicate that, historically, human nutrition developed from an early dependency upon a wide variety of foods rich in vitamins and minerals as well as dietary fiber. Archeological records indicate that early peoples were nomadic hunters and gatherers, following the herds and eating primarily nuts, berries, seasonal fruits, and other wild foods and game.

When agriculture was developed, a shift occurred from the wild and varied (and sometimes none too plentiful) diet to one that included cultivated grain products such as maize (a corn ancestor). With this came the ability to keep grain reserves, which in turn allowed cities to develop, a social order to evolve, and a complex human culture and society to flourish.

We have come a long way from our original legacy of a diverse and rich, unrefined dietary intake of animal- and vegetable-based products high in vitamins and minerals.[4] The highly processed diet we consume today contributes to selected micronutrient insufficiencies and may lead us into the gray area of malnutrition, or borderline vitamin and mineral deficiency, which produces diffuse symptoms not often recognized by medical practitioners.

This modern transition to highly processed, "empty" foods, in conjunction with a migration from the farms to the cities since 1910 that has fostered a more sedentary, less active lifestyle, is a major contributor to the change in disease patterns in our culture. The sedentary lifestyle and the nutrient-depleted diet are major factors in the erosion of health and the increased prevalence of certain degenerative diseases in our society today.

Marginal Undernutrition

A number of questions concerning the relationship of marginal vitamin and mineral intake to human health or disease go beyond questions commonly asked by most nutritionists. These questions can be summarized as follows:

1. Is there a state of optimal nutrition beyond that which is considered adequate?

2. Does marginal vitamin deficiency have any clinical significance and, if so, what is it?

3. Are there links between behavior and nutrition?

4. How widespread are the marginal vitamin and mineral deficiencies in the population at large?

There is considerable difference of opinion today among health and nutrition professionals regarding the concept of optimal versus adequate nutrition. Traditionally, nutritionists and doctors have presumed that the absence of clinical signs of classic deficiency diseases such as scurvy, pellagra, beriberi, rickets, kwashiorkor, or marasmus indicates that the individual must be adequately nourished. These doctors consider people to be healthy until proven diseased; however, this assumption may not necessarily be true.

Putting it another way, we can say that the absence of disease does not mean optimal wellness. Marginal vitamin deficiency may be the middle ground between adequate nutritional status and optimal states of health. Because there are no specific textbook symptoms associated with marginal deficiency, this intermediate stage of depletion may not be apparent to the medical practitioner. In common terms, it may be that you are just feeling less than your best or "under the weather."

As will be discussed in the following chapters, there is now strong evidence suggesting that vague symptoms such as lethargy, irritability, insomnia, and difficulty in concentrating may in many cases reflect an underlying marginal nutritional deficiency. Beyond that, a marginal deficiency may even be reflected in the body's lowered ability to resist disease and infection, its lowered ability to recover from surgery or stress or disease, or even the lowered ability of the brain to function at a high level.

Recognizing Your Nutritional Status

As will be discussed throughout the remainder of this book on the implementation of the Nutraerobics Program, greater attention is now being placed on the area of identifying marginal deficiencies using biochemical, anthropometric, and dietary information and managing them before they actually produce the signs of diagnosable diseases such as heart disease, diabetes, or cancer. Experience has shown that detecting and treating these deficiencies at an early stage, rather than waiting for clinical signs, is highly beneficial and may be a much more cost-efficient path toward health-care improvement.

What then is a marginal deficiency and how can we define it in you? **Marginal deficiency** is a state of gradual vitamin or mineral depletion in which there is evidence of lack of personal well-being associated with impaired physiological function.[5] Many of the symptoms you indicated on your Symptoms Evaluation Questionnaire are related to such marginal deficiency symptoms, although you may never have considered them to be related to your diet or lifestyle at all.

Depletion of the body's reserve of vitamins or minerals goes through several stages. An asymptomatic preliminary stage progresses into a stage of biochemical alteration at the cellular level not normally detected by most health assessments or physical examinations. A third stage, called the psychological stage, shows nonspecific symptoms such as loss of appetite, depression, irritability, anxiety, or insomnia and passes into a clinical stage which, left untreated, finally becomes an anatomical stage in which a disease is recognized.

Most people are not suffering from the latter stages of this sequence, but they may be in the throes of the early stages of it at the physiological or biochemical level. This marginal vitamin depletion can have a significant effect on functions such as your body's ability to properly handle drugs, alcohol, or exposure to environmental chemicals, and it can influence your immunity to disease.[6]

Given this information, there does appear to be a state of optimal nutrition beyond that which is merely adequate. It can be defined and measured by following through the questionnaires in Chapter 2, which can help you learn how to achieve that optimal state.

Some marginal vitamin deficiencies do have clinical significance; they affect behavior by producing changes in mood, mind, memory, and personality. These deficiencies may be reasonably widespread in the public-at-large which consumes the average American diet.

You may find by completing the design of your Nutraerobics Program that selected nutritional supplementation may be desirable in your basic daily program. If so, it is important to evaluate any potential adverse side effects that may come from excessive intake of vitamins or minerals. We need to know how to evaluate toxic effects and what level of nutrient intake may produce any apparent toxicity.[7]

Toxicity of Vitamins

Chronic intestinal problems, headaches, or nervous system disorders are signs of vitamin toxicity. The vitamins most likely to lead to such symptoms, when consumed in excessive quantities, are those that can accumulate in the body. These are the fat-soluble vitamins, particularly vitamins A and D.

A recent report[8] discusses cases of possible vitamin A toxicity in individuals who consumed a diet of normal food sources and vitamin A supplements where the total vitamin A intake was between 50,000 to 60,000 units per day. The symptoms of toxicity in these individuals were headaches, dryness of the mucous membranes, and liver problems. A total intake of 50,000 to 60,000 units a day of vitamin A would not be considered excessive for most individuals, however—only for those who may have compromised liver function or other unique features of their biochemistry.

Another study reports the symptoms of vitamin A toxicity as hair loss, headaches, intestinal upset, and liver function problems, and points out that these are reversible upon removal from the diet of the vitamin A.[9] It is much more the exception than the rule that individuals taking 30,000 units per day would have any toxic reaction to vitamin A; to be safe, however, the level of vitamin A suggested for normal intake is 2,500 to 10,000 units.[10]

The problem surrounding vitamin D excesses may be more significant, however. Vitamin D in excess quantities leads to calcium deposition in muscles and other soft tissue, a problem that is not reversible.[11]

It is also possible that excessive vitamin D may present itself as a factor actually contributing to hardening of the arteries and heart disease.[12] Levels of vitamin D exceeding 1000 units per day in the adult may be considered excessive, except for specific cases where vitamin D is required in therapeutic quantities, such as in the treatment of osteoporosis, discussed in greater detail in Chapter 10.

Vitamin E, another of the fat-soluble family, has not been demonstrated in controlled studies to cause a problem with long-term administration of 1000 units per day or less. There may be some isolated examples of people who react unfavorably to vitamin E in enhanced quantities with headaches or an increase in blood pressure, but again these are very exceptional cases. One report suggested that vitamin E in supplemental doses produced adverse side effects,[13] yet a number of follow-up reports indicated that this suggestion was ill-founded and not justified from clinical research, and that vitamin E is a safe substance to employ in supplemental doses for long periods of time.[14]

Again, it should be recalled that any substance, including water, when given in excessive quantities can be toxic. The question then, in evaluating toxicity, is what the safety margin is with regard to its use in supplemental doses. For vitamin E, as for vitamin C and the B-complex vitamins, the margin of safety is quite large, as there are no known, well-established, either short-term or long-term toxicity effects for these supplements when given at normal supplementary levels.

There have been reports that vitamin C in large quantities supposedly causes kidney stones, or produces a type of anemia called pernicious anemia, due to the destruction of vitamin B-12.[15] Further research has shown that these reports are more hypothetical than clinically accurate. A recent study indicated that consumption of 10,000 milligrams of vitamin C a day led to no greater output of oxalic acid in the urine than what one would get from a normal diet, therefore arguing against the proposition that oxalate kidney stones may be a result of vitamin C supplementation.[16] In another series of studies investigators found that vitamin C, when fed in large quantities with a meal containing vitamin B-12, did not lead to destruction of the B-12 and did not produce pernicious anemia.[17]

Similarly, adverse side effects from consumption of the B vitamins in very large quantities are virtually negligible. They are excreted very rapidly and do not build up in the body and produce cumulative, long-term toxic effects. Consumption of the B vitamins at ten to a hundred times the Recommended Dietary Allowance levels will not produce any significant adverse side effects, except in the case of niacin (vitamin B-3), which may produce extensive flushing, a feeling of

warmth, and redness of the body when given in larger than 50-milli-
gram quantities, due to dilation of the small blood vessels causing
pooling of the blood in the skin. There is no known hazard to this
reaction, other than the discomfort of the hotness of the skin. This will
not happen if a form of vitamin B-3 called niacinamide is used.

Most trace minerals also are reasonably safe in supplemental
doses, due to their water solubility and rapid excretion if consumed in
excessive quantities. There are some notable exceptions, however.
Chromium, selenium, copper, and manganese, if consumed in excessive quantities, can lead to direct toxicity symptoms, including intestinal disorders and liver and central nervous system problems.

The levels of vitamins and minerals generally accepted as safe for
daily use are as indicated in Table 2. The ranges given in this table for
each of the nutrients can safely be used by individuals on either a
maintenance or a therapeutic program.

Nutrients as Therapeutic Agents

Throughout the remainder of the book we will be discussing the
use of various nutrients as therapy for specific genetically inherited
needs or to manage certain health-related problems. The concept of the
use of nutrients in large quantities as therapy is a reasonably new
branch of nutrition entitled **nutritional pharmacology**. Much of the
information covered in the following chapters may not be standard
knowledge to many contemporary nutritionists or medical doctors.
The concept of using nutritional substances in amounts above and
beyond those you would get in the average diet to help promote improved human function is only recently becoming better understood
and more accepted by the scientific community.

Gerald Spiller discusses the philosophy of nutritional pharmacology in his recent book by that title and concludes, "Nutritional
pharmacology is the study of substances found in foods that might
have a pharmacological effect when fed in higher concentrations than
normally found in the diet and/or chemically modified form. These

Table 2

**Ranges of Safe Daily Intakes of
the Essential Vitamins and Minerals**

Water-Soluble Vitamins
Vitamin C	100–6,000 mg
Vitamin B-1	5–100 mg
Vitamin B-2	5–100 mg
Vitamin B-3	10–1,000 mg
Vitamin B-6	10–1,000 mg
Vitamin B-12	10–1,000 mcg
Biotin	50–400 mcg
Pantothenic Acid	10–1,000 mg
Folic Acid	400–1,000 mcg

Fat-Soluble Vitamins
Vitamin A	2,500–10,000 IU
Vitamin D	200–1,000 IU
Vitamin E	50–1,000 IU

Trace Minerals
Iron	10–30 mg
Copper	2–5 mg
Zinc	10–30 mg
Manganese	2–10 mg
Chromium	50–200 mcg
Selenium	50–200 mcg
Vanadium	50–100 mcg
Molybdenum	50–200 mcg

Macrominerals
Sodium	3,000–6,000 mg
Potassium	3,000–6,000 mg
Calcium	500–1,200 mg
Magnesium	300–600 mg
Phosphorus	1,000–1,600 mg

compounds might not be essential nutrients per se."[18]

The term **essential nutrients** refers to those substances known to be necessary for human function in all individuals. There are a number of natural food substance concentrates, discussed in this book as they apply to specific therapies, that are not considered essential nutrients for all people but that may prove to be useful therapeutically, such as lecithin, inositol, taurine, carnitine, dimethylglycine, specific nonessential amino acids, vegetable gums, garlic concentrate, saponins, various dietary fibers, bioflavonoids, beta-carotene, and specific oil concentrates. These substances may be classed as **accessory nutrients.** They are useful for individuals who have a biochemical need for them, but they are not considered essential nutrients for the population at large and will not appear in standard textbooks on nutrition.

An inspection of your own unique biotype, as defined from the questionnaires in Chapter 2 and modified in future chapters, will point you toward accessory nutrients you may have need for at a level beyond that which you get in diet or are able to manufacture in your own body.

The Test of Success

The test, of course, of the usefulness of a nutritional substance is whether it has been proven safe and effective.[19] As you pattern your own specific program through use of the material in this book, you will note that the information provided is documented and referenced as to the safety and effectiveness of the nutrients in controlled studies. If you have interest in pursuing any topics beyond the material covered in the text, please do seek out the original literature by following through the references provided in the notes.

Now let's go back and review your self-analysis from Chapter 2. By tracing through your particular responses to the questions, you can identify what areas you may want to concentrate on and in which you have the greatest biochemical sensitivity. You undoubtedly identified a number of specific nutrients as being related to some of your symptoms. If certain nutrients crop up a number of times, it gives greater support to the fact that you may need to supplement your diet with these nutrients for optimal function. Although it's often confusing, remember that what may be adequate for someone else, may be inadequate for you. The concept of biochemical individuality is the overriding feature of the Nutraerobics Program and is the cornerstone in designing an approach to your own optimal nutrition.

This concept of unique need, genetically determined nutritional requirements that are above those provided by the average diet, has also been termed "justification theory."[20] The author of this theory points out that there are a number of people who have been found to not necessarily be deficient in any nutrient by population standards such as the Recommended Dietary Allowances, but who have chronic health disabilities that are alleviated by consuming certain substances in higher quantities. In fact, there may be substances that are not generally considered essential at all that are needed by specific individuals in therapeutic quantities due to their unique genetically determined biochemistries. It should be emphasized that if you have continuing symptoms of a deficiency of a specific nutrient, even if you are getting what would generally be considered adequate levels of that nutrient from your diet, you may need therapeutic administration of that nutrient for your own optimal biochemical state.[21]

Now, spend some time going back over your responses to the questionnaires in Chapter 2 and see if you can define what nutrient or areas of nutrition you seem to need to concentrate on the most, and what your symptoms-versus-nutrition relationships are. From that analysis, you should then be pointed toward specific chapters where you will be designing your individualized program based upon your biochemical need. You may have to sit down with a pencil and paper and actually make a list of the places where redundancy exists in your responses to the questions, so that you will see where identical nutrient deficiency symptoms come up several times.

Once you have completed this analysis and have identified areas where you are sure you need to concentrate, we are ready to move on into the next chapters of the book which will give you the specific design of a Nutraerobics nutrition and exercise program tailored to your needs. From here on, you can either read the book a chapter at a time, or skip around and pick out those areas that you feel are most important for your specific situation. By the time you complete this book, you should have been able to identify the components of your own Nutraerobics Program, which we will put into action in Chapter 14. Good luck, and let's have at it!

Notes

1. *Recommended Dietary Allowances,* 9th rev. ed. (Washington, DC: National Academy of Sciences, 1980).

2. *Dietary Goals for the United States* (Washington, DC: U.S. Government Printing Office, 1976).

3. L. Page and B. Friend, "The Changing U.S. Diet," *BioScience, 28,* 192(1978).

4. "Chemical Methods Reveal Diet of Early Humans," *Chemical and Engineering News* (28 January 1982):31.

5. M. Brin, "Dilemma of Marginal Vitamin Deficiency," *Proceedings of the 9th International Congress on Nutrition, Mexico, 1972, 4,* (Basel: Karger, 1975).

6. A.E. Axelrod, "Immune Processes in Vitamin Deficiency Status," *American Journal of Clinical Nutrition, 24,* 265(1971); L.R. Horn, and L.J. Macklin, "Drug Metabolism and Hepatic Hemeproteins in the Vitamin E Deficient Rat," *Archives of Biochemistry and Biophysics, 172,* 270(1978).

7. T. Jukes, "Meganutrients and Food Fads," in *Nutrition: Metabolic and Clinical Applications* (London: Plenum Press, 1979).

8. V. Herbert, "Toxicity of 25,000 I.U. Vitamin A Supplements in Health Food Users," *American Journal of Clinical Nutrition, 36,* 185(1982).

9. M.Y. Jenkins, in *CRC Handbook Series in Nutrition and Food, Section E: Nutritional Disorders* (West Palm Beach, FL: CRC Press, 1978), pp. 73–85.

10. D. Davis, "Nutritional Needs and Biochemical Diversity," in *Medical Applications of Clinical Nutrition* (New Canaan, CT: Keats, 1983).

11. R.S. Goodhart and M.S. Shils, *Modern Nutrition in Health and Disease,* 5th ed. (Philadelphia: Lea and Febiger, 1973), pp. 163–165.

12. F.A. Kummerow, "Nutrition Imbalance and Angiotoxins as Dietary Risk Factors in Coronary Heart Disease," *American Journal of Clinical Nutrition, 32,* 58(1979).

13. H. J. Roberts, "Toxicity of Vitamin E," *Journal of the American Medical Association, 246,* 129(1981).

14. J. Archer, "Vitamin E," *J. Amer. Med. Assoc., 247,* 29(1982).

15. V. Herbert, "Facts and Fictions About Megavitamin Therapy," *Resident and Staff Physician* (December, 1978):44–49.

16. K. Schmidt and G. Rutishauser, "Urinary Oxalate Excretion After Large Intakes of Ascorbic Acid in Man," *Amer. J. Clinical Nutr., 34,* 305(1981).

17. S. Ekvall and R. Bozian, "The Effect of Supplemental Ascorbic Acid on Serum Vitamin B-12 Levels in Myelomeningocele Patients," *Amer. J. Clinical Nutr., 34,* 1356(1981).

18. G. A. Spiller, *Nutritional Pharmacology* (New York: Alan Liss, 1982).

19. V. Herbert, "The Vitamin Craze," *Archives of Internal Medicine, 140,* 173(1980).

20. S. P. Bessman, "Justification Theory," *Nutrition Reviews, 37,* 209(1978).

21. R. J. Williams and G. Deason, "Biochemical Individuality," *Proceedings of the National Academy of Sciences U.S.A., 57,* 1638(1968).

4

The Aging Process: Life After 30

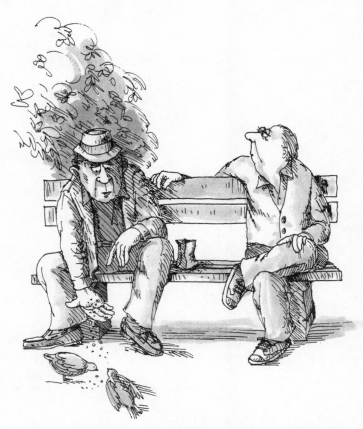

IF I'D KNOWN I WOULD LIVE THIS LONG, I'D HAVE TAKEN BETTER CARE OF MYSELF.

If you are over 30 years of age:

1. Do you have short-term memory loss?

1	2	3	4
No	Occasionally	Frequently	Always

2. Do you have nocturnal leg cramps?

1	2	3	4
No	Occasionally	Frequently	Always

3. Do you have pain in your hands and feet?

1	2	3	4
No	Occasionally	Frequently	Always

4. Do you have low back pain?

1	2	3	4
No	Occasionally	Frequently	Always

5. Do you get winded easily, or have pains in your legs when walking?

1	2	3	4
No	Occasionally	Frequently	Always

6. Do you suffer from depression?

1	2	3	4
No	Occasionally	Frequently	Always

7. Do you gain weight easily and have difficulty taking it off?

1	2	3	4
No	Occasionally	Frequently	Always

8. Do you have chronic constipation?

1	2	3	4
No	Occasionally	Frequently	Always

If your score exceeds 25, then you may have accelerated aging due to lifestyle misadjustments and you need to concentrate on this chapter.

There is life after 30. Your health can even improve after 30. The question is not **whether** we get older in number of years, but how we experience those years. Will it be with health or increasing debilitation? As we age we generally tend to get sicker, but getting sicker is not necessarily an absolute requirement of the aging process.[1]

In young adult life, we have reserves of capacity in each of our organ systems from four to ten times that required to just sustain life. This is called **organ reserve** and enables us to cope with stress such as illness or trauma and return ourselves to good health. After the age of 30, however, we tend to lose our organ reserve. As organ reserve decreases, so does our ability to maintain ourselves and defend ourselves against disease, so that eventually even the smallest stress we're exposed to can no longer be accommodated by our organ reserve, and we end up with a diagnosed disease.

The loss of organ reserve is associated with declining function and increased biological age. **Biological age** is the measurement of the functional capacity that you possess at any chronological age. As you probably know, there are some people who are chronologically 60 years old, but biologically 40; and there are other people who are chronologically 40 and biologically 60. A person in the latter group is at much greater risk to disease than one in the former. Your biological age is based to a great extent upon what you have been doing to yourself. If you have been involved in a Living Life Insurance Program, you have been investing in a lower biological age from which you can draw dividends as you get older. The organ reserve you are maintaining is there when you need it, which keeps you vital and reduces your risk to disease.

It is true that the average lifespan has risen from 47 to 73 years during this century, but the maximum lifespan has not increased, and, in fact, people who are living longer are not necessarily living healthier lives. For a person 40 years of age or older, life expectancy has increased relatively little over the past seventy years, and for those 75 years old and over the increase in lifespan is barely perceptible. The key, then, is increasing your probability of living a long and healthy life after the age of 40. People who are young and vital and setting world records in sports or athletics at the age of 20 may not necessarily be healthy specimens at the age of 40 who can contribute productively throughout the remainder of their lives free from debilitating illness. The Nutraerobics Program, as designed by you for you, will not necessarily guarantee you an infinitely long life, but it will greatly increase the probability of a higher-quality life with decreased illness and decreased biological age.

In essence, what your Nutraerobics Program should allow you to do is to "rectangularize" your survival curve.[2] What this means is that by implementing your program you should be able to reduce the eroding factors of degenerative disease that could plague you from midlife on. These factors are too common in older years, preventing you from living a life to the fullest of your biological potential.

Gerontologists are now suggesting that the biological lifetime potential of the human is between 90 and 120 years and should be associated with reasonably good health and functional capacity. If we are able to optimize our potential, your Nutraerobics Living Life Insurance Policy will help you secure that goal.

To help you appreciate the many factors that can contribute to your keeping healthy from age 30 on, spend a few minutes responding to the following questionnaire, **Testing Your Lifestyle.**

Rank your responses to each of the questions as follows: 1 if you feel the question relates strongly to you; 0 if it doesn't relate to you at all or you have the negative or opposite response; and .5 if you are somewhere in between.

1. Work. Does it meet your needs? Is it something you look forward to? If so, give yourself a 1. If it's something you dread or you're not able to do, give yourself a 0. If you're in between, give yourself .5. _____

2. Recreation and hobbies. If you know how to relax, enjoy your leisure time, and have adequate recreation and hobbies, give yourself a 1. If you hate vacations, don't know how to occupy your leisure time, and have no recreation, give yourself a 0. In between, .5. _____

3. Pain or suffering. If you are free from pain or suffering, give yourself a 1. If you are significantly debilitated by pain or suffering, give yourself a 0. In between, .5. _____

4. Mental suffering, worry, or unhappiness. If you are free from these, give yourself a 1. If you are laboring with considerable unhappiness, worry, tension, and grief, give yourself a 0. In between, .5. _____

5. Communication. If you are able to communicate orally, in writing, and nonverbally to your satisfaction with other people, give yourself a 1. If you feel frustrated by lack of communication, that people don't listen to you and you can't get things off your chest, give yourself a 0. In between, .5. _____

6. Sleep. Are you able to get six to eight hours of regular, uninterrupted sleep each night? If so, give yourself a 1. If your sleep is spotty, interrupted by insomnia, then give yourself a 0. In between, .5. _____

7. Dependency on others. If you are reasonably able to make your own decisions and are operating independently in the world, give yourself a 1. If you feel highly dependent upon other people and are unable to make decisions for yourself, give yourself a 0. In between, .5. _____

8. Nutrition. Do you eat a good diet from the seven fundamental food groups each day and maintain an adequate weight-to-height ratio? If so, give yourself a 1. If your diet is more convenience-oriented, high in sugar and fats, give yourself a 0. In between, .5.

9. Excretion. Do you have regular bowel and bladder habits and no problem with constipation? If so, give yourself a 1. If, however, you are chronically constipated and need laxatives or have a urinary problem, give yourself a 0. In between, .5.

10. Sexual activity. Does your sexual life meet your needs, so that there are no apparent psychological problems? If so, give yourself a 1. If, however, you have apparent sexual problems and/or inadequacy, give yourself a 0. In between, .5.

                                                                    Total

Once you've totaled up your ranking of the answers to this short questionnaire, you should have a number from 1 to 10. What does this number mean in terms of your health and a prescription for middle age?

This questionnaire has been given to over 180 patients and the following relationships between the scores of these patients and their health were found:[3]

If the patient's score was:	the medical diagnosis was found to be:
8.5–10	benign health conditions (at worst)
6.5–8.5	chronic degenerative diseases in the early phase
4.0–6.5	diagnosed health problems such as gout, diabetes, low back pain, alcoholism
2.5–4.0	acute disease syndromes such as heart failure, cancer, and kidney stones

What does this questionnaire tell you about your general health and biological age? First of all, you'll notice that the questions seem to have no direct relationship to one's health. They are certainly not the topics that would be considered most essential in a medical school curriculum for the training of doctors. Yet we now find that the way people live in their environment and the way they treat themselves in their lifestyle seem to have a significant impact on their health. We will be discussing later in this chapter the way that stress can have an impact upon your health and erode your energy level.

If you came up with a reasonably high score on this questionnaire, from 8.5 to 10, you are doing very well in your adjustment to your world and your environment and contributing to a state of mind that promotes health and wellness. If, however, your score was very low (4.0 or lower), it indicates that there are certain aspects of your lifestyle that need considerable moderation and improvement to both decrease your biological age and improve your general level of health and vitality.

Most of us don't spend very much time thinking about how our work, recreation, communication with others, sleep patterns, or feelings of independence affect our general level of physical functioning, but each of these areas can be either an eroding or a supporting factor in the way that we operate in the world. Areas where you scored low on this questionnaire are areas you want to concentrate on in developing your Nutraerobics Program.

Does Function Decline with Age?

Possibly at this point you are saying that aging is something that is an inevitable feature of living and there is nothing we can really do about it. We're going to get sicker as we get older anyway, so shouldn't we just live with the accelerator to the floor and enjoy it while we've still got it? You can use as a justification for this philosophy the information provided in Figure 2, which shows the loss of lung and respiratory function as a measure of the decrease in mean vital capacity with age. You'll notice that the curves indicate a distinct loss of func-

Figure 2

Declining Lung Capacity with Age

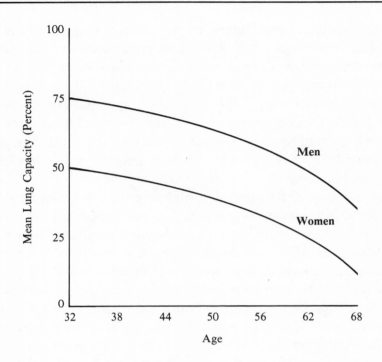

tion for men and women after the age of 32; similar declines in for many other functional capacities after 32 have also been observed. However, it should be pointed out that although these curves represent what happens to average people in our society today, they do not necessarily represent what happens to **all** people after the age of 32.

A good example of this is the case of a man of 39 who came to the Bellevue-Redmond Medical Facility in Seattle, Washington, a number of years ago: he was experiencing headaches, was 35 pounds overweight, was on high-blood-pressure medication, and was so tired when he got home after work that he could do nothing but sit like a zombie in front of the TV until he retired to bed at 10 or 11 o'clock in the evening. His wife complained that it was a major chore just to get him to do the yard work on the weekend; he had only enough energy to sit and watch sports on TV. He arrived at the clinic very concerned about his health and had his status evaluated by the same types of tools that we are discussing in this book. He was found to have a biological age not of 39, but of 52, after a comprehensive evaluation in the clinic. Needless to say, this scared him greatly. Who likes to learn that his or her biological function is 13 years older than the number of birthdays?

He dedicated himself to a rigorous health improvement program, applying the Nutraerobics concepts and tailoring his program to meet his biological needs. He was a model patient and committed himself totally to the program. At the age of 42, some three years later and much improved, he was retested at a human performance laboratory in a large medical center and was found to have the fitness level of a fit 17-year-old—in a short three years he had turned around his biological age, thereby increasing his vital and functional capacity tremendously. He had not put hair back on his head, nor seen the loss of those seasoned wrinkles around his eyes, but he had improved his general level of functioning and his ability to perform at a high level of productivity in his job and at home. And he had more organ reserve to draw upon under stressful conditions. At the age of 42 he was now competing in running races, was actively involved in his children's sports and recreational programs, had become politically active, and was much more productive on his job. He is a classic example of what can happen when people take an aggressive approach toward improving their level of wellness.

Considerable literature has been written over the past several years on the mechanisms by which people age. Almost all of these mechanisms point us to one important conclusion—the aging process is the result not only of our genes, but also of how we treat ourselves by the way we live. People can deliberately alter the rate at which they biologically age by the way they treat themselves.[4] The Nutraerobics Program that you're designing will allow you to facilitate a reduction in your biological age.

Table 3

Assessing Your Biological Age After 30

Make the following adjustments to your chronological age to get your biological age: if the factor is present add the number of years in the right column; if the factor is absent, add 0 (no change); if you meet the requirements listed, subtract the number of years in the left column.

Subtract this number of years if:	Factor	Add this number of years if present:
	Fatness (reduced lean body mass)	3.0
	Smoking (more than half a pack/day)	2.0
	Alcohol (more than 2 drinks/day)	0.5
Less than 180, 1.0	Elevated blood cholesterol (greater than 250)	1.0
Less than 130/75, 2.0	High blood pressure (greater than 140/90)	2.0
Excellent, 1.0 (in good shape)	Poor exercise tolerance (recovery after exercise)	1.0
	Reduced red blood cell count and hemoglobin levels (anemia)	0.5
No history of chronic illness, 2.0	Reduced immune status (white blood cell activity)	1.0
	Poor digestive function (long bowel transit time or constipation)	1.0
Not easily winded, 1.0 (no asthma or other breathing problems)	Reduced vital capacity of lungs (easily winded or fatigued for age)	1.0
Less than 60, 1.0	Elevated resting pulse rate (greater than 80 beats/minute)	0.5
	Poor short-term memory for age	1.0
	Protein spill in urine	2.0
No vision problem, 1.0	Difficulty with close vision	0.5
	Sexual dysfunction	0.5

Determining Your Own Biological Age

You would probably like to determine your own biological age. From Table 3, you'll notice that there are at least fifteen different things that can be taken into account in the crude approximation of your biological age. The right column of this chart shows the number of years to add to your chronological age if you have the problem listed. On the left are the number of years you subtract from your chronological age if you do not have that particular problem and your value falls within the listed range. You'll note that if you are 40, are a smoker, are overweight, have an elevated blood cholesterol level with elevated blood pressure and poor exercise tolerance, your biological age is more like 50. If, however, you're chronologically 40 and you are of ideal weight, a nonsmoker, and have low blood cholesterol and reduced blood pressure with an excellent exercise tolerance, and no history of chronic illnesses, your biological age is 34, making the difference between the two some sixteen years.

By implementing the Nutraerobics Program designed for you, you will be able to shift those risks on the right column to protective factors on the left, thereby reducing your biological age, increasing your organ reserve, and reducing your risk to disease throughout the remainder of your life.

Your View of Yourself and Your Health

How you manage your lifestyle as you age may dictate how fast you truly do increase your biological age. As recently pointed out by one health professional, "Behavioral factors contribute to much of our burden of illness. Half of the mortality from the ten leading causes of death in the United States is strongly influenced by lifestyle. Known behavioral risk factors include cigarette smoking, excessive consumption of alcoholic beverages, use of illicit drugs, certain dietary habits, insufficient exercise, reckless driving, nonadherence to medication regimens, and maladaptive responses to social pressures."[5]

What type of health-care system, then, can offer a form of preventive care that takes these things into consideration to keep you healthy after the age of 30? If one judges investments by the returns they bring, the American health-care industry as it is now defined is excellent in delivering disease care, but poor in helping people keep healthy. The concentration of dollars and time is on the treatment of disease and not on the early-warning recognition of potential disease at a stage where your lifestyle can be modified appropriately to meet your biochemical need, thereby preventing disease.

The system, as it is now operating, assures payment or reimbursement through third-party insurance payers for medical care people receive in health crises. The system does not reimburse patients or doctors for services rendered in promoting health. This approach encourages an ever increasing demand for ever more expensive interventive hospital services to treat disease. The system is basically a sickness system designed to treat illness, not keep people healthy.[6]

The Medical Profession and Prevention

Is it reasonable for us to look to the medical profession for better delivery of preventive medicine? Or as one doctor has said about his profession, "If we're so good, why aren't we better?"[7] Patients are asking different things of their doctors today than they were twenty years ago. First, far more people are interested in knowing more about their health problems. Fewer and fewer are of the "Don't tell me about it, just fix me up, Doc" mentality. Most patients want to be treated as individuals working with the doctor, rather than objects receiving unexplained treatments.

Second, patients also now wish to receive more health care, as opposed to disease care. Larger numbers of practicing physicians are now moving into the area of health maintenance, while medical school curricula still lag behind in this area. It was out of this dilemma that the Nutraerobics Program was born, as a self-help program that starts you along the way toward assessing your own lifestyle needs and then brings this information to a level where you and your health practitioner can do something about it.

Another doctor commented recently, "If a national comprehensive preventive health program is to be implemented and succeed, it must have enthusiastic support of the medical profession . . . which must cooperate with the government in this effort; and of the individual who must accept a greater responsibility for his or her own well-being and exert the self-discipline required in modifying lifestyle habits. With such a partnership a true health-care-promoting system can be created for the generation and those who follow."[8] The Living Life Insurance Program that you're developing through reading and implementing the concepts in this book is a first step in changing the level of understanding about preventive medicine and putting the pressure on the health-care delivery system not to give up what we have traditionally done well, and that is to deliver quality disease care, but to simultaneously embrace the new paradigm of health promotion called preventive medicine.

Preventive medicine is based on the basic strategy we have been working with in the first three chapters of this book—**early warning risk factor intervention**. Risk factor intervention is a technique whereby the symptoms, genetic history, and characteristics of an individual are closely evaluated, just as you have done already in establishing your biotype, and this information is allowed to paint a picture of the relative risks to later-stage health problems for that person. We may not be able to define from this material precisely what disease you might get or at what specific age, but we should be able with reasonable accuracy to talk about your relative risks to various disease families and what you can do to reduce your risks.

As one doctor observes, "The present situation regarding risk factors, including the potential for intervention, is somewhat analogous to the situation that existed when polluted water became known as a causative factor of infections such as cholera and typhoid before their actual mechanism of illness was demonstrated bacteriologically."[9] This means that we do not yet know precisely how your lifestyle may produce disease, but we do know there are many lifestyle habits that increase your risk to disease, and if those habits are improved, your probability of aging at an accelerated rate will be much lower. By looking at the complicated features of your lifestyle, assigning your biological age, and looking at your dietary and genetic uniquenesses, we are starting to develop a program specifically tailored for you that has identified certain risks and will put you on the path to minimizing these risks, so that health after the age of 30 becomes a reality and not just something to be talked about.

We can summarize this situation with a quote from Dr. Gio Gori, former director of the National Cancer Institute: "Over the last three decades, the United States has invested an unprecedented portion of its national income in the study and care of disease, but the health and longevity of Americans during that time have not shown commensurate improvement; a 1967 study suggested that neither a rise nor a decline in disease care expenditures would have a further impact on life expectancy . . . but evidence accumulated during the last twenty years indicates that the most important of modern diseases are caused by a variety of factors, most significantly by reckless personal and social habits suggesting that at least partial prevention of important diseases may be possible."[10]

If for no other reason, the motivation to accept the principles outlined in the Nutraerobics Plan may be derived from economics. The rate of inflation operative in the disease care sector suggests that we have only three alternatives to stem the tide of what is an ever increasing potential bankruptcy of our economy because of the major focus on disease care. These alternatives are:

1. Delivery of high-quality disease care only to those who can afford to pay for it;

2. Delivery of less costly, mediocre care to everyone; or

3. The embracing of an alternative preventively focused program that helps keep people healthy, so that the funds for disease care will be available to those who need it.

Of these three alternatives, both the most humanistically and economically justifiable seems to be the third option, that is, the embracing of a more effective approach toward preventive care balanced with the excellence of disease treatment.

Nutraerobics and Aging

Now, what characteristics define the Nutraerobics preventively focused approach that we're designing for you? First of all, we are not so interested in identifying specific disease processes through comprehensive testing, because what we're looking for are the warning signs and symptoms of declining organ reserve. This is prognosis, **not** diagnosis. The focus then is on finding in you as an individual any early warning markers to subsequent disease, so that we can design a program to minimize your risks.

Second, this preventive program should still provide a range of choice about your lifestyle. Not all people enjoy the same things. The Nutraerobics Program you are designing has options. This approach is also low technology and cost-efficient, utilizing materials that are readily available and understood by you.

Third, this approach at worst causes no harm; it upholds the Hippocratic Oath. Not only, at worst, does it do no harm, but preventive approaches using nutritional and lifestyle intervention have been demonstrated to be effective in reducing the risks to all diseases of public importance today.

As was pointed out by Dr. William Connor in his outgoing presidential address before the American Society of Clinical Nutrition, the need to implement preventive early warning medical assessment techniques is no longer of idle academic interest. It is a challenge that must be addressed by the public and health practitioners now. He went on to say, "I know full well that these dietary treatment modalities aren't going to be taken up first by the cardiologists, or indeed by any subspecialist of medicine. Here is a vast arena for the talents of the clinical nutritionist to be expressed if he would so incline himself."[11] I would go on to say that this is also a vast arena for the talents of the person who knows the most about you, and that is **yourself**. By properly reading your physical signs and symptoms, looking critically at your performance and level of wellness, and accomplishing the Nutraerobics Assessment Program in Chapters 2 and 3, you can start charting your own path toward a higher level of health.

As one physician aptly points out, "The busy practitioner does not have the time to muster the necessary skills to effect significant changes in the well-ingrained bad habits of the patient."[12] If this is true, then it is time for us to take the responsibility for assessing our own health needs and designing our own programs. This is exactly what we are about to do in discussing how to implement a program for your own individualized biotype.

Vitamins and Minerals and the Aging Process

What role do vitamin or mineral supplements have in implementing your Nutraerobics Program after 30? Clinical studies have indicated that groups of individuals who consumed higher than average dietary intakes of vitamins A and C had lower overall mortality rates.[13] The specific way in which vitamins and minerals are related to the reduction of risk to disease, however, is not yet clearly established.

In a recent report, a group of 233 men and 256 women who were at least 65 years of age and were users of vitamin supplements was studied. The individuals in this study were health-conscious individuals, based on data from self-reported questionnaires in 1974 and 1977. These people were primarily nonsmokers, although about 50 percent of them formerly smoked cigarettes. Most of them ate meat, poultry, or fish, but did so in moderation, and they consumed only modest amounts of alcohol, whole milk, white bread, salt, and sugar. Based upon comparisons of the number of deaths in this group over a six-year follow-up compared with the 1977 U.S. average mortality for individuals in this group, it was found that the health-conscious group had significantly fewer deaths and better health than would have been expected in the standard population. For both sexes combined, the reduction in cancer mortality was 14 percent, for heart disease and other vascular disease, 38 percent, and for all other causes of death, 27 percent. No clear prolongation of life or reduction in disease could be attributed to the vitamin regime alone, but inactivity, smoking, previous heart trouble, and either very high or very low intakes of vitamin E were associated with shortened life expectancy, according to this study. The conclusion of the study was "For this highly selected group of health-conscious, older individuals, it appears that a high-vitamin, improved-nutrition lifestyle is a healthy one, but there is no clear indication of reduction in total illness or death because of high levels of vitamins alone."[14] In general, then, we can say that vitamin supplementation may accompany a total lifestyle improvement program, based upon a person's need as indicated from the initial health index that started this chapter and his or her biotype.

What particular vitamin and mineral problems reflecting specific needs are not being met for the older-age individual? Many older individuals lose their sense of taste, which then results in altered appetite and the consumption of lower-quality foods. Taste alone is responsible for certain dietary preferences. Basically, there are only four taste perceptions: sour, sweet, salt, and bitter. It has been found that a zinc deficiency in the aged individual can lead to loss of taste sensitivity and discrimination between sweet, sour, and salt perceptions.[15] Some investigators feel that the loss of taste perception after the age of 50 is the result of the aging process itself; however, recently there is more and more evidence that the loss of proper taste perception in the aged individual comes more from a zinc deficiency rather than from the natural aging process.

Other reports confirm that some aged individuals of low income have marginal to deficient intakes of zinc and exhibit depressed taste acuity for sweet and salt taste.[16] Poor taste acuity due to a zinc deficiency can lead to intake of poor-quality foods, which results in reduced nutrition and increases the rate of loss of organ reserve, the biological age, and the risk to disease. Zinc intake may need to be 15 to 30 milligrams a day to restore taste acuity, or even as high as 50 milligrams in some individuals, if they have been zinc-depleted for some period of time.

Zinc is just one of a number of trace elements found to be reasonably poor in the diets of aged individuals;[17] iron, copper, and chromium are others. A copper deficiency is known to increase the risk to heart disorders and lead to degeneration of the heart muscle in many animal species. Abnormalities associated with copper deficiency can include anemias that are not iron-responsive, disorders of the bone with increased bone loss, nervous system disorders, reproductive failure, inability to tan, and kinky, coarse texture of the hair.[18] Copper intake may need to be 5 milligrams a day in some older individuals to promote proper balance and lead to improved tanning, bone formation, and blood and heart function.

A deficiency of chromium in aged individuals may result in an abnormal control of blood sugar, leading to the symptoms of adult-onset diabetes or poor fat metabolism, with weight gain of unknown origin. It appears likely that the consumption over a long period of time of highly refined foods characteristically low in chromium is an important factor in the declining levels of chromium in the tissues observed in older people in the United States.[19] A number of investigators have reported that supplementation with chromium from chromium-enriched brewer's yeast at the level of 200 micrograms a day improved blood sugar tolerance and lowered blood cholesterol in elderly women and men subjects.

A research study done with women aged 40 to 75 years at Lincoln University in Missouri indicated that a supplement of 5 grams of brewer's yeast extract containing chromium given daily for three months led to improved blood sugar control and decreased blood cholesterol.[20] Similar results were reported in a study where brewer's yeast was given to subjects who averaged 78 years of age. In order to get 200 micrograms a day of chromium in the diet, it is almost essential to supplement with a chromium-rich brewer's yeast or a trivalent chelated chromium supplement or consume liver, whole grains, and yeast-risen products. More will be said about the importance of these trace elements in future chapters.

Memory Loss and Nutraerobics

How about the loss of memory that seems to sometimes come along with aging? In the extreme case, this condition of presenile dementia is termed Alzheimer's disease. This condition has recently been shown to be responsive to increased levels of dietary choline (a B-complex vitamin), which is best administered in the form of high-quality lecithin, that is, lecithin with phosphatidyl choline constituting at least 60 to 70 percent of its total makeup. Most low-grade nutritional lecithin does not provide adequate levels of phosphatidyl choline to be therapeutically useful. Read the label of the lecithin bottle to make sure it is high in phosphatidyl choline. The dose of high-quality lecithin required to help improve memory in the individual with presenile memory loss is between 20 and 100 grams daily (administered half in the morning and half in the evening).

Lecithin has also been found useful in the treatment of a variety of nervous system disorders, some of which may coincide with aging, such as Huntington's disease with its problems with equilibrium and balance, and tremors.[21] The substance phosphatidyl choline from lecithin works by delivering to the brain high levels of choline, which is used by the brain to manufacture acetylcholine. The deficiency of acetylcholine in the nervous system has been associated with the problems in older individuals just discussed.[22] Recent work indicates that there is no clinical difference in response to either egg- or soy-derived lecithins as long as they are of high (at least 70 percent) phosphatidyl choline content.[23]

Many people feel that loss of memory is a natural consequence of the aging process. However, in a recent study, old mice, when given high levels of dietary choline, had retention of learning superior to choline-deficient young mice; the conclusion was that manipulation of dietary choline can significantly alter behavior in ways that are similar to those occurring across the lifespan of an individual. It may be that behavioral and intellectual changes suggested to occur with age might be modified through appropriate dietary control of such nutrients as choline or lecithin.[24]

Aging Pigments and Nutraerobics

Another feature associated with aging is the accumulation of aging pigments, called ceroid or lipofuscin pigments, in such areas as the intestinal tract, the skin, the brain, and in epithelial tissues. These aging pigments are a result of accumulated damage to cells over your lifespan; they have been suggested to be involved in declining tissue function in the aged individual and may contribute to increased biological aging. Recently it was found that these aging pigments accumulate much faster in vitamin E–deficient than in adequately vitamin E–nourished persons. This is presumably a result of vitamin E's ability to scavenge or soak up the molecular time bombs that produce these aging pigments before they have a chance to do their destructive work on the cell.[25] Vitamin E supplementation above normal dietary levels in animal studies did lead to decreased accumulation of these aging pigments.

The human need in aged individuals for vitamin E may be between 100 and 400 units per day for optimal defense. The form of vitamin E that seems best in preventing pigmentation on a milligram-per-milligram basis is natural vitamin E, or d-alpha tocopherol.

The B Vitamins and Aging

Other symptoms associated with aging are insomnia, mental confusion, and various anemias. Studies in which supplemental doses of vitamins B-1, B-2, and B-6 were administered to older-age patients were able to not only demonstrate improved tissue function, but also

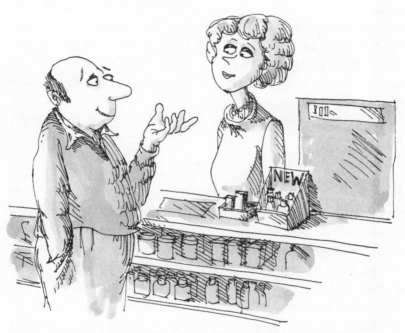

THE DOCTOR GAVE ME A LIST OF VITAMINS THAT WILL HELP
MY MEMORY, BUT I CAN'T REMEMBER WHERE I PUT IT.

to show alleviation of these symptoms that were associated with aging. Many of these symptoms may not have been recognized as vitamin deficiency symptoms by most medical evaluators.[26] Vitamin levels used in these studies were 20 milligrams per day of B-1, 10 milligrams per day of B-2, and 20 milligrams per day of B-6. Most individuals would need a B-complex supplement to achieve these levels.

One common orthopedic problem associated with aging is that of carpal tunnel syndrome, in which the individual loses the contractability of the carpal ligament resulting in wrist pain, poor grip, and reduced finger flexibility. Historically, this condition has been treated surgically, yet recent work indicates that in many cases this syndrome may be a result of a vitamin B-6 deficiency in the aged individual.[27] Alleviation of the carpal tunnel syndrome was produced by administering 100 milligrams a day of vitamin B-6, an amount far in excess of the Recommended Dietary Allowance level of 2 milligrams a day. This dosage did, however, have to be continued for eleven to twelve weeks to achieve therapeutic results. Why such a high level of the vitamin is needed may have to do with both its absorption and utilization, which seem to be impaired in certain aged individuals. Not all patients with carpal tunnel problems responded, but for those who did, the impact was considerable.

Immunity and Aging

Other problems associated with reduced flexibility of the limbs commonly accounted for as part of aging are conditions called arthritis or bursitis, where joints become inflamed and swollen and movement is painful. Apparently the immune system suffers defects as a result of aging that may lead to an increased risk to arthritic ailments. We will discuss the immune system and the Nutraerobics Program in more detail in Chapter 11, but, in general, achievement of an ideal body weight-to-height ratio, removal of food allergens wherever possible, and daily supplementation with zinc (20 mg), vitamin B-6 (50 mg), vitamin C (1000 mg), and niacinamide (500–2,000 mg), along with essential fatty acids such as linseed oil or MaxEPA (a fish oil derivative), may be helpful in reducing the symptoms of age-related arthritis.[28] The amino acid D,L-phenylalanine has recently been suggested to be very helpful in reducing the pain of arthritis when given as a nutritional supplement. Doses that are effective yet nontoxic range between 100 and 300 milligrams per day.[29]

Toxic Minerals and Aging

Two last interesting observations seem pertinent to specific therapeutic approaches toward reducing the decline in function associated with increased biological age. The first is the recent observation that aluminum accumulation in the body may be correlated with such neuromuscular conditions as amyotrophic lateral sclerosis (ALS) and Parkinsonism-like syndrome.[30] Aluminum can come to be concentrated in the body from a variety of sources, most predominantly from aluminum-containing antacids, which are used frequently by older individuals to treat what they believe to be hyperacidity of the stomach or heartburn. Other sources of aluminum are from cooking acid foods in aluminum cookware for many years, and from water treated with certain types of aluminum-containing water softeners. The actual effect of aluminum on the brain and other nervous system tissues is not fully understood, but there is a strong implication that excessive accumulation of aluminum may be a risk factor to such conditions as ALS and Parkinsonism-like syndrome and may contribute to the loss of calcium from bone associated with old age. The best way to remove aluminum from the body appears to be by displacing it with calcium, magnesium, and vitamin D in the diet and using a vitamin C supplement.

Blood Pressure and Aging

Conditions of elevated or reduced blood pressure in the aged individual have been found responsive to salt restriction and supplementation with an amino acid called tyrosine.[31] Tyrosine administration, at 6 grams per day in three doses of 2 grams each, one hour before each meal, was found to increase blood pressure in those who had low blood pressure and decrease it in those who had elevated blood pressure. Tyrosine may therefore be useful therapeutically in conditions characterized by alteration of blood pressure due to adrenaline imbalances in the bloodstream.

In summary, in this chapter we have identified specific factors within the lifestyle of individuals beyond the age of 30 that will help improve their probability of leading a long, healthy life out to the limits of their biological lifespan. What they can look forward to, then, is "natural death," where they just "wear out," rather than the prospect of degenerative disease that strikes in midlife and leads to years of declining organ reserve and rapidly increasing biological age. By implementing the principles discussed in this chapter and applying them directly to your biotype as determined in Chapter 2, you should start along the road toward living your Living Life Insurance Program. Undoubtedly there will more modification required depending upon specific genetic sensitivities and tendencies to be discussed in subsequent chapters, but at this point you should have started developing a comprehensive approach using therapeutic nutrition, early warning risk factor intervention, and preventive medicine as powerful tools to help you move to higher levels of wellness.

Let's now explore specific modifications of the basic Nutraerobics Program as they relate to your specific biochemical needs and such things as fatigue, sleep disorders, or mood swings.

Notes

1. J. F. Fries, "Aging, Natural Death and the Compression of Morbidity," *New England Journal of Medicine, 303,* 130(1980).

2. A. Comfort, *The Biology of Senescence,* 3rd ed. (New York: Elsevier, 1979).

3. A. W. Grogono and D. J. Woodgate, "Index for Measuring Health," *Lancet* (6 November 1971):1024–1025.

4. J. A. Miller, "Making Old Age Measure Up," *Science News, 120,* 74 (1981).

5. D. A. Hamburg, "Health and Behavior," *Science, 217,* 455(1982).

6. M. Kristein, C. B. Arnold, and E.L. Wynder, "Health Economics and Preventive Care," *Science, 195,* 457(1977).

7. D. Detmer, "If We're So Good, Why Aren't We Better?" *J. Amer. Medical Assoc., 243,* 930(1980).

8. Kristein, Arnold, and Wynder, "Health Economics and Preventive Care," *Science, 195,* 457(1977).

9. L. Breslow, "Risk Factor Intervention for Health Maintenance," *Science, 200,* 908(1978).

10. G. Gori and B. J. Richter, "Macroeconomics of Disease Prevention in the United States," *Science, 200,* 1124(1978).

11. W. E. Connor, "The Case for Preventive Nutrition," *Am. J. Clin. Nutr., 32,* 1975(1979).

12. P. L. White, "Nutrition and the New Health Awareness," *J. Amer. Medical Assoc., 247,* 2914(1982).

13. R. B. Shekelle, M. Lepper, S. Liu, and A. H. Rossof, "Vitamin A and C Consumption and Mortality Rates," *Lancet,* ii, 1185(1981).

14. J. E. Erstrum and L. Pauling, "Mortality Among Health-Conscious Elderly Californians," *Proceedings of the National Academy of Sciences U.S.A., 79,* 6023(1982).

15. S. K. Kamath, "Taste Acuity and Aging," *Amer. J. Clin. Nutr., 36,* 766(1982).

16. H. H. Sandstead, "Zinc Nutrition in the United States," *Amer. J. Clin. Nutr., 26,* 1251(1973).

17. J. W. Nordstrom, "Trace Mineral Nutrition in the Elderly," *Amer. J. Clin. Nutr., 36,* 788(1982).

18. L. M. Klevay, "Coronary Heart Disease and the Zinc/Copper Hypothesis," *Amer. J. Clin. Nutr., 28,* 764(1975).

19. H.A. Schroeder and I.H. Tipton, "Abnormal Trace Metals in Man's Chromium," *Journal of Chronic Diseases, 15,* 941(1962).

20. V. J. K. Lin and R. Dowdy, "Effect of High Chromium-Yeast Supplementation on Glucose Tolerance in Older Women," *Federation Proceedings, 36,* 4509(1977).

21. G. S. Rosenberg and K. L. Davis, "The Use of Cholinergic Precursors in Neuropsychiatric Diseases," *Amer. J. Clin. Nutr., 36,* 709(1982).

22. S. H. Zeisel, "Dietary Choline: Biochemistry, Physiology and Pharmacology," *Annual Review of Nutrition, 1,* 95(1981).

23. S. G. Magil and R. J. Wurtman, "Effects of Ingesting Soy or Egg Lecithins on Serum Choline, Brain Choline and Acetylcholine," *Journal of Nutrition, 111,* 166(1981).

24. R. T. Bartus, R. L. Dean, and A. S. Lippa, "Age Related Changes and Modulation with Dietary Choline," *Science, 209,* 301(1980).

25. J. D. Manwaring and A. S. Csallany, "Fluorescent Compounds in Liver, Heart and Brain of Vitamin E Deficient and Supplemented Mice, *Journal of Nutrition, 111,* 2172(1981).

26. R. K. J. Hoorn, J. P. Flikweert, and D. Westerink, "Vitamin B-1, B-2, and B-6 Deficiencies in Geriatric Patients," *Clinica Chimica Acta, 61,* 151(1975).

27. K. Folkers and J. Ellis, "Biochemical Evidence for a Deficiency of Vitamin B-6 in the Carpal Tunnel Syndrome," *Proceedings of the National Academy of Sciences USA, 75,* 3410(1978).

28. D. F. Horrobin, "Loss of Delta-6-Desaturase Activity as a Key Factor in Aging," *Medical Hypotheses, 7,* 1211(1981).

29. R. C. Balagot and J. Greenberg, "Analgesia in Mice and Humans by D-phenylalanine," *Advances in Pain Research and Therapy,* vol. 5 (New York: Raven Press, 1983).

30. D. P. Perl and C. J. Gibbs, "Intraneuronal Aluminum Accumulation in Amyotrophic Lateral Sclerosis and Parkinsonism of Guam," *Science, 217,* 1053(1982).

31. J. C. Aghatanya and R. J. Wurtman, "Changes in Catecholamine Excretion After Short-Term Tyrosine Ingestion," *Amer. J. Clin. Nutr., 34,* 82(1981).

5

Emotions, Fatigue, or Lack of Sleep Got the Best of You?

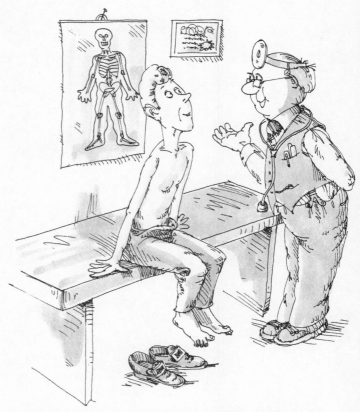

A SLIGHT CHANGE IN YOUR BIOCHEMICAL BALANCE MAY HELP YOUR INSOMNIA, MR. VAN WINKLE.

1. Do you have a low energy level?

1	2	3	4
No	Occasionally	Frequently	Always

2. Is muscle weakness a problem for you?

1	2	3	4
No	Occasionally	Frequently	Always

3. Do you have sleep disturbances, insomnia, or recurring bad dreams?

1	2	3	4
No	Occasionally	Frequently	Always

4. Do you have constipation or diarrhea or both alternating?

1	2	3	4
No	Occasionally	Frequently	Always

5. Do you have a craving for sweets?

1	2	3	4
No	Occasionally	Frequently	Always

6. Do you get shaky before meals?

1	2	3	4
No	Occasionally	Frequently	Always

If your total score exceeds 15 you may have a specific undernutrition or blood sugar problem and you should concentrate on information in this chapter.

Everyone has blue days, tired periods, episodes of insomnia, mood swings, and transient anxieties leading to personality changes, but what happens if one or more of these become the rule, instead of the exception?

We know that psychological disturbances are some of the earliest symptoms of nutritional inadequacy.[1] Evidence is now accumulating to suggest that better brain chemistry can be achieved through better living, and better brain chemistry means clearer thinking, the smoothing out of mood highs and lows, and sunnier emotional days. Let's see how applying the understanding of your Nutraerobics biotype may help you right the ship of emotional upheaval and put some needed energy back in your life.

Your mood, mind, memory, and behavior are controlled by the master shop boss of your body—the brain. The functioning of the brain is dependent upon its ability to properly metabolize its food, which is blood sugar (glucose), into usable forms of energy for its various portions responsible for such activities as thinking, control of hormones, regulation of involuntary functions such as respiration and heartbeat, control of motor activity, and sense perception. The proper manufacture of energy in your brain from blood sugar is dependent upon an adequate supply of the helper substances, vitamins and minerals. The proper functioning of the brain is more dependent upon adequate levels of these nutrients, in fact, than any other organ in your body.

The breakdown of blood sugar in your brain to produce energy, which is facilitated by the proper level of vitamins and minerals, leads to the production of a series of chemical messenger substances called *neurotransmitters*. These neurotransmitters act like chemical intercoms in your nervous system, delivering messages from one portion of the body to another and ultimately regulating mood, mind, memory, and behavior.

There are approximately thirty different substances that are known or suspected to be neurotransmitters in the brain, and each has a characteristic ability to either excite or inhibit brain function. These transmitters are not randomly distributed throughout the brain; they are localized in specific clusters, which then control the specific functions of the various regions of the brain. Behavioral disorders, neurological problems, and seizure disorders may be related to various aspects of poor regulation of these neurotransmitters in specific regions of the brain. The brain controls the release of these neurotransmitters in part by proper production of energy through the breakdown of blood sugar in brain tissue. Although the brain represents only 2 percent of the total body weight, it accounts for over 20 percent of the total utilization of oxygen and 15 percent of blood sugar. The brain is obviously voraciously hungry and is dependent upon your nutritional status for its function.

Tissue such as muscle is able to function for short periods of time in the absence of proper levels of sugar and oxygen, but the brain cannot; it must continually metabolize blood sugar into energy in the presence of proper levels of oxygen and vitamins and minerals. If your brain goes hungry for more than ten minutes, it dies or suffers irreparable damage.

Neurotransmitters and Diet

The brain is also unique in that it is insulated from the rest of the body by what is called the blood–brain barrier. The **blood–brain barrier** is a membranous sac that covers the brain tissue and prevents substances in the blood from automatically entering into the brain. Nutrients and other substances can enter the brain only by way of **selective transport** across the blood–brain barrier.

The production of a number of the brain neurotransmitters is directly tied to the uptake of substances from the blood, across the blood–brain barrier, into the brain. For example, the essential amino acid tryptophan, when it crosses the blood–brain barrier, can be converted into the neurotransmitter serotonin. The amino acid phenylalanine, derived like tryptophan from dietary protein, can lead to the production of a class of neurotransmitters called the dopamine family, which includes adrenaline and noradrenaline.[2] Some neurotransmitters —like the dopamine family—are neuroactivating transmitters and others—like gamma-aminobutyric acid (GABA)—are neuroinhibitory transmitters.

Different types of mental illness are related to serious imbalances of these various neurochemicals, and less extreme imbalances may produce behavioral and personality changes. Recent research indicates that dietary intake can lead to alterations and imbalances in these neurotransmitter substances, thereby having an impact upon brain chemistry and ultimately behavior. Special nutritional requirements based on biochemical uniqueness may, in fact, create specific emotional or psychological problems. These observations have led drug companies to attempt to develop antipsychotic and tranquilizing drugs that mimic the brain's normal neurotransmitters or block imbalanced ones in attempts to reestablish proper balance or deactivate an overactivated pathway.[3]

Even learning and memory may be closely tied to the processes of brain neurotransmitters and neurochemicals. Studies have been done in which animals were trained to certain avoidance tasks, such as being afraid of the dark. The animals were then sacrificed, their brains extracted, and a chemical substance derived from them injected into the brains of animals not trained to be afraid of the dark. The result was immediate fear of the dark in the treated animals.

These studies, along with the recent human studies on the effect of diet on neurotransmitters, have opened up tremendously exciting new approaches toward the management of behavior disorders and personality problems beyond psychological counseling and drug therapy. Eight of the common neurotransmitter substances that regulate behavior have been found to be closely related to certain patterns of dietary intake.[4] Such symptoms as memory loss in the aged, fine motor shaking of the hands, nervous tics, aspects of uncontrolled blood pressure (both high and low), depression, and even certain forms of schizophrenia may all be related to imbalances of these nutrition-related neurotransmitters.

Two dietary amino acids have been found to be helpful in managing certain forms of nervous system disorders, when given in therapeutic amounts: tryptophan, which has been used to help manage insomnia in individuals deficient in the neurotransmitter serotonin, which is derived from tryptophan in the brain; and tyrosine, which has been used successfully to control both high and low blood pressure.[5] Tyrosine, which comes from phenylalanine, is converted in the nervous system to the neurotransmitters adrenaline or noradrenaline. The uptake of these amino acids into the brain is also influenced by the proportion of carbohydrate in the diet. With improved carbohydrate intake there is an increase in the uptake of tryptophan and proportionately an increased serotonin synthesis in people who may have insomnia or depression problems. Levels of tryptophan used were between 1 to 3 grams per day.

It is also found that one of the B-complex vitamins, choline, can serve as a template in the brain from which another neurotransmitter called acetylcholine is manufactured. As was discussed in Chapter 4, this substance prevents such conditions as presenile memory loss, moderates the aging disease called Alzheimer's disease, and may be useful in treating such neurological problems as Huntington's disease and tardive dyskinesia (a disease characterized by fine motor shaking and tremors which are side effects found in 50 percent of the patients taking antipsychotic medications).

The author of this research is optimistic about the direction his research will take in terms of therapy for patients suffering from a number of central nervous system disorders and brain biochemical problems. "Is it possible," he suggests, "that old people in whom the brain has lost many of the neurons that release neurotransmitters might benefit from a routine diet enhanced with tyrosine, tryptophan, or lecithin (choline)? If they might, should their continued reliance on normal but unenriched diets be construed as constituting poor nutrition?"[6] This is another excellent expression of the concept of biochemical individuality—that what is normal for one person may be suboptimal for another—and that as we age we may undergo changes in our ability to transport nutrients across the blood–brain barrier that necessitate augmented supplies of certain of these substances for proper neurotransmitter balance to be achieved and proper mood, mind, memory, and behavior to result. This is an exciting area of application of the concepts we have been discussing in the development of the Nutraerobics Program. The application of this approach leads us into a more detailed discussion of what may constitute brain biochemistry difficulties resulting in disorders of personality, some of which may be entitled schizophrenia.

Personality Disorders and Diet

Schizophrenia can really be thought of as a cluster of behavior and personality disorders whose symptoms relate to disorders of emotion, perception, thinking, and motor behavior. The diagnosis of this syndrome is based upon somewhat arbitrary clinical evidence, as there is probably no single cause of schizophrenia, but rather many different potential causes, a number of which are related to the inability of the nutritional support or lifestyle of patients to meet their genetic needs. Medical scientists now agree that schizophrenia, or behavior disorders that resemble perception problems, is a syndrome of diverse causes with very different kinds of genetic and environmental influences.[7] As one doctor says, "The nature-versus-nurture controversy is becoming as obsolete in the study of schizophrenia as it is in the rest of medicine. It is no longer which is involved, but how much, and what specific biologic and psychosocial factors operate in the continuous interaction between genetics and environment to produce those disorders of mental state and behavior that we perceive as abnormal."[8] It is obviously of great importance for people who have personality or psychological problems to identify the various environmental factors or unique nutritional requirements that could help them improve their brain biochemistry.

Orthomolecular Psychiatry

The field of orthomolecular psychiatry is that branch of psychiatry using substances natural to the human body to treat deficiency states and to produce a normal brain biochemistry. It was developed by two-time Nobel prize laureate Dr. Linus Pauling in the 1970s in response to the the theory that some mental disorders are caused by an inability to properly control natural substances within the brain. More conventional psychiatric circles, in contrast, use unnatural substances—drugs such as thorazine and haldol—to manage behavior. As Dr. Pauling points out, "Orthomolecular psychiatry is the treatment of mental disease by the provision of the optimal molecular environment for the mind, especially the optimal concentrations of substances normally present in the body."[9]

Extensive work over the last decade has demonstrated that emotional or psychological problems, usually associated with early warning signs of physical disease, may result from low intake from the diet —and therefore a low amount in the brain—of vitamins B-1, B-3, B-6, B-12, biotin, vitamin C, and folic acid. There is also evidence that mental function and behavior are affected by changes in the concentration in the brain of a number of other substances such as the amino acids L-glutamine and taurine, and the B vitamin choline. Inasmuch as the functioning of the brain and nervous tissue is more sensitively dependent upon the intake of essential nutrients than the functioning of other organs or tissues, it is not surprising that one of the first signs of nutrient insufficiency in an individual might be behavioral or nervous system problems.

We know that in acute deficiencies of vitamin B-1, significant nervous system disorders can develop, and a vitamin B-3 deficiency can lead to a frank case of dementia or psychotic behavior. We also know that individuals deficient in vitamin B-12 develop forms of mental illness well before the acute physical symptom of B-12 inadequacy, called pernicious anemia (a blood disorder), is recognized. A very low concentration of vitamin B-12 has been found in the blood of a much larger number of patients with mental illness than in that of the general population.

There have been a number of studies reported on the treatment of certain forms of mental illness with vitamin B-3 in doses much larger than the RDA levels, ranging in therapy from 300 milligrams to 3000 milligrams per day. Dr. Abram Hoffer, a well-known orthomolecular psychiatrist, has pioneered the work using B-3 in the treatment of certain forms of schizophrenia.

In one study, vitamin B-3 was used in the treatment of twenty-nine patients with severe psychiatric symptoms when none of these patients had physical symptoms of the acute deficiency disease of vitamin B-3, called pellagra. With this particular treatment, marked improvements over what had been previously accomplished by standard therapies were achieved.[10]

More recently, a number of studies have been done utilizing vitamin B-3 and its derivative niacinamide in the management of behavior and personality disorders; it has been found safe, inexpensive, and highly successful in large doses as a therapeutic agent.[11] The one drawback to niacin (B-3) therapy in the treatment of mental disorders is the flushing redness and hot feeling it produces in those who take it in large doses. This is not necessarily unsafe, but the reaction is unpleasant to many people. Niacinamide will not produce flushing, but it is also not as successful a treatment substance and may result in adverse effects upon the liver if taken at levels of 1000 to 5000 milligrams for a prolonged period of time.

Similarly, vitamin C has been used by a number of investigators in doses from 1,000 to 10,000 milligrams a day to manage certain behavior disorders. Vitamin B-6 has also been used in doses from 100 to 1,000 milligrams a day.

Strengths and Weaknesses of the Orthomolecular Model

The field of using natural substances to help activate certain biochemical pathways in the brain that promote optimal behavior is built upon the recognition that some individuals have genetically determined higher requirements for certain nutrients in the brain than other, "average" individuals. The recognition of symptoms associated with the insufficiency of various vitamins and minerals in your diet may uncover effects that have an impact not only on general health, but more specifically on your brain chemistry. If you are chronically depressed, tired, fatigued, or weak, you should consider the impact of your diet and lifestyle on your brain chemistry.

Orthomolecular psychiatry is not for every person who is suffering from emotional or mental illness, but it is for many people a successful alternative to psychotherapy, chemotherapy, or electroshock, the standard methods of managing psychiatric illness. Even if only one out of every ten emotionally or psychologically disturbed individuals responded to the orthomolecular psychiatric approach, it would be a considerable reduction of the burden upon our health-care system, not to mention a reduction in anguish suffered by those individuals. The reasons for and solutions to emotional problems are often not easy to find by standard Freudian or Jungian psychological models alone. The brain biochemical model provides a very attractive alternative to these approaches and leads to new clinical directions.

One of the most interesting theories relating vitamin and mineral factors to improved brain function and behavior is the **transmethylation theory.** This theory suggests that certain neurotransmitters in the brain become chemically converted, due to genetically determined unusual biochemical reactions in the brain, to substances that resemble hallucinogenic drugs such as mescaline. Certain vitamins, B-3 for example, when given in sufficient doses, can block these unusual biochemical reactions and prevent the druglike substances from being formed.

It has also been found that decreased rates of the metabolism in the brain of the neurotransmitter dopamine can be related to certain behavior disorders, and once again certain nutritive factors may help facilitate the increased conversion of dopamine to nontoxic waste products.[12] This theory is at least a working hypothesis as to how certain genetic uniquenesses contribute to altered brain biochemistry, leading to behavior disorders, and how the intake of specific levels of nutrients, sometimes far in excess of what would normally be considered adequate, may be necessary for normalizing the brain chemistries of afflicted individuals.

The brain functions by virtue of a very subtle balance between the substances that excite brain activity and those that inhibit it. Certain individuals may have excessive quantities in the brain of the mood excitatory substances leading to "hyper" personalities; this biotype may require substances that reduce brain overactivity, such as vitamin C, iron, copper, and vitamin B-2. Clinical symptoms associated with this biochemical type are a tendency toward alcoholism, chronic forms of schizophrenia, and manic depression. This syndrome may also require a higher quantity of the trace element manganese, vitamin B-3, and the amino acid tryptophan.

Other individuals may have excessive quantities of mood inhibitory substances, leading to the clinical symptoms of depression and possibly acute schizophrenia-related disorders; these people might respond better to higher quantities of vitamin B-12, folic acid, vitamin B-6, and zinc.

A Case Study of Orthomolecular Control

A 13-year-old girl was admitted to the hospital because of progressive withdrawal, hallucinations, the inability to eat, and tremors. Her early growth and development had been normal, and she was characterized as a sweet, shy girl who preferred to be alone. She had done average work in regular school until the age of 11 when her family moved to another area. Within the next year, she had considerable difficulty concentrating and was found upon retesting to have an IQ of 60. At this point she was placed in a special education program and began to fight with other children and have severe temper tantrums. When punished, she became withdrawn, stopped eating, and lost weight. It was found upon detailed medical evaluation that she had an elevated level in the blood of the amino acid homocysteine, which may be related to a vitamin B-6 or folic acid deficiency. She was treated with very high levels of vitamin B-6 (300 mg; the RDA is 2 mg per day) and her mental status improved within four days. At that point folic acid was also administered at a dose of 20 milligrams per day by mouth (RDA, .4 mg per day). In response to the folic acid along with the vitamin B-6, there was a marked improvement in her function, an increased intellectual capability, and a decrease of homocysteine in her blood. Over the next two years it was found that every time she went off the vitamin therapy, the condition started again almost immediately. Resuming the vitamin therapy led to clinical improvement and she became free of hallucinations and was able to feed herself and recognize her family. On continued maintenance of the vitamin supplements, this young woman has been free of psychotic manifestations for several years, but she continues to require the megavitamin intake to stabilize her mental health.[13] Such an example illustrates the powerful effect that orthomolecular treatment can have on those people who need a high-level vitamin intake to promote proper brain biochemistry.

Your Biotype and Personality Disorders

The future is very bright for orthomolecular psychiatry, for new tests are being developed that will allow doctors to assess what specific types and levels of biochemical support a patient with mental illness may require for improved functioning. We have been talking here about examples of extreme mental illness; what about the less extreme examples, the minor personality and behavior modifications often called "personality disturbances of unknown origin"? The early warning signs of many of these disturbances may be such symptoms as recurrent bad dreams, insomnia, muscle weakness or easy fatigue, mood swings, inability to concentrate, and personality disorders, as well as depression.

From your analysis of the questionnaires in Chapter 2, you have determined some of your specific sensitivities and needs for these various nutritive factors to promote optimal brain biochemistry and to alleviate symptoms. This concept doesn't mean, however, that if taking a few vitamins is good, then taking a whole lot at high levels must be better. We are still specifically addressing the concept of individualizing the approach to your needs. Not all people with behavior disorders require high levels of one or more nutrients to promote optimal mental health. There are many other factors that contribute to emotional stability. But if we could look seriously at orthomolecular concepts in context with the other psychosocial and environmental factors that contribute to mental health, it would lead to considerable improvement in therapeutic success in the treatment of psychological and behavior disturbances.

Learning Ability and Nervous System Disorders

In the chronic cases of learning and memory problems in children we now recognize that a higher-vitamin, higher-mineral dietary intake has a direct relationship to the improvement of such things as achievement in school, intelligence, and mental functioning. It has recently been found that in children a diet high in refined sugars, which means a diet low in vitamins and minerals, negatively affects intellectual functioning.[14] It was also found in this study that children who consumed diets of poor quality with low vitamin and mineral content tended to concentrate cadmium, a toxic mineral, in their bodies more readily. Cadmium displaces the essential mineral zinc, which is required by children and adults alike for normal brain and body function. Interestingly, zinc is also essential for growth in children, so a poor-quality diet may also contribute to growth retardation in children. The study concluded that a poor diet may significantly contribute to childhood learning disorders, and once again points to the importance of matching the quality of the nutritional intake with the brain's need for nutrients for optimal mental functioning.

Another trace mineral found to produce toxic effects upon the nervous system is vanadium. Although vanadium may be required at low levels for health, at high body burden levels it has been found to result in manic-depressive illness.[15] Large doses of vitamin C (3000 mg per day) resulted in elimination of the excess vanadium from the individuals affected and a reduction in the severity of their depressions.[16]

Cerebral Allergy

Amino acids, vitamins, and minerals are not the only food substances responsible for modulating brain function. Recently, behavior disorders have been related to food allergy and what are called cerebral allergic effects. It is well known that chronic schizophrenics often improve when placed on a wheat- or milk-free diet and relapse when the wheat or milk is returned to their diet. This was one of the first links discovered between nutritional factors and mental disorders. Recently, one researcher has found that after partial digestion, certain allergic foods may enter the blood as foreign proteins and cause a brain allergy to result.[17] These **incomplete protein breakdown** products (IPBs) can leave the intestinal tract unchanged, be delivered into the blood circulation, and have allergic effects upon the brain and other tissues.

It has been found that these incomplete protein breakdown products may have a similarity in the body to the class of very active hormones called endorphins.[18] Endorphins have a chemical activity similar to that of morphine and other analgesics, or pain killers. If diet could be responsible for substances that had activities similar to these endorphins, produced by incomplete digestion of certain food proteins delivered to the blood, it could account for the adverse behavioral effects certain people experience after eating allergy-producing foods like wheat, corn, milk, yeast, coffee, tea, chocolate, peanuts, beef, eggs, or citrus products. Incomplete digestion products of these food proteins may have an effect on central nervous system activity. These IPB's have been called **exorphins** because they come from outside the body and are a result of dietary factors in sensitive individuals.[19]

If food allergic substances can, in fact, produce behavioral changes, it is of obvious importance to evaluate the potential for allergy in patients who have chronic behavior disorders and also display food allergy–related symptoms such as intestinal upset, headaches, tiredness after eating, or skin problems. A more lengthy discussion of these allergy problems occurs in Chapter 11.

Depression Management

We have already learned that depression, which is one of the symptoms associated with a brain that is not working correctly, may be related to certain genetically determined characteristics. There is some recent evidence indicating that certain people may have what one author terms "melancholic genes," that is, genes that give them a predisposed, significant risk to depression disorders. These are individuals who may need strict attention to certain dietary and environmental supports to avoid the expression of their tendency toward depression.[20]

With a genetic sensitivity toward depression, you may be sensitive to being triggered into a depressive episode by a variety of different stimuli. We know that stress can induce the production of certain brain neurochemicals such as endorphins, which can be related not only to the reduction of pain, but also to behavioral changes and depression.[21] People who carry this genetic tendency should be very careful to adjust their daily lifestyle to avoid distressful situations and to provide proper time for relaxation, exercise, and leisure-time activity.

Hormones and Behavior

It is interesting to note that even certain medications used by a mother during pregnancy may stimulate increased risk to behavioral disorders in her offspring. In a recent study seventeen females and eight males who where exposed during gestation to synthetic hormones

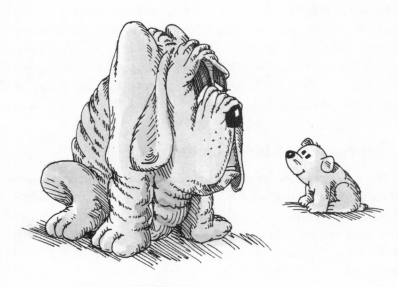

WHAT CAN I DO ABOUT IT?
I'VE GOT MELANCHOLY GENES.

taken by their mothers showed a significantly higher potential for aggression than their matched, unexposed brothers and sisters.[22] The observed influence of these synthetic hormones during gestation on later behavior suggests that some differences in the frequency of behavior disorders may be related to exposure of the fetus to natural hormones prior to birth. We know that women under high stress during pregnancy have very different hormone levels than women under low to normal stress; these high hormone levels could have a modulating effect on the developing nervous system of the child, which could influence his or her brain biochemistry and needs throughout life.

The hormones related to behavior are secreted by the glands of the endocrine system: the hypothalamus, pituitary, thyroid, and adrenals. If you tend to be cold all the time, have trouble managing your weight, have constipation periodically, have poor wound healing, and

poor exercise tolerance, it may indicate that you are also more susceptible to certain emotional disorders due to low thyroid gland output.
This may even be more of a problem if you tend to be very allergic,
very sensitive to loud noises, or have a "hyper" personality. These
latter symptoms are often associated with excessive function of the
adrenal glands. It has been found that when the adrenal glands and the
thyroid gland are not working correctly, people may have more depression and behavior disorders.[23]

One other master gland that regulates the activity of other hormone-secreting tissues is the pineal gland, which sits deep within your
brain. This gland is activated by exposure of your eyes to full-spectrum
sunlight. Exposure to sunlight stimulates the release of a hormone
from the pineal called melatonin, which helps regulate some of the
activity associated with depressive symptoms. If you spend all of your
day behind window glass or sunglasses or prescription lenses, then you
are not getting proper exposure of your eyes to full-spectrum sunlight.
This may also be a problem if you spend most of your time indoors
working under fluorescent lights, which are generally not full spectrum
and may not stimulate proper secretions of this important hormone,
melatonin. Use of zinc, vitamin B-6, vitamin C, and full-spectrum light
may be very helpful in stabilizing the pineal gland and the thyroid-
adrenal axis and improving your endocrine gland biochemistry.

What we have learned so far is that the subtle chemistry of the
brain profoundly affects your behavior and that there are a number of
factors under your control that may have direct impact upon this
chemistry. If you have a specific genetic need, as indicated by your
biotype, for increased levels of certain nutrients, satisfying that need
may be extremely helpful in modulating behavior or personality problems, as well as improving general health.

Blood Sugar and Mood

Another factor of obvious concern in any discussion of brain
chemistry is the regulation of the food that the brain consumes—blood

sugar. Too much or too little blood sugar can cause the brain to have interrupted performance and lead to distinct symptoms of personality change. Depression, anxiety, rapid mood swings, shaking, dizziness, confusion, lack of mental alertness can all be related to the brain's inability to receive proper levels of glucose. The conditions of high and low blood sugar are commonly called **hyperglycemia** and **hypoglycemia,** respectively. We know that individuals whose glandular system—the pancreas, pituitary, thyroid, and adrenal glands—is not operating properly have difficulty in controlling blood sugar and that they are very sensitive to excessive dietary sugar, which amplifies the problem of blood sugar control in their body.

Blood sugar, or glucose, can be made from either dietary sugar (sucrose, dextrose, etc.) or dietary starch (carbohydrate), but starch may be digested and absorbed into the blood at a much slower rate than sugar. Starch is digested and absorbed over several hours, whereas sugar is absorbed in a matter of tens of minutes. To demonstrate this significance between starch and sugar, a study was done on men and women from 35 to 55 years of age on two types of diets for six weeks. One was composed of foods high in sugar and the other of foods high in starch; the number of calories was the same in each diet. The results of the studies indicated that there were significant increases in the hormone insulin secreted by the pancreas in the individuals who were consuming the high-sugar diet, compared to when those same individuals were on the high-starch diet. This insulin secretion causes the blood sugar levels to fall rapidly and can result in hypoglycemia, which results in the brain suffering for lack of "food." They also had much higher levels of a hormone that stimulates appetite, meaning that the high-sugar diet is also an appetite-enhancing diet.[24] It has even been found that certain dietary sources of starch have less effect upon blood sugar than other sources of starch. Rice and corn have been shown to cause a less rapid rise and fall in blood sugar than do potatoes and wheat.[25] Therefore, brown rice and corn may be preferable sources of starch for the individual susceptible to reactive hypoglycemia than potato or wheat sources of starch.

The amount of sugar in the diet can also have a significant impact upon blood sugar and stress on the endrocrine system. Twenty-two percent of the calories in the average American diet are in the form of sugar. Recently, common abnormalities in blood sugar control were seen in individuals who had consumed 18 percent or more of their dietary calories as sugars, and it was concluded that "sucrose intake at levels now commonly consumed in the American diet by sugar-sensitive individuals can lead to abnormalities in blood sugar control."[26]

The ability of a high-sugar diet in sugar-sensitive individuals to produce adverse behavioral effects may be most important for understanding certain behavior abnormalities seen in children. A recent study indicated that in the 5-to-12-year-old age group, the younger children are, the greater a percentage of their total body weight is the amount of food consumed in sugars. If we believe that sugar in excessive quantities exerts a pharmacological effect upon the brain, then it is not surprising that these sugar-rich diets may have a greater impact on younger children who are consuming as sugar a greater percentage of their total weight each year than older, heavier children.[27]

Ninety-five percent of the sugar consumed by these children was found in six groups of food items: sweetened beverages and soft drinks; candy and confectionary goods; cookies, cakes and pies; ice cream; sugared cereals; and salty and caramel snacks. Diets composed of these high-sugar, low-protein items were recently found in animal studies to be associated with aggressive behavior and altered brain-wave activity.[28] Another study has also found that children who have been classed as learning disabled often show abnormal responses to low blood sugar, and these conditions are aggravated by diets high in refined sugars.[29]

The results of these studies and other clinical observations are quite clear. If you are one of the individuals who is sugar sensitive, if you have developed the symptoms of mood swings, aggressive personality changes, depression, anxiety, confusion or lack of mental alertness after a period of not eating or after having a sugar-rich meal, then improving your intake of complex starches and reducing your dietary

Figure 3

Brown and White Rice Bread
Enriched with Vegetable Gum

---

2 tsp sugar ½ c water	*Dissolve in small bowl.*
1 package dry, active yeast	*Sprinkle over sugar water. Set aside for 10 minutes.*
1½ c water ¼ c shortening	*Combine in saucepan. Heat until shortening melts. Cool to lukewarm.*
1 c brown rice flour 2 c white rice flour (long-grain, if possible) ¼ c sugar 3½ tsp guar gum or glucomannan ⅔ c nonfat dry milk powder 1½ tsp salt	*Combine in mixing bowl.*
	Add yeast mixture. Blend well.
	Add shortening/water mixture. Blend well.
2 large eggs	*Add. Mix at highest speed of mixer for 2 minutes. Pour dough into greased bowl. Let rise in warm place until doubled, approximately 1 to 1½ hours.*
	Return to mixing bowl. Beat 3 minutes.
	Pour dough into 2 small or 1 large greased loaf pan(s). Let rise until dough is slightly above top of pan. Bake at 400°F. for 10 minutes. Place foil over bread and bake 50 minutes more.

Note: Measure ingredients *very* carefully. The dough looks more like cookie dough than bread dough, so don't be alarmed. Bread structure is a little better if bread is baked in 2 small loaf pans. Store gum tightly sealed in cool, dry place.

Yield: 1 large or 2 small loaves.

sugars would significantly help to restore proper brain biochemistry. Consumption of breakfast and regular meals throughout the day rich in complex carbohydrates from corn and rice, and secondarily from beans, legumes, potatoes and whole wheat, is very beneficial in establishing proper slow release of sugar from your diet into your blood to help you stabilize the delivery of sugar to your brain as a source of energy.[30]

The Use of Dietary Gums and Fibers

It has been found that any food substance that helps slow the release of sugar across the intestinal membranes into the blood will help stabilize blood sugar, putting less demand on your endocrine system and giving your brain a more constant supply of energy.[31] Even dietary gums such as apple pectin or guar gum can be very helpful in slowing your blood sugar response after eating.[32] These gums can either be taken as a supplement with the meal or can be gotten naturally by eating more unrefined carbohydrate sources. Substances such as glucomannan have been found useful as a meal supplement (1–3 teaspoons) in slowing the release of sugars from the meal into the blood and reducing the demand upon the endocrine system. These substances are thickening agents and should be taken with adequate fluids with the meal. The bread recipe in Figure 3 incorporates one of these gums into an easily consumed product.

Chromium and Its Effect
on Blood Sugar

One important trace element for the stabilization of blood sugar is chromium.[33] The function of chromium in the body is directly tied to that of the hormone insulin which helps cells absorb sugar from the blood. A chromium deficiency results in a resistance of various cells in the body to insulin and prevents sugar from being properly stabilized. Chromium is found in high quantities in whole-grain cereal products, but nearly 90 percent of it is removed when the grains are milled for white-flour products. Also, chromium can be depleted from the soil when standard chemical fertilizers are used, but because chromium is not essential for plants as it is for humans, the plants may not show the chromium deficiency. (The same thing happens with iodine; loss of iodine from the soil can lead to iodine-poor foods that produce goiter in humans, but the plants grown in the soil may be perfectly healthy and produce a high yield.)

A number of studies indicate the important role chromium plays in helping the body better use blood sugar. A recent double-blind crossover experiment used seventy-six men and women ranging in age from 21 to 69 years. Half were put on 200 micrograms of chromium and half on a suitable placebo for three months. At the end of three months, the two groups were switched and it was found that on chromium supplementation fifty-eight out of the seventy-six participants exhibited improved control over blood sugar; and this effect was even more profound in those who started the study with hyper- or hypoglycemic problems.[34]

In another study, twenty-four men and women 63 years of age or older were fed a high-chromium brewer's yeast supplement or a chromium-deficient torula yeast supplement. It was found in this study that blood sugar was again stabilized, and there was an enhanced state of wellness while supplementing with the high-chromium brewer's yeast.[35]

In a group of twenty college-age subjects, chromium supplementation was again found to improve the control of blood sugar and reduce the demand on the pancreas to secrete insulin.[36] Chromium is best gotten in a high-chromium brewer's yeast product that contains the chromium compound called **glucose tolerance factor (GTF)**. GTF forms of chromium are much more absorbable and are better at stabilizing blood sugar than a standard chromium supplement or inorganic chromium that might come from drinking water.

A recent report indicated that chromium at the level of 200 micrograms a day in a high-chromium brewer's yeast supplement is useful for a number of health problems including a tendency toward diabetes, hypoglycemia, and a host of behavioral and psychological problems such as depression that come from lack of blood sugar controls.[37] A balanced, varied diet from unprocessed foods is likely to furnish the chromium requirement, whereas the high-fat, high-sugar, high-alcohol diet commonly consumed by the average person would not.

Putting glucose-tolerance-factor chromium together with a program to manage blood sugar through the restriction of dietary sugars and the increase in unrefined starches from whole grains, legumes, corn, and brown rice is an excellent way of flattening out those blood sugar highs and lows which have attendant mood swings, behavior problems, and psychological disorders.

Long-Term Effects
of Poor Blood Sugar Control

Long-term difficulties with control of blood sugar can lead to a maturity-onset form of diabetes that will need medical treatment.[38] Evidence now exists that there may be a long prediabetic period associated with poor blood sugar control and psychological problems well before an individual has been diagnosed as having the disease diabetes, requiring insulin therapy. This may even be true in children and once again suggests that by the use of the Nutraerobics Program to optimize health at an early stage there is every opportunity to avoid later-stage, more significant diseases such as diabetes. If you have lost or gained weight rapidly in the recent past, had difficulty healing wounds or cuts, have abnormally large thirst, night shakes, or frequent urination, then you may be in a prediabetic situation and need administration of this program as outlined.

The irony of the story is that both hypoglycemia and hyperglycemia, or diabetes, are manifestations of the same problem—the inability of your body to properly handle blood sugar. This situation is a result of poor hormonal control of the uptake of sugar by various tissues and can be stabilized by improved diet, exercise, weight management, and stress reduction. Heeding these by using your biotype correctly and recognizing any physical or psychological symptoms you may have of poor hormonal control of blood sugar, you can avert recurrent feelings of the blues, inability to concentrate, or mood swings.

Toxic Elements and Brain Chemistry

Throughout this discussion of brain biochemistry and its effect on behavior, the subtle relationship between how the brain operates and how one feels has been stressed. Recently, it has become obvious that not only are there substances that help promote proper brain function and normalize mood and emotions, but subtle exposure to low-level toxic substances may produce abnormal brain function and behavior. One such example is the toxic metal family, including mercury, lead, and aluminum (aluminum has only recently been discovered to be potentially hazardous). Exposure to these toxic elements can occur in a variety of different places, in many of which the exposure is not at all apparent to the average person. Studies have indicated that dentists and dental technicians who have been exposed to mercury through the use of materials used in the filling of teeth have high levels of tissue mercury in their bodies and that 30 percent of the individuals with an elevated mercury body burden had developed chronic impairment of their neurophysiology.[39]

Aluminum has been traditionally considered a nontoxic element, but there is now ever increasing information indicating that it may be accumulated in the nervous system and can be a potentially toxic substance. Recently, some residents of Guam have been evaluated who have a nervous system disorder that has been diagnosed as amyotrophic lateral sclerosis (ALS), or a Parkinsonism-type disease. They lose muscle control, speech, and equilibrium. In examining individuals who have died from these conditions, it was found that their brains and nervous systems were very high in aluminum. Preliminary analysis of environmental samples indicated that the regions where these individuals lived have soils and local water supplies rich in aluminum but virtually devoid of calcium and magnesium. Calcium and magnesium are known to be the antagonists of aluminum; therefore, on a diet or water supply high in aluminum and low in calcium and magnesium, it may be possible to accumulate aluminum in the nervous system over a long period of time, leading to its impairment.[40]

Aluminum can be obtained through the use of antacids, water that has been softened with aluminum ion exchange resins (water softeners), food that is contaminated with aluminum and is low in calcium and magnesium, and cooking of acid or alkaline foods in soft aluminum cookware.[41] The extent to which aluminum accumulation contributes to neurological disorders is not yet fully understood, but there is strong evidence to suggest that conditions such as memory loss with aging and certain nervous system diseases may have at least a relationship to increased aluminum accumulation. Therefore, the best protection would be a diet adequately rich in calcium and magnesium and elimination of the obvious sources of aluminum.

Seizure Disorders and Taurine

What about the cases in which demonstrated brain biochemical problems lead to such disorders as epilepsy, which is characterized by overactivity in certain portions of the brain and seizures? There has been a considerable amount of work done in the past several years indicating that seizure disorders are a result of imbalances in neurotransmitters that regulate activation and deactivation of certain portions of the brain. When there is an excess of the excitatory neurotransmitters or a deficiency of the inhibitory neurotransmitters the brain can be in a state of heightened chemical activity leading to seizure problems. Some inhibitory neurotransmitters that can be deficient are gamma-aminobutyric acid, glycine, and taurine. Recent studies have indicated that dietary taurine may be useful in managing seizure problems when given in supplementary doses. Taurine is a naturally occurring amino acid which is found in the brain and in heart tissue in high levels and has the important role of modulating certain aspects of brain biochemistry.

When taurine was used in controlled studies with epileptics, it was found that 50 percent of the patients seemed to respond with improved management of their seizure problems.[42] Taurine levels in the brain have been found abnormal in epileptics, and oral taurine can be used to increase brain taurine levels in many epileptics and to manage regions of the brain that may be suffering from deficiency of this inhibitory neurotransmitter.[43] This is another example of biochemical individuality: we all manufacture taurine in our own bodies, but it may be that certain people are not capable of manufacturing enough to meet their daily needs, causing them to show unique brain chemistry abnormalities.

Interestingly, there is another substance not usually considered an essential nutrient that has shown usefulness in the management of a seizure disorder, a substance natural to the body called N, N-dimethylglycine (DMG). It has been pointed out that, despite the development of many new anticonvulsion agents in recent years, many epileptic patients continue to have seizures. There was one case of a 22-year-old man who had presented himself to researchers with long-standing mental retardation and seizure problems that had not been controlled by medication. His mother was instructed to give him a twice-daily dosage of DMG (90 mg); after one week his seizure frequency had dropped to three per week, and attempts to withdraw the DMG resulted in dramatic increases in seizure frequency. This may make good brain biochemical sense in that dimethylglycine is a close relative to the neuroinhibitory amino acid glycine which works along with taurine in the brain. As the researchers point out, "although no definite conclusions can be drawn from this single patient's apparent response to DMG, the results suggest that this relationship certainly warrants further studies to determine whether this substance may work with taurine and other natural substances in restoring proper brain biochemistry in patients with seizure disorders."[44]

Another substance receiving considerable attention for its potential therapeutic benefit in nervous system or seizure disorders is wheat germ oil concentrate (prometol), which has high levels of the natural substances octacosanol, triacantanol, and myristanol. This concentrate was originally shown to improve endurance and reduce muscle fatigue in athletes studied at the University of Illinois but has more recently been suggested to be useful in treating a variety of organic brain syndromes.[45] The dosage used in these therapies ranges from 2500 to 5000 micrograms of octacosanol from wheat germ oil concentrate. Studies are now under way to determine the mechanism by which this substance stimulates nervous system and brain function, and the future for its application to coma patients, seizure disorders, and nervous system problems appears bright.

Conclusions of Your Biotype

The conclusions that can be drawn from all this information are far-reaching and very exciting. They suggest that much of what may be termed behavior disorders of unknown origin may, in fact, be related to alterations in brain biochemistry that can be modified by altered dietary intake and lifestyle. This new working hypothesis in psychiatry opens up tremendous new doors for therapy beyond traditional psychological counseling and medications. By reading your subtle psychological symptoms and by being better in tune with your biotype, you should be able to design an appropriate program to normalize your brain biochemistry and improve your mental functioning. Even in the cases of fairly extreme neurological disease there may be hope for improvement by utilizing the concepts of biochemical individuality and essential nutrient support. The tremendous progress made the past few years in understanding the relationship of diet to brain biochemistry only whets our appetite for what in the future may prove to be a major therapeutic tool for managing a whole host of behavioral and psychological disorders that have previously been un-amenable to standard therapies.

A second common problem area associated with vertical disease is that of proper weight management. There are twenty-five to thirty million Americans who at any one time are on weight loss diets and countless others who are underweight to the point where they are suffering from reduced health and vitality. There are so many heavily marketed weight management programs that frequently people are so confused about which is the safest and most effective program that they end up on potentially hazardous fad diets. As you will see in the next chapter, knowing your biotype will allow you to put together a safe, effective weight management program if you need to either gain or lose weight.

Notes

1. Myron Brin in L. Iversen, "Chemistry of the Brain," *Scientific American* (June 1980):139–149.

2. Iversen, "Chemistry of the Brain."

3. J. Fox, "Scientists Face Explosion of Brain Compounds," *Chemical and Engineering News* (19 November 1979): 30–32.

4. L. Iversen, "Neurotransmitters and Central Nervous System Disease," *Lancet* (23 October 1982):914–918.

5. R. J. Wurtman, "Nutrients That Modify Brain Function," *Scientific American* (June 1982):50–59.

6. Ibid.

7. M. E. Lewis, "Biochemical Aspects of Schizophrenia," *Neurochemistry and Neuropharmacology, 4,* 1(1980).

8. D. Kety, "Affective Personality Disorders: A Look at Their Causation," *Psychological Reviews, 12,* 327(1967).

9. L. Pauling, "Orthomolecular Psychiatry," *Science, 196,* 212(1970).

10. V. P. Sydenstricker and H. M. Cleckley, "Nicotinic Acid Therapy in Schizophrenia," *American Journal of Psychiatry, 99,* 83(1941).

11. A. Hoffer, *Niacin Therapy in Psychiatry* (Springfield, IL: C. C. Thomas, 1962).

12. J. L. Sullivan, C. E. Coffey, and J. O. Cavenar, "Metabolic Factors Affecting Monoamine Oxidase Activity," *Schizophrenia Bulletin, 6,* 308(1980).

13. "Folate-Responsive Homocystinuria and 'Schizophrenia,' " *Nutrition Reviews, 40,* 242(1982).

14. M. L. Lester, R. W. Thatcher, and L. Monroe-Lord, "Refined Carbohydrate Intake, Hair Cadmium Levels, and Cognitive Functioning in Children," *Nutrition and Behavior, 1,* 3(1982).

15. G. J. Naylor and A. H. W. Smith, "Vanadium: A Possible Etiological Factor in Manic-Depressive Illness," *Psychological Medicine, 11,* 249(1981).

16. R. E. Hodges, "Vanadium, Vitamin C and Depression, *Nutrition Reviews, 40* 293(1982).

17. W. A. Hemmings, "Dietary Proteins Reach the Brain," *Orthomolecular Psychiatry, 6,* 309(1977).

18. C. Zioudrou and W. Klee "Opioid Peptides Derived from Food Proteins," *Journal of Biological Chemistry, 254,* 2246(1979).

19. Ibid.

20. W. Herbert, "Melancholic Genes," *Science News, 121,* 108(1982).

21. J. C. Willer and J. Cambier, "Stress-Induced Analgesia in Humans," *Science, 212,* 689(1982).

22. J. M. Reinisch, "Prenatal Exposure to Synthetic Progestins Increases Potential for Aggression in Humans," *Science, 211,* 1171 (1981).

23. L. Wetterberg and F. Unden, "Melatonin and Cortisol in Psychiatric Illness," *Lancet* (10 July 1982):100.

24. S. Reiser and T. M. O'Dorisio, "Effect of Isocaloric Exchange of Starch and Sugar on Gastric Inhibitory Polypeptide," *Amer. J. Clin. Nutrition, 33,* 1907(1980).

25. A. Coulston and G. Reaven, "Effect of Source of Dietary Carbohydrate on Plasma Glucose in Normal Subjects," *Amer. J. Clin. Nutrition, 33,* 1279(1980).

26. S. Reiser and J. Hallfrisch, "Blood Lipids and Their Distribution in Lipoproteins in Subjects Fed Three Levels of Sucrose," *Journal of Nutrition, 111,* 1045(1981).

27. K. J. Morgan and M. E. Zabik, "Amount and Food Sources of Total Sugar Intake by Children Ages 5–12 Years," *Amer. J. Clin. Nutrition, 34,* 404(1981).

28. K. Kantak and B. Eichelman, "Low Dietary Protein and Its Facilitation of Defensiveness and Aggression in Adult Rats," *Nutrition and Behavior, 1,* 47(1982).

29. H. Powers, "Dietary Measurements to Improve Behavior and Achievement," *Academics and Therapeutics, 9,* 203(1973).

30. S. Reiser and E. S. Prather, "Serum Insulin and Glucose in Hyperinsulinemic Subjects Fed Three Different Levels of Sucrose," *Amer. J. Clin. Nutr., 34,* 2348(1981); A. Coalston and G. M. Reaven, "Effect of Differences in Source of Dietary Carbohydrate on Insulin Responses in Patients with Impaired Carbohydrate Tolerance," *Amer. J. Clin. Nutrition, 34,* 2716(1981); D. J. A. Jenkins and S. R. Bloom, "Slow Release Dietary Carbohydrate Improves Second Meal Tolerance," *Amer. J. Clin. Nutrition, 35,* 1339(1982).

31. G. Collier and K. O'Dea, "Effect of Physical Form of Carbohydrate on the Postprandial Glucose, Insulin, and Gastric Inhibitory Polypeptide in Type 2 Diabetes," *Amer. J. Clin. Nutrition, 36,* 10(1982).

32. T. Poynard and G. Tchobroutsky, "Pectin Efficacy in Insulin-Treated Diabetes," *Lancet* (18 January 1980):158.

33. W. Mertz, "Chromium: An Essential Micronutrient," *Contemporary Nutrition, 7,* 3(1982).

34. V. J. K. Liu and R. P. Abernathy, "Chromium and Insulin in Young Subjects with Normal Glucose Tolerance," *Amer. J. Clin. Nutrition, 35,* 601(1982).

35. M. McCarty, "The Therapeutic Potential of Glucose Tolerance Factor," *Medical Hypotheses, 6,* 1177(1980).

36. E. G. Offenbacher, "Beneficial Effect of Chromium-Rich-Yeast on Glucose Tolerance and Blood Lipids," *Diabetes, 29,* 219(1980).

37. V. J. K. Liu and R. Dowdy, "Effect of High Chromium Yeast-Extract on Serum Lipids, Insulin and Glucose Tolerance in Older Women," *Federation Proceedings, 36,* 1123(1977).

38. A. N. Gorsach and A. G. Cudworth, "Evidence for a Long Prediatetic Period in Diabetes Mellitus," *Lancet* (26 December 1981):1363.

39. J. M. Shapiro and P. Bloch, "Neurophysiological and Neuropsychological Function in Mercury-Exposed Dentists," *Lancet* (22 May 1982):1147.

40. D. P. Perl and C. J. Gibbs, "Intraneuronal Aluminum Accumulation in Amyotrophic Lateral Sclerosis and Parkinsonism-Dementia of Guam," *Science, 217,* 1053(1982).

41. S. E. Levick, "Dementia from Aluminum Pots?" *New England Journal of Medicine, 299,* 164(1980).

42. R. J. Huxtable and A. Barbeau, *Taurine in Neurological Disorders* (New York: Raven Press, 1979).

43. H. O. Goodman and M. Resnick, "Taurine Transport in Epilepsy," *Clinical Chemistry, 26,* 414(1980).

44. E. S. Roach and L. Carlin, "N,N-dimethylglycine for Epilepsy, *New England Journal of Medicine, 307,* 1081(1982).

45. S. K. Ries and R. A. Levitt, "Triacontanol and Increased Plant Growth," *Science, 195,* 1339(1977); T. Cureton, *Physiological Effect of Wheat Germ Oil Concentrate in Human Subjects* (Springfield, IL: C. C. Thomas Publishers, 1972).

6

Overweight or Underweight?

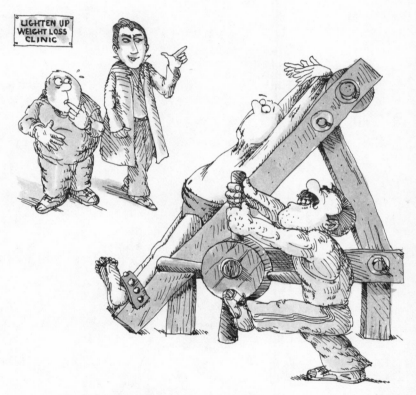

AND AS YOU CAN SEE, WE HAVE ALL THE LATEST METHODS FOR
ADJUSTING YOUR WEIGHT-TO-HEIGHT RATIO.

Have you ever been on a diet to lose or gain weight and had one or more of the following problems?

1. Lightheadedness upon standing

0	1
No	Yes

2. Heartbeat changes

0	1
No	Yes

3. Constipation

0	1
No	Yes

4. Joint or muscle pain

0	1
No	Yes

5. Cold intolerance

0	1
No	Yes

6. Dry skin

0	1
No	Yes

7. Menstrual irregularities

0	1
No	Yes

8. Anemia

0	1
No	Yes

9. Prolonged sleep tendency

0	1
No	Yes

10. Hair loss

0	1
No	Yes

11. Nervousness

0	1
No	Yes

12. Muscle loss

0	1
No	Yes

If your score exceeds 4 you have been experiencing the first signs of a poor weight management program with adverse side effects. It is not losing or gaining weight itself that affects your health, but how that weight change is effected.

In this chapter we are going to explore why certain people have a tendency to be overweight or underweight and what the development of your Nutraerobics Program according to your biotype can do to help stabilize your proper weight-to-height ratio.

Genetics and Weight Problems

Is being overly fat or overly thin a genetically inherited condition? There is a considerable amount of evidence suggesting that a tendency toward a weight problem runs in families. All of us have seen overweight children whose parents have their own problem with weight management. And it is known from animal studies that various strains of animals can be genetically predetermined to be obese and have extremely voracious appetites, high blood cholesterol, and the diseases associated with obesity.

There is also limited evidence from human studies that when one parent is obese, the children have a 40 percent chance of obesity, and that when both parents are obese, the probability is greater than 80 percent. Children of nonobese parents have only about a 14 percent probability of having a weight problem. This, of course, doesn't prove that parental obesity genetically determines childhood obesity; it may just suggest that the environment in which the children are living may dispose them toward obesity.

To really test whether children inherit their parental biological disposition toward obesity, studies have been done with identical twins who have been adopted by different families. The results of these studies are somewhat conflicting but, basically, the suggestion from studying 256 families is that body fatness does not directly correlate with the biological parents but seems to correlate more with the family who raised the child; however, there was a biological parental disposition towards obesity that was passed on to the child and could be expressed as a weight problem if the child's eating environment was not properly managed.[1]

Detailed medical studies have now identified several genetic alterations that could dispose an individual toward a weight problem. One of these is a possible genetic defect in an enzyme called sodium-potassium ATPase.[2] This enzyme is important for maintaining a proper sodium and potassium balance within the cells. If it is not working correctly, it may lead to the accumulation of fluid, a weight increase, and the inability to properly excrete sodium, which could contribute to high blood pressure and weight problems.

Again, a disposition toward a particular problem does not necessarily mean that the problem will be expressed if nutrition and lifestyle are properly adjusted to compensate for it. In the case of a genetic disposition to a problem with sodium-potassium ATPase, a low-sodium diet and avoidance of foods that have been demonstrated to impair the enzyme can encourage both proper sodium balance and fluid maintenance.[3] Foods with the substance that seems to inactivate this enzyme include tea, cocoa, red wines, cucumber, turnip greens, and cabbage, and avoiding these may allow better maintenance of sodium levels within the genetically inclined individual. Symptoms of this problem include fluid retention, swelling of the ankles, and puffiness of the face.

Designing a Weight Control Program

We all have predispositions toward certain variations in metabolism, some of which may result in weight difficulties. But we can use our biotype and the newest information on metabolic control to design our own Nutraerobics Program that may even prevent the continual need for hard-to-follow diets.

Let's first talk about problems associated with being overweight or obese. A nationwide survey completed in 1974 indicated that 15 percent of the men and and 25 percent of the women aged 20 to 74 years were 20 percent or more overweight, which is considered the definition of obesity. When people are more than 50 percent above their optimal weight-to-height ratio they are said to be morbidly obese, meaning that their obesity contributes directly to the decline in their health with increasing risk to many of the degenerative diseases and certainly a shortened lifespan. Conditions associated with morbid obesity include increased risk to coronary heart disease, high blood pressure, diabetes, osteoarthritis, susceptibility to infection, and kidney problems.[4]

The attempt to control obesity has led to the birth of a tremendous industry in which over \$3.5 billion is spent per year on weight control. The major thrust of this industry is to help people lose weight; but, again, the *way* in which the weight is lost is of utmost importance. You can lose weight by shedding fat, muscle, or water. Many quick weight loss diets work by muscle or water loss, not proper fat loss, and are undesirable in any case because either weight is regained easily or your health is compromised.

As we explore the management of weight, the major emphasis will be on developing a safe, controlled, fat-wasting (losing), muscle-sparing weight loss method that will not produce diuresis, or fluid loss, leading to dehydration or the loss of excessive quantities of potassium, magnesium, or calcium in the urine.

Some Causes and Effects of Obesity

A number of suggested causes of obesity have to do with genetic predisposition: improper functioning of the thyroid and/or adrenal glands, brown fat metabolism problems, psychosocial problems with food intake regulation (eating behavior and appetite theories), and the most recent concept of set-point theory (the theory that the body has a particular, somewhat hard to control, set weight it tries to maintain).[5] We will be talking about some of these causes as we work on designing a program for successful weight management.

We now recognize that by maintaining a proper weight-to-height ratio a person can reduce the risks to most of the major killer diseases. Elevated blood pressure can be brought closer to a safe level upon weight loss in the obese individual.[6] The heart has to work less hard to pump blood to tissues without the extra burden of the 100 miles of additional capillaries necessary for every pound of fat stored in the body.[7] Even the risk to certain types of cancer, particularly of the breast, ovary, prostate, and intestine, goes down with reduced body fatness.[8]

One of the most enlightening and potentially most useful new bits of information concerning the impact of obesity on health is the finding that women who are upper-body heavy (meaning that they carry the bulk of their extra weight above the waist) have an eight times greater likelihood of developing adult diabetes than do women who have a normal weight-to-height ratio. A study of 15,000 overweight women indicated that approximately 25 percent were upper-body heavy and suggested that as many as six million American women already may have some clinically diagnosable diabetes that they are unaware of.[9] The good news is that the health of these women can be improved by restoring the proper weight-to-height ratio.

Given the scope of the health problems associated with excessive weight and the fact that it is the number one nutritionally related health problem in our culture today, how do we approach the management of this difficult problem?

Approaches to Weight Loss

Three major approaches to weight loss are now being explored by contemporary medicine. The first of these, which has been debated hotly in the past year, is the surgical rerouting of the intestines or stapling of the stomach so that nutrients cannot be absorbed as easily and the individual can eat without retaining the calories.[10] Although this procedure is useful in losing weight (it seems to lead predominately to fat loss, not muscle loss), there is some concern about its long-term safety. Certain doctors believe that these procedures are still in their developmental stage and should not be performed as frequently as they are today. Many thousands of these operations have been performed over the past few years and some surgeons do as many as five to seven of the gastric stapling procedures a week. Yet these procedures have a 41-percent failure rate, where failure is defined as a patient's not losing at least 15 percent of his or her starting weight.

The second procedure, also very experimental, is a so-called lipectomy. This procedure is one done on obese infants, young children, or adults in which much of the subcutaneous fat (fat deposits near the surface, just under the skin) is removed surgically; the idea is that if there is no place for storage of fat, it cannot be stored and the adult will be able to maintain weight better.[11] Again, this procedure is considered highly experimental and may have wide-ranging adverse side effects in the adult.

Third, the pharmaceutical approach toward weight management uses drugs to dull the appetite or to speed up the metabolism. It should be recalled that no medication is without side effects, and some of these drugs have wide-ranging and long-term adverse side effects in people who are dependent upon them for weight control. This is true even for such medications as the over-the-counter appetite suppressant phenyl-propanolamine, which is used in many nonprescription weight loss products.[12] Several recent reports describe adverse reactions to phenyl-propanolamine, including headaches, fever, nausea, vomiting, weakness, and severe muscle tenderness.

What about highly popularized diets that are receiving much consumer support these days? They are not all that effective and many of them, as we will discuss later in this chapter, may be actually hazardous to your health in the long term. There is no simple answer to the difficult question of maintenance of proper body weight other than to try to learn more about your specific metabolism and direct your diet and lifestyle toward your unique genetic requirements. By the end of this discussion you should know what types of things you need to concentrate on to develop your own safe and effective weight management program, whether you need to decrease the tendency to gain weight or put on muscle mass if you are underweight.

Thermodynamics of Weight Loss

To control your weight, the number of calories you take in each day from your food must equal the number of calories that you expend in energy, as shown in Figure 4. One part of this equation is extremely important, as it is the thrust of the whole Nutraerobics weight manage-

Figure 4

The Metabolic Weight Equation

Take: Total calories
                  consumed in food.

Subtract: Calories expended
                  in metabolic and
                  active energy.

The remainder: Zero means weight
                  control: calories consumed
                  equal calories expended.

                  More than zero means
                  weight gain.

                  Less than zero means
                  weight loss.

ment program. The calories that you expend each day are a combination both of your activity units **and** your basal metabolic rate, or the "idle speed" of your "engine." Your body is just like an engine that needs fuel in combination with oxygen to give rise to productive energy. If you take in fuel, or food, and are not able to properly burn it under appropriate metabolic control (if your "idle" is too slow), then your engine is working inefficiently and "carbon can develop on the spark plugs." We call that fat deposition or weight gain.

One of the major goals of the Nutraerobics Program is to find ways of tuning up your engine or making your basal metabolic rate more efficient. Doesn't it seem contradictory that people who are apparently taking in more energy from their food than they need, because they are gaining weight and becoming fat, have the symptoms of not getting enough energy, for they are tired, weak, easily fatigued, and apparently energy deficient? They have what may be termed a **switched metabolism.** They are taking in calories as food, but they are not properly turning them into the energy of activity because their metabolism is switched and their metabolic engine is not working correctly.

Given this concept, we might ask if obesity in many individuals is not really a metabolic problem.[13] Certainly excessive food intake will lead to weight gain, but inefficient metabolism of the calories taken in will also encourage fat storage. This metabolic inefficiency is, however, modifiable through improved nutrition and lifestyle.

Lean Body Mass

The Nutraerobics Program tries to find ways of improving the efficiency of your metabolism so that fat is lost while muscle is maintained, so that your lean body mass improves. *Lean body mass* is defined as the percentage of your total weight that is made up of muscle and bone as opposed to that of fat. Most researchers feel that the ideal lean body mass is 85 percent for men and 80 percent for women, meaning that men should be no more than 15 percent and women no more than 20 percent fat. Finding the key to unlock the metabolic efficiency of your body's machinery so that muscle can be properly maintained without storing excessive fat will be somewhat like doing detective work, but you already have learned a number of clues about yourself that we will use in coming to the final solution.

First let's calculate your lean body mass so we know whether you are overweight or underweight. An easy method to use is the body mass index. On Figure 5 connect a straight line between your weight and your height. In the middle that line will intersect your body mass index.[14] Now from your body mass index, you can determine approximately how many pounds you need to lose or to gain. Women have ideal body mass indices from 3.2 to 3.7; men, from 3.4 to 3.9. If your number determined from Figure 5 is above these ranges, you have excessive body fat and you need consider a fitness improvement program; if your number is lower, you need to gain weight and you should consider some of the suggestions at the end of the chapter.

Figure 5

Nomogram for Calculating Body Mass Index

Connect a straight line from your weight to your height. Where it crosses the middle line is equal to your body mass index.

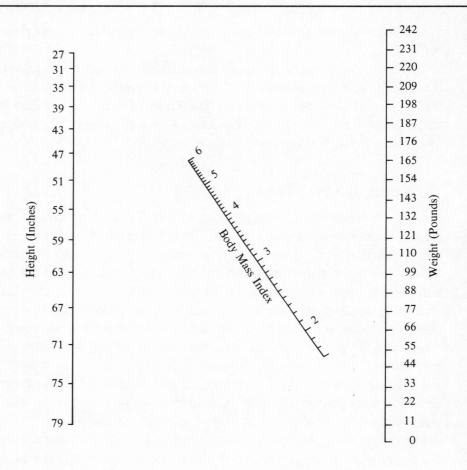

Source: A. E. Roche and P. Webb, "Grading Body Fatness from Antropometric Data," *American Journal of Clinical Nutrition, 34,* 2831(1981).

Keeping the Weight Off

If you are overweight and have determined the amount of weight as fat you are worried about, how can you lose it safely and effectively? First, we should recognize that the majority of the weight programs available have very poor short-term success and even more discouraging long-term success. Of one hundred people who go on the average weight loss programs, only eight of them achieve short-term success in meeting their ideal weight, and less than one out of the hundred has long-term success, meaning that for a year after they have been on the diet they have maintained optimal body weight.[15] Given these statistics, it's obvious that an alternative is needed to the standard weight management approaches, an alternative developed around improving metabolic efficiency, controlling appetite naturally, and improving lifestyle according to biochemical individuality.

We know that individuals can vary significantly in their metabolic energy expenditure, even among those with the same body size, shape, sex, age, and work energy expenditure.[16] Recent evidence indicates that our weight may be controlled by a set-point mechanism—a "thermostat" in the brain dictates what weight we're supposed to be and controls our food intake and hunger appropriately to maintain that weight. The unfortunate thing is that as we grow older, our set-point seems to get higher, so that what we weighed at age 17 may become 20 pounds heavier at age 37 and 10 or 15 pounds heavier yet at age 50. We know how that the set-point is controlled in part by the activity of a very interesting kind of fat, which most people are not too familiar with, called brown fat.

Brown Fat

Brown fat is metabolically very active and is quite different from yellow fat, the majority of the fat in your body and the kind you can see deposited in cosmetically obvious areas. Brown fat is bound to the skeleton, is concentrated in the neck and back, and is responsible for producing body heat. It is brown because it is filled with tiny chemical powerhouses called mitochondria and cytochromes, which are what the biochemist knows as the energy-producing portions of your cells. These tissues act as minifurnaces to generate heat and burn away unneeded calories.[17]

Brown fat is thermogenically responsive ("thermo," heat; "genesis," producing) meaning that when you take in an excessive number of calories, your body compensates in part for the extra calories by producing more body heat and burning them off. If you've had the experience of going to bed right after eating a meal and you've found you were hot all night long, this is a result of your body trying to compensate for the extra calories you've consumed by burning them off as heat rather than storing them as fat. Your body is attempting to normalize weight by means of this brown fat tissue.

Unfortunately, in many individuals as they grow older, the brown fat seems to become less active and less thermogenically responsive, meaning that extra calories, rather than being lost as heat, are stored now as extra fat.[18] The concept of brown fat activity may explain why some people can overeat and remain slim, while other people just think about eating and they tend to gain weight. This concept may also explain the subtle onset of weight gain as individuals grow older, suggesting that thermogenesis in brown fat becomes less functional as we age.

It is clear, then, that to turn down the set-point so that weight is maintained at a lower level, brown fat should be activated. A number of factors are known to contribute to the activation of brown fat, all of which are important in designing the Nutraerobics Program toward weight management. But remember, what may be important for another, may not be for you, so you should tailor your program to your needs as indicated by your biotype.

If you have been truly trying to control your food intake and sticking to a low-calorie diet, but you still maintain extra body weight, you may be one of the candidates for increased brown fat activation. It was recently shown that in a study of women aged 26 to 67 years

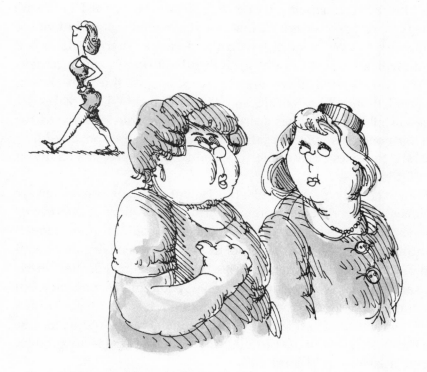

SO SHE'S THIN, BIG DEAL.
WHAT'S SO GREAT ABOUT HOT BROWN FAT?

who could either not lose weight on most diets or keep the weight off, there was considerable evidence to support the fact that their brown fat was not responding thermogenically and that it was in part related to underactive parts of their endocrine system, particularly the thyroid and adrenal hormones.[19]

Thyroid and Weight Gain

The thyroid gland, at the base of the neck, is the master gland that controls your metabolic rate; it gets its signals from the pituitary and hypothalamus glands, deep in the brain. The thyroid secretes hormones that activate specific tissues like brown fat toward increased thermogenic responsiveness. At first it was assumed that an individual with inactive brown fat must have an underactive thyroid gland and thyroid medication was prescribed. Recently, however, evidence indicates that the thyroid gland may be working just fine, but that in nonthyroid tissues like muscle and liver there is a lack of proper conversion of the hormones secreted by the thyroid gland into the active hormones that affect basal metabolic rate. These converted hormones are the ones responsible for producing the proper activity of brown fat.[20]

Now metabolic problems like this lack of adequate conversion are not managed properly by just administering one or more of the thyroid hormones; it is far better to stabilize proper thyroid hormone conversion through nutritional support and exercise. This conversion or activation of the thyroid hormones is controlled in part by adequate levels of zinc and copper. Once again, individual requirements may vary, but in general levels of zinc from 15 to 30 milligrams and copper from 3 to 10 milligrams are considered in the acceptable range. Iodine may be needed also at levels of 100 to 300 micrograms per day to produce adequate active thyroid hormones.

Diet, Exercise, and Brown Fat

Another factor that seems to increase brown fat activity is higher complex carbohydrate, moderate protein, low fat meals.[21] Foods that are too high in fat or protein, both of which figure predominantly in the average American diet, may tend to "poison" the brown fat and prevent it from being as thermogenically responsive as it might be to a higher-carbohydrate diet. This may account for the success of some of the recently popularized high-carbohydrate diets such as the Pritikin diet in improving proper weight-to-height balance in obese individuals.[22] Diets higher in complex starches from whole grains, beans, and legumes and lower in highly processed, sugar- and fat-rich foods encourage better thermogenic responsiveness.

Certain amino acids may also be responsible for increasing activity of the brown fat, one of which is tyrosine. Tyrosine has been shown to increase certain activity of the endocrine, or hormone-producing, system and might prove useful in activating under responsive brown fat in some individuals at doses of 1 to 3 grams per day.[23]

As far as dietary fats are concerned, light vegetable oils are far preferable for activating brown fat than animal fats or partially hydrogenated vegetable oils.[24] Corn, peanut, sunflower seed, soy, sesame, or safflower oil should be used in the diet in preference to animal or other vegetable fats. Again, fat in the diet should account for no more than 20 to 25 percent of the daily calories while a person is on a program to activate brown fat.

Natural sugars, such as the fruit sugar fructose, appear to be better than refined sugars in activating brown fat.[25] Natural sugars should be gotten in whole food that is not highly processed, food rich in unrefined starches, moderate in protein, and low in fat.

One interesting ingredient that seems to activate brown fat and improve the thermogenic or heat-producing effect is caffeine.[26] The amount of caffeine required to promote this effect, however, is only equivalent to approximately two cups of mildly brewed coffee per day and levels of caffeine beyond that have no additional therapeutic benefit on improving brown fat metabolism. Caffeine is not necessarily prescribed as an aid to brown fat activity, but it can be employed at an intake of no more than 100 to 200 milligrams per day in whatever form it is consumed.

A more important therapeutic means of activating brown fat is appropriate aerobic exercise. Not only does aerobic exercise help promote proper brown fat activity but it also encourages appetite regulation. Considerable progress has been made in understanding why certain people have voracious appetites and how these appetites may be decreased by variations of diet and exercise.

Appetite and Appetite Problems

Recently, pharmacologists have found receptors in the brain that appear to control appetite.[27] Appetite here means hunger rather than taste. We have four basic taste perceptions: bitter, salty, sweet, and sour; these along with our senses of smell and texture give rise to the palatability of various foods. Foods taste good to us because of biochemical and learned responses to them; hunger, however, is a biochemical manifestation in response to a control mechanism within the brain called the **appestat,** or the "thermostat," that controls the amount of calories our body requests that we eat each day.

The appestat or appetite control area is located in that portion of the brain called the hypothalamus, which is in part regulated by the neurotransmitters adrenaline, serotonin, and dopamine, all of which have been previously discussed as mood, mind, and memory regulators. It is known that drugs that alter these neurotransmitters may also alter appetite: some medications used to treat depression produce hunger and cause patients to gain weight due to the increased amount of noradrenaline in their brains; L-dopa, used in the treatment of Parkinson's disease, turns off the appetite control mechanism and causes individuals to eat less.

Investigators have also found that anxiety, stress, and psychological disturbances can cause the release of appetite-stimulating substances and cause people to eat compulsively and, therefore, gain weight. And it has been found that certain hormones secreted by the stomach travel in the blood to the brain and cause a feedback inhibition of appetite. So diet can affect some of the substances produced within the brain that regulate appetite; that's why an empty-calorie diet deficient in protein may cause significant increases in appetite.

Foods high in sugar and fats and low in quality protein can encourage overeating. Recent experiments have found that when sugar is increased in the diets of animals, it stimulates hunger.[28] The average American eats, per year, more than 100 pounds of refined sugar, 55 pounds of fats and oils, 300 cans of soda pop, 200 sticks of gums, 18

pounds of candy, 5 pounds of potato chips, 7 pounds of corn chips, 63
dozen doughnuts, 50 pounds of cakes and cookie, and 20 gallons of ice
cream. This may indicate why we have such weight and appetite regulation problems in our society.[29]

Food manufacturers spend $3.8 billion per year advertising these
high-calorie, low-nutrition foods, and studies indicate that 50 percent
of our food purchases are done on impulse rather than for quality
nutrition. When the majority of the calories that a person takes in are
from these empty-calorie foods, the body is unable to properly metabolize those calories to energy, due to its chronic deficiency of vitamins
and minerals; it therefore stores these calories for a rainy day that never
comes—as fat.

The Use of Fiber to Control Appetite

Another part of the problem is that most of the foods we consume
so routinely are calorie-rich foods due to their high degree of processing and a few mouthfuls can provide an excessive number of calories.
Less processed foods, which are high in natural dietary fiber, dilute the
calories and give the individual the opportunity to eat more mouthfuls
for fewer calories. Most of us don't want to give up taking mouthfuls
because eating is enjoyable and part of our cultural heritage; what we
really want to do is reduce the number of calories per mouthful so we
can enjoy eating without gaining weight. So eating more unrefined
foods with more dietary fiber means we can eat virtually twice as many
mouthfuls for the same number of calories. In this case, the jaw gets
tired chewing before the body deposits fat.

Nutrients and Appetite

When foods are very low in vitamins and minerals, the liver
becomes depleted of these nutrients and signals to the brain that it is
hungry for more nutrition. Therefore, lack of adequate vitamins and
minerals can turn on the appetite mechanism.[30]

Recently, another group of dietary substances has been implicated in the regulation of appetite, the nucleic acids such as adenosine, inosine, and guanosine found in foods such as yeast, liver, and sardines.[31] These substances, called purines, when taken in adequate quantities in the diet, turn off the appetite center in the hypothalamus of the brain and seem to play a regulatory role in reducing fat tissue accumulation. They have been proven in animal studies to markedly suppress spontaneous food intake. There is the suggestion that these are the substances actually secreted within the body that help turn off the appetite control center in the brain.[32]

Other substances that suppress appetite are neurotransmitters secreted by the brain called endorphins. These substances are also important for reducing pain.[33] It is interesting that these substances are secreted after exercise, which may explain the appetite suppression characteristics of an appropriate exercise program. I am sure you've had an occasion when you've been famished and felt that you just had to eat, and then you got up to do something you found that your hunger seemed to have gone away. Conversely, sometimes when we are the most sedentary and would seem to need to eat the least, we are the most hungry. The control of appetite by the secretion of appetite-suppressive substances may be stimulated by proper exercise; a sedentary lifestyle will decrease their secretion and increase appetite. As will be pointed out later in this chapter, proper aerobic exercise is a mandatory part of a good weight management program, both for the increase in metabolic energy expenditure and for the appetite-suppression characteristics of the exercise.

So, in conclusion, appetite suppression may be accomplished through the use of a diet moderately rich in protein, high in fiber, complex carbohydrates, vitamins, and minerals, and low in empty-calorie convenience foods, a diet properly balanced with the substances that stimulate the appetite-suppression neurotransmitters (such as dietary tyrosine and tryptophan) and the purines (inosine, guanosine, and adenosine), and adequate aerobic exercise.

The "Diet"

What type of therapeutic diet should you consider if you want to lose weight quickly and safely so that you can then go on a dietary maintenance program to preserve your proper weight-to-height ratio? Should you fast, or take starch blockers, or drink liquid proteins, or eat a lot of fat and protein, or take meal replacement protein powders, or go on a mixed-food, lower-calorie diet? The way you answer this question may, to a great degree, dictate how good you feel on the diet, how effective it is in selectively losing fat while maintaining muscle, and set the stage for how effective your long-term weight management will be.

What about fasting as a way of losing weight? Recently, the effects of fasting on eighteen healthy but obese patients who fasted for twenty-one days were investigated. It was found that in these patients a protein called fibronectin, which is associated with the proper function of the liver and immune system, was decreased throughout the fasting period. The authors of the study conclude "the starvation-induced decrease in fibronectin may suggest a serious mechanism associated with physio-logical insults of fasting."[34] This, of course, is long-term fasting for weight loss purposes, not short-term fasting, which may be done for other therapeutic reasons and which may be much safer under con-trolled conditions.

Fasting has been found to produce a significant lowering of blood pressure and reduced heart activity, as well as suppression of the mood-elevating hormone endorphin release.[35] Fasting has also been found to produce hypothyroidism (low thyroid activity), which can actually encourage slower weight loss than consuming a few hundred calories a day.[36] Fasting can also lower blood sugar levels, thereby increasing the appetite and resulting in excessive hunger after the fast is concluded.

A modification of the total fast is the Beverly Hills Diet, which was very popular a couple of years ago. Individuals on this diet were to depend upon certain fruits for their dietary calorie intake, which supplied no more than about 300 calories a day. Its low-protein, low-calorie content did encourage weight loss, but its high-acid and high–fruit sugar content led to serious adverse side effects including diarrhea, muscle weakness, or dizziness after the first week. Prolongation of the diet led to protein deficiency states associated with hair loss and even a small degree of muscle loss.[37]

It is probably true that any strange, extremely limited diet will lead to weight loss, because you can only eat so much of any one thing alone before you lose your appetite and the thought of eating becomes repulsive. This doesn't mean, however, that such a diet properly controls the way you lose weight so that it comes preferentially from fat and not from muscle and so that it does not produce imbalances of specific nutrients.

Another recent diet claim is that people can eat all the carbohydrates they want and still lose weight as long as they take starch blockers. Starch blockers are derived from beans; their active ingredient is an enzyme called amylase inhibitor. This substance prevents the breakdown of starches in the intestine and keeps them from being absorbed into the body.

Starch blockers have been purified and utilized in England under the prescription name Acarbose in the management of blood sugar problems in diabetics, where some side effects have been associated with them. The side effects include intestinal gas, digestive disorders due to the fermentation by bacteria of the undigested starch in the lower intestine, and pancreas problems where the pancreas tries to compensate for the undigested material by secreting more digestive enzymes.

The position of the Food and Drug Administration (FDA) on starch blockers is summarized by one official when he states, "One does not go around interfering with digestion unless you know what you're doing. These potential problems with starch blockers are not trivial issues." The conclusion, once again, is that weight management is not just a matter of taking a pill and having complete control and safety result. Substances that prevent the absorption of calories can lead to a whole host of nutritionally related problems and other side effects, many of which may be very serious.[38]

Next we come to the highly popularized liquid protein diets or protein powder replacement diets, whose link with heart problems and even death has recently been explored.[39] A while ago the FDA received reports of sudden and unexpected deaths in relatively young, apparently healthy individuals in the United States and Canada during or shortly after rapid weight reduction using very low-calorie, liquid protein diets. The deaths followed a pattern: nearly all occurred in females age 25 to 44 years of age; all had died after adhering strictly to a liquid protein diet for an average of five months and had lost extensive amounts of weight, averaging over 80 pounds; and all had been under the regular care of a physician and felt generally well. Lightheadedness and/or fainting had prompted hospitalization in some individuals. The immediate cause of death seemed to be heart problems due to what is called ventricular arrhythmia, or heartbeat changes.

The protein products used were mostly liquid-based substances made of collagen derived from predigested animal hides; over fifty name brands were then commercially available. These products are a very poor mixture of protein substances and have been proven unable to sustain human function for an extended period of time. Individuals on these diets were suffering from protein starvation throughout the whole course of the diet and may have been actually slowly losing protein from the heart muscle.[40]

Many doctors who are doing research on weight loss diets, however, urge us not to completely dismiss protein-based diets because individuals on some of them that were poorly designed have had medical problems; not all protein-based diets are hazardous. The protein-sparing modified fast, or PSMF, has been used under appropriate control very successfully in the management of mild obesity (twenty to eighty pounds overweight).

The Protein-Sparing Modified Fast

On a **protein-sparing modified fast** people are taking in enough calories as protein each day to replace the amount of protein that is being broken down in their muscles but not enough to contribute excessive calories to their dietary intake and lead to fat accumulation. This diet is reasonably low in total fat, moderate in carbohydrate, and high in protein. This protein must be of high quality (meaning it has the proper balance of the essential amino acids) to stimulate the body's remanufacture of any muscle that is broken down in the body.

In theory, the PSMF is extremely attractive because it leads to the beneficial effects of a low-calorie diet without the hazards of causing muscle loss. It selectively encourages fat loss while maintaining blood sugar levels and energy. A number of questions need to be asked about the safety of these protein diets, however.[41]

How does the PSMF or low-calorie protein diet differ from other diets? The basic premise is that by eliminating dietary fat and most of the carbohydrate, hunger will be reduced and body protein (muscle stores) will be maintained.

What is the evidence of greater success for the PSMF versus other low-calorie diets? In a number of controlled studies, it has been found that the protein-sparing modified fast leads to safe and effective three to six pounds of primarily fat loss per week when properly designed. Other diets may result in more weight loss, but most of this weight loss may actually be a result of muscle wasting and water loss.

What caused the deaths reported for patients on the liquid protein diets? The evidence suggests that three factors contributed to the deaths: first, the protein products used were of low quality and contributed to actual loss of protein from organs such as the heart muscle; second, the protein products were low in specific trace elements, notably copper and magnesium, which may have contributed to heart irregularities; third, there may have been deficiencies of the essential amino acid methionine which enables the heart to properly hold on to potassium and so maintain proper heart rhythm.

How should the PSMF be used in the management of obesity?
The recommended number of calories per day is 600 to 800. A high-quality protein product, balanced in vitamins and minerals, replaces two meals; the third is a mixed high-protein, low-fat, moderate-carbohydrate meal. Dilute fruit juice and vegetable juices should be consumed during the diet and exercise should be a regular accompaniment.

How do you evaluate the safety of a protein product? First of all, the label should read that the majority of the protein comes from the animal materials lactalbumin and/or casein, not from soy or collagen, which are incomplete proteins. Even supplementation of soy protein formulas with selective amino acids still leaves them of less quality than complete proteins like casein and lactalbumin.[42] The amino acids methionine and cystine should represent 3 percent, and tryptophan should be at least 1 percent of the protein. The protein efficiency ratio, or PER, of the product, shown on the label, should be at least 2.6 to sustain human nutrition adequately, and trace minerals should be included.

The amino acid methionine is necessary in the product in adequate balance to stimulate the manufacture in your heart of a substance called taurine. Taurine is responsible for holding on to potassium in the heart for proper heart rhythm.[43] There has been some suggestion that individuals who died on the protein diets did so because they were on low-methionine protein products which led to taurine depletion and potassium wasting even though they were supplementing with potassium. The heart was unable to hold on to this potassium adequately, which contributed to the observed heart irregularities.[44]

It is extremely important that the trace element copper be included in adequate quantities in a protein-sparing modified fast to prevent heart irregularities. It was found upon examination of commercially available protein powders used for weight loss that not a single product tested was adequate with regard to any of the trace elements, including copper. The product should contain at least 3 milligrams of copper per day to maintain adequacy.[45]

The Safe Approach to Dieting

What, then, is a safe therapeutic weight loss program? Use of the low-calorie protein based diet has been proven safe when administered correctly. In one study, patients who had been on a 600–800-calorie-per-day protein-sparing modified fast for a prolonged period of time were monitored twenty-four hours a day; no evidence of any clinically important heart problems were found.[46] These results have been confirmed by other studies in which additional benefits of PSMF were found: lower blood cholesterol, lower blood sugar levels in diabetics, and lower blood pressure in hypertensive patients.[47]

Adequacy in this diet seems to be achieved with 60 to 70 grams of high-quality protein and about 60 to 70 grams of carbohydrate a day; the carbohydrate should be balanced between whole-grain starch and unrefined sugars such as fructose from fruit and vegetable juices. The protein can come either from lean meats, cheese, fish, or—possibly more ideally—from a well-balanced protein powder. Minerals should be at the level of 800 milligrams of calcium, 2000 milligrams of potassium (mostly from fruits and vegetables), 400 milligrams of magnesium, and 1400 milligrams of phosphorus per day. If an individual is not taking the protein powder in skim milk, the need for calcium supplementation may be present because it is difficult to get 800 milligrams of calcium from nondairy products on this diet unless the protein powder is already calcium fortified.

There should be enough bulk in the diet to promote proper intestinal regularity so that constipation does not occur. If constipation does result, it indicates that there is not enough fiber or bulk like the vegetable gums in the diet.

Exercise and Dieting

Exercise is a mandatory component of the dietary program. It was recently found that obese women put on a weight management program had much better compliance and lower appetite when they exercised than when they did not. If the diet does not allow you enough energy to exercise, then it is inappropriately designed to meet your metabolic needs. The study actually indicated that women who participated in a long-term, moderate exercise program while losing weight did not compensate for their exercise by increased calorie intake; it actually contributed to appetite suppression, presumably through the endorphin-release mechanism.[48]

The exercise should be aerobic, that is, one in which you work to move oxygen through your cardiovascular system. To make sure that you are exercising aerobically, monitor your heart rate during your exercise and hold it at approximately 180 beats per minute minus your age in years (this is your training level). Whatever exercise can get your pulse rate into that range and keep it there for fifteen minutes is a suitable exercise. Not everyone needs to or should be a jogger. People who have very significant body mass above ideal may actually do their joints harm by trying to jog. Remember, each time your heel comes down when you're running, you can put several tons of force onto your joints, depending on how heavy you are.

For individuals not suited to jogging, some alternatives are dancercise, aerobic exercises, trampolining, or stationary bicycling, all at a rate vigorous enough to get your heartbeat up into your training zone. Swimming is another excellent way to increase your aerobic fitness; its advantage is that it works almost all muscles of the body in a reasonably trauma-free environment (the water supports your body so that, for example, joints don't get the concentrated force they do in jogging.

Raising your pulse rate into your training level each day for fifteen minutes is mandatory, not optional, on the appropriate fitness and weight management program. Remember, by aerobically tuning yourself up, you are activating your brown fat to work for you twenty-four hours a day; you are also increasing the number of mitochondria, those little powerhouses in each cell, two- or threefold. This is like increasing the number of furnaces that can burn fat for you and do the work for the rest of your life in maintaining proper body weight.

The Plateau

It is not uncommon for individuals to achieve plateaus—stretches of time during which no weight is lost—while on weight management programs. These plateaus are generally a result of the body restoring differing levels of water balance as you lose fat. It is important to recall that water is actually heavier than fat per unit volume and, therefore, you may lose fat but actually hold weight until your body reestablishes a new water balance. Don't weigh yourself too frequently while on the program or you may be discouraged by the small subtle plateaus occurring as your body reestablishes a new water and muscle balance each time. The ultimate aim of the program is to decrease fat while maintaining muscle and, therefore, the real test of the program is not necessarily the number of pounds lost, but your increased level of fitness.

Vitamins and Minerals

Remember also that your dietary program should be adequate in vitamins and minerals as well. One vitamin is extremely important in normalizing the metabolism of fat in a weight loss program is biotin, which is not found in adequate quantities in many products. Biotin should be consumed at the level of at least 100 to 400 micrograms a day while on a weight management program, along with the other B-complex vitamins, and 1000 milligrams of vitamin C.

When you are on a weight loss program and taking in a low number of calories, all your vitamins and minerals must be derived from the small amount of food you are eating. The intake of these nutrients, however, should still be at the level comparable to what you would be taking in if you were eating a normal diet. The reason many people on weight loss diets develop vitamin or mineral deficiency symptoms is that they are not accommodating the lower-calorie intake by increasing the levels of vitamins and minerals in the remaining portions of their diets, or by supplementing. This is one of the advantages of using a properly designed protein powder; it contains adequate levels of vitamins and minerals to prevent deficiency problems.

Underweight Problems

As with overweight, underweight is a general symptom of metabolic problems in need of balancing. A number of factors can contribute to an underweight condition, including a maldigestion-malabsorption syndrome where dietary calories are not being properly assimilated, an overly active thyroid hormone output, the consumption of low-nutrient foods, energy expenditure through exercise and activity that is not met by adequate food intake, and reduced appetite due to a zinc deficiency which may actually be associated with eating disorders like anorexia nervosa or bulimia. Psychological anxieties can also play an important role in anorexia nervosa. Compulsive running in young males seems to be associated with the same psychological profile of hard-driving, high achievement as anorexia nervosa in young women.[49]

Underconsumptive eating disorders may actually be manifestations of the same problem as overconsumptive ones—metabolic switching. Consumption of higher-nutrient unrefined foods with adequate vitamin and mineral content, proper exercise, and the elimination of excessive alcohol intake and cigarette smoking can all contribute to improved weight management for the underweight individual.

Excessively high protein diets (where dietary protein exceeds 150 to 200 grams a day) may be considered hazardous to individuals who are not exercising very vigorously or who do not have large body sizes. It is suggested that underweight individuals increase weight by consuming more of the foods discussed to manage overweight problems. This diet, which leads to optimization of quality weight gain, contains 70 to 100 grams of dietary protein, 350 grams of carbohydrate of which 90 percent is unrefined starches and whole grains and 10 percent natural sugars, and about 50 to 60 grams of dietary fat predominantly from unsaturated vegetable oils with a smaller percentage from saturated animal fats.

This dietary breakdown, in conjunction with the minerals and vitamins suggested for your biotype, will help normalize your biochemistry and improve quality weight gain. Exercise is mandatory and the use of digestive enzymes may be required as an oral supplement if there is a maldigestion syndrome.

Individuals who have appetite disorders and are not hungry are not eating enough calories to keep their body weight at ideal levels. They should consider the consumption of several smaller meals throughout the day.[49] These foods should be rich in zinc (30 mg), vitamin B-1 (10 mg), and B-2 (10 mg). The practical application of these concepts in their administration to your own unique biotype should allow for normalization of body weight-to-height ratio through improved muscle mass and decreased fat stores while contributing to improved aerobic competency and reduced risk to many of the major killer diseases.

Health problems closely associated with excess weight are increased risk to heart disease, high blood pressure, and stroke. The early warning signs of heart disease, which the Nutraerobics Program is able to positively influence, include high blood cholesterol and blood pressure, shortness of breath, leg pain after walking, and rapid heartbeat. A heart attack may come after years of increasing debilitation due to vertical disease, and the next chapter will show you how to recognize these early warning signs and help you design your program of management.

Notes

1. G. B. Forbes, "Is Obesity a Genetic Disease?" *Contemporary Nutrition 6,* No. 8, (1981).

2. M. A. Mir and P. J. Evans, "Erythrocyte Sodium-Potassium ATPase and Sodium Transport in Obesity," *New England Journal of Medicine, 305,* 1264(1981).

3. D. M. Harlan and G. J. Mann, "A Factor in Food Which Impairs Na-K-ATPase *in vitro,"* *Amer. J. Clinical Nutr., 35,* 250(1982).

4. T. B. Van Itallie and J. G. Kral, "The Dilemma of Morbid Obesity," *J. Amer. Medical Assoc., 246,* 999(1981).

5. J. Hirsch and B. Batchelor, "Adipose Tissue Cellularity in Human Obesity," *Clinics in Endocrinology and Metabolism, 5,* 299(1976).

6. E. H. Sims and P. Berchtold, "Obesity and Hypertension," *J. Amer. Medical Assoc., 247,* 49(1982).

7. F. H. Musserili, "Cardiovascular Effects of Obesity and Hypertension," *Lancet* (27 May 1982):1165.

8. A. Tannenbaum, "The Dependence of Tumour Formation on the Composition of the Calorie-Restricted Diet," *Cancer Research, 5,* 616(1945).

9. T. H. Maugh, "A New Marker for Diabetes," *Science, 215,* 651(1982).

10. R. W. A. Check, "Bad and Good News on Gastroplasty," *J. Amer. Medical Assoc., 248,* 277(1982).

11. P. G. Lindner, "Future of Obesity," *Obesity and Bariatric Medicine, 11,* 110(1982).

12. W. M. Bennett, "Hazards of the Appetite Suppressant Phenylpropanolamine," *Lancet* (7 July 1979):42.

13. W. P. T. James and R. T. Jung, "Is Obesity Metabolic?" *British Journal of Hospital Medicine* (December 1980):1140–1145.

14. A. E. Roche and P. Webb, "Grading Body Fatness from Limited Anthropometric Data," *Amer. J. Clinical Nutr., 34,* 2831(1981).

15. W. Bennett and J. Gurin, "Do Diets Really Work?" *Science 82* (March 1982):43.

16. P. V. Sukhatme and S. Margen, "Autoregulatory Homeostatic Nature of Energy Balance," *Amer. J. Clinical Nutr., 35,* 355(1982).

17. R. Rawls, "Obesity Linked to Metabolism in Brown Fat," *Chemical and Engineering News* (16 February 1981):25.

18. J. Elliott, "Blame It All on Brown Fat Now," *J. Amer. Medical Assoc., 243,* 1983(1980).

19. P. S. Shelly, R. T. Jung, and B. A. Callingham, "Post Prandial Thermogenesis in Obesity," *Clinical Science, 60,* 519(1981).

20. A. R. Glass, K. D. Burman, and T. M. Boehm, "Endocrine Function in Obesity," *Metabolism, 30,* 89(1981).

21. Z. Glick and G. Brag, "Brown Adipose Tissue: Thermic Response Increased by a Single Low Protein, High Carbohydrate Meal," *Science, 213,* 1125(1982); S. D. Moulopoulos, "Metabolic Insufficiency as a Limiting Factor in Obesity," *Hormones and Metabolic Research, 13,* 477(1982).

22. L. Landsberg and J. B. Young, "Diet-Induced Changes in Sympathoadrenal Activity: Implications for Thermogenesis and Obesity," *Obesity and Metabolism, 1,* 5(1981).

23. Ibid.

24. N. Baba and S. A. Hashim, "Enhanced Thermogenesis and Diminished Deposition of Fat in Response to a Diet Containing Medium Chain Triglyceride," *Amer. J. Clinical Nutr., 35,* 678(1982).

25. N. Sharif and I. MacDonald, "Differences in Dietary-Induced Thermogenesis with Various Carbohydrates in Overweight Men," *Amer. J. Clin. Nutr., 35,* 267(1982).

26. M. A. Hollands and M. A. Cawthorne, "A Simple Test for Energy Expenditure in Humans: The Thermic Effect of Caffeine," *Amer. J. Clinical Nutr., 34,* 2291(1981).

27. G. Kolata, "Brain Receptors for Appetite Discovered," *Science, 218,* 460(1982).

28. P. L. Geiselman and D. Novin, "Sugar Infusion Can Enhance Feeding," *Science, 218,* 490(1982).

29. M. S. Lasky, *The Complete Junk Food Book* (New York: McGraw-Hill, 1977).

30. P. E. Sawchenko and M. I. Friedman, "The Liver and Its Control of Energy Metabolism," *American Journal of Physiology, 236,* R5(1979).

31. M. C. Capogrossi and M. DiGirolamo, "Suppression of Food Intake by Adenosine and Inosine," *Amer. J. Clin. Nutr., 32,* 1762(1979).

32. A. S. Levine and J. E. Morley, "Purinergic Regulation of Food Intake," *Science, 217,* 77(1982).

33. J. E. Morley and A. S. Levine, "The Role of the Endogenous Opiates as Regulators of Appetite," *Amer. J. Clinical Nutr., 35,* 757(1982).

34. R. L. Scott and M. G. MacDonald, "The Effect of Starvation and Repletion on Plasma Fibronectin in Man," *J. Amer. Medical Assoc., 248,* 2025(1982).

35. D. Einhorn and L. Landsberg, "Hypotensive Effect of Fasting: Possible Involvement of Sympathetic Nervous System and Endogenous Opiates," *Science, 217,* 727(1982).

36. B. T. Walsh, "Hormonal Responses to Semi-starvation States," *Journal of Clinical Endocrinology and Metabolism, 53,* 203(1981).

37. W. B. Mirkin and R. N. Shore, "The Beverly Hills Diet," *J. Amer. Medical Assoc., 246,* 2235(1981).

38. D. Jenkins and H. Fielder, "Low Dose Acarbose Without Symptoms of Malabsorption in the Dumping Syndrome," *Lancet* (9 January 1982):109.

39. H. E. Sours, V. P. Frattali, and C. D. Brand, "Sudden Death Associated With Very Low Calorie Weight Reduction Regimens," *Amer. J. Clinical Nutr., 34,* 453(1981).

40. W. R. Ayers and A. M. Altschul, "Severe Calorie Restriction," *Amer.J. Clin. Nutrition, 34,* 2855(1981).

41. P. Felig, "Four Questions About Protein Diets," *New England Journal of Medicine, 298,* 1025(1978).

42. S. J. Fomon and B. B. Edwards, "Methionine Supplementation of a Soy Protein Formula Fed to Infants," *Amer. J. Clinical Nutr., 32,* 2460(1979).

43. J. H. Thurston and E. F. Naccarato, "Taurine: Possible Role in Osmotic

Regulation of Mammalian Heart," *Science,
214,* 1373(1981).

44. J. R. Darsee and S. B. Heymsfield,
"Decreased Myocardial Taurine Levels," *New
England Journal of Medicine, 304,* 129(1981).

45. A. O. Lee Jones and J. H. Gould,
"Elemental Content of Predigested Liquid
Protein Products," *Amer. J. Clinical Nutr.,
33,* 2545(1980).

46. D. L. Singer, "24 Hour Monitoring Fails
to Find Significant Cardiac Arrhythmias in
Patients on a PSMF," *Obesity and
Metabolism, 1,* 159(1981).

47. B. R. Bistrian and G. L. Blackburn,
"Metabolic Changes During a PSMF," *Amer.
J. Clinical Nutr., 36,* 833(1982).

48. R. Woo and F. X. Pi-Sunyer,
"Voluntary Food Intake During Prolonged
Exercise in Obese Women," *Amer. J. Clinical
Nutr., 36,* 478(1982).

49. J. J. Wurtman and S. H. Zeisel,
"Carbohydrate Craving in Obese People,"
International Journal Eating Disorders, 1,
4(1982).

Heart Disease and Nutraerobics

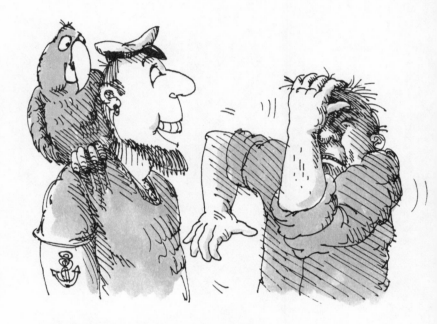

EVER SINCE I PUT MY PARROT ON HER LOW
CHOLESTEROL DIET, I CALL MY POLLY UNSATURATED.

1. Do you have elevated blood cholesterol?

1	2		4
No	Somewhat		Yes, it's too high

2. Do you have high or low blood pressure?

1	2		4
No	Somewhat		Yes, it is a problem

3. Do you have a sedentary lifestyle?

1	2		4
No	Somewhat		Yes, definitely

4. Do you like salty foods?

1	2		4
No	Somewhat		Yes, I salt foods frequently

5. Is your diet high in cheese, whole milk, meats, and eggs?

1	2	3	4
No,	Somewhat high	Reasonably high	Yes

6. Do you smoke?

1	2	3	4
No	Less than 1 pack per day	1–2 packs per day	More than 2 packs per day

7. Are you overweight?

1	2	3
No	Somewhat	Significantly

If your score exceeds 17, the information in this chapter may be very helpful in reducing your risk to the major killer disease—heart disease.

About heart disease there is both good news and bad news. Over the past thirty years, the United States has seen a reduction in heart disease death by over 30 percent, with over 60 percent of this decrease occurring between 1970 and 1980. This is certainly good news. The bad news is that heart disease still strikes 3,400 Americans each day as a heart attack and approximately 1,600 people each day as a stroke. The leading cause of death in the United States is still heart disease; it was responsible for 650,000 deaths in 1978, 150,000 of which were in people less than 65 years old. The total economic cost of heart disease is estimated to be in excess of $60 billion annually. This accounts for more than 20 percent of the total cost of illness in the United States. Heart disease robs many young people under 50 years of age of years of productive contributions.[1]

The attempt to understand how a 40-year-old, seemingly healthy individual can suddenly be struck down by a fatal heart attack is in the forefront of cardiovascular research. The evidence is beginning to show that the answer is related to the individual's lifestyle and genetic predisposition. Approximately one-third of all the deaths of people from the age of 35 to 64 are due to coronary heart disease. To reduce the incidence of this condition in younger individuals, the emphasis should be on the recognition of early warning signs and risks to heart disease, and then on modification of the lifestyle and nutrition through application of a personalized Nutraerobics Program.

Determining Heart Disease Risk Factors

On assessing risks to heart disease, it is interesting to note that certain portions of the United States have much higher incidence of heart disease than others. Figure 6 shows the incidence of heart disease on a state-by-state basis. In general, heart disease is highest in the South, moderate in the East and West, and low in the farm belt of the Midwest. This distribution suggests that there may be lifestyle and dietary relationships associated with the incidence of heart disease.

Figure 6

Incidence of Heart Disease by State, 1978

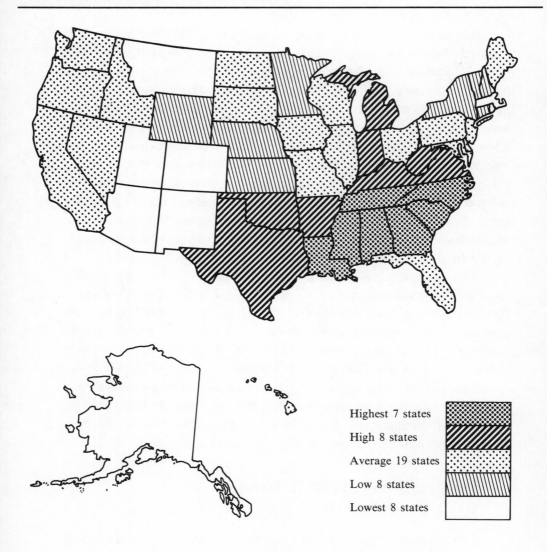

Highest 7 states
High 8 states
Average 19 states
Low 8 states
Lowest 8 states

To find out just which factors do correlate with heart disease, a study called the Framingham Study was done a number of years ago in which the health of individuals in Framingham, Massachusetts, was followed for some twenty-five years. The results of this study led to the development of the so-called cardiovascular risk factors, which related certain lifestyle and personality traits to increased risk to heart disease. Factors such as a sedentary lifestyle, a family history of heart disease, smoking, elevated blood cholesterol, elevated weight-to-height ratio, and high blood pressure were all associated with increases in the risk to heart disease.[2] For instance, if you are a man, age 40, with a sedentary lifestyle and a family history of heart disease, who smokes two packs a day and is 20 percent above his ideal body weight for height, you would have over a fivefold higher risk to heart disease than a nonsmoking, 40-year-old male with a vigorous lifestyle, no family history of heart disease, and an ideal body weight-to-height ratio.

Since then, the recognition that there are a number of dietary and lifestyle factors associated with increasing risk to heart disease led to a very impressive public information program to confront people with the fact that what they do in their lifestyles may have an impact upon their later developing heart disease. Dr. R. I. Levy, ex-director of the National Heart, Lung and Blood Institute, has suggested that the remarkable decline in heart disease death we have seen in the past two decades is primarily not a result of better medication, surgical intervention, coronary care units in hospitals, or training in resuscitation techniques, but rather of improved lifestyle on the part of the informed American public.[3]

Lifestyle Changes and Heart Disease

The American public is changing its view of health care. Ten years ago we did not see men and women in the morning out jogging up and down our city streets, or the frequency of seafood and vegetarian entrees served in the finest restaurants, or the popularity of yogurt as a light meal substitute, or natural food sections in the major food chain stores. These are all indications of a great wave of consumer interest in lifestyle modification and keeping healthy, which Dr. Levy feels is one of the major contributors to the decline in heart disease. The most exciting conclusion drawn from this recent information is that heart disease is not an inevitable consequence of aging or genetic makeup; it can be prevented.

The MRFIT Study

In one attempt to look at the causes of heart disease, especially their relationship to lifestyle, the National Heart, Lung and Blood Institute sponsored a large ten-year, $115-million study called the Multiple Risk Factor Intervention Trial (MRFIT). In this study certain individuals were asked to decrease their blood cholesterol by changes in their diets, to lower blood pressure, and to reduce cigarette smoking, three major factors associated with increasing risk to heart disease; they were then compared to a group of comparable age who were not asked to reduce these risk factors. The results were not what was expected—basically, they were inconclusive. The group of men in the study who were consulted to reduce their risk factors did **not** have a lower mortality rate than the control group, so on the surface it appeared that risk factor reduction was not beneficial. On further examining the results of the study, however, it was found that, due to the great consumer interest in health improvement and the general knowledge that certain lifestyle factors are related to the increasing risk of heart disease, **both** the treatment group and the control group in the MRFIT study reduced their risk factors, confusing the results of the study considerably. Those in charge of the study could not prevent the control group from changing their eating and exercise habits, even though they gave them no formal medical advice on doing so.

It was also found that the treatment group received medications to reduce their blood cholesterol that may have had adverse side effects and actually contributed to slightly increased mortality from heart disease in this group.[4] Because of the uncertainty in the interpretation of the data, one cannot utilize the information from the 12,866-person MRFIT to draw sweeping conclusions as to the benefit or lack of benefit that reduction of risk factors has upon heart disease.

One conclusion that can be drawn from this study, however, is the possibility that the use of drugs for the management of heart disease risk factors may not be the most beneficial way to handle the problem. It seems that natural lifestyle modification procedures through application of the Nutraerobics Program may prove much more successful without adverse side effects.

Can ordinary people, then, be persuaded to change their eating and living habits to meet their own biological sensitivities and reduce their risk to heart disease? The history of the past ten years tells us yes, they can and will if properly informed. A number of studies in various countries around the world have all come to the conclusion that once people have been educated and provided with alternatives that reduce their risk factors to heart disease, they are willing to modify their lifestyles as long as these particular changes do not constrain them to unusual or confusing habits or behaviors.

A study done in Oslo showed that advice to follow a diet lowering blood cholesterol and to stop smoking was well accepted and led to a large drop in heart disease in men 40 to 49 years old. Results from a collaborative World Health Organization–sponsored study demonstrated that in 49,781 men, aged 40 to 59, working in 88 factories in England, Belgium, Italy, and Poland, who were educated as to cardiovascular risk factors, there was an 11 percent reduction in heart disease risk compared to a control group that did not get the educational program.[5] The conclusion is obvious—people will change their lifestyles if there is a reason to do so.

Target of the Nutraerobics Program

Studies in twelve countries around the world all come to the same conclusion—elevated blood cholesterol is associated with an increased incidence of heart disease. Given this observation, a major target of a heart disease risk reduction program is to reduce blood cholesterol. This does not mean approaching the problem solely by cutting cholesterol-rich foods out of your diet. Dietary cholesterol accounts for only about 10 percent of your total blood cholesterol. The remaining 90 percent is manufactured in your body by your liver and intestines from fats, protein, and sugars in your diet.

The Nutraerobics Program seeks to reduce blood cholesterol by implementing ways of reducing your body's synthesis of cholesterol and improving your body's excretion (elimination) of excess blood cholesterol. In order to design a program for you that will lower blood cholesterol, we need to know what a "healthy" or optimal blood cholesterol level is. Recently, a number of investigators have found that individuals with low incidence of heart disease have blood cholesterol levels between 160 and 180 milligrams percent, which is far below the 225 milligrams percent for the average American.[6] Your doctor will generally tell you that if your blood cholesterol is between 150 and 300, you are "normal." Normal means that you have a blood cholesterol level within the range of 96 out of a 100 people tested. It is possible, however, to have a "normal" blood cholesterol level and actually have an increased risk to heart disease; that is, it is possible to be normal in a sick population. "Normal" does not necessarily mean "well"—it just means like most everyone else.

There is one confusing part of the blood cholesterol story. Some people who have high levels of one form of blood cholesterol called high-density lipoprotein cholesterol (HDL) actually have low risk to heart disease.[7] This HDL form of cholesterol serves as an arterial garbage collector, picking up cholesterol in places where it might be deposited and actually reducing the risk of atherosclerosis (hardening of the arteries). In general, most people who have elevated blood cholesterol do not have elevated HDL's and, therefore, are at increased risk to heart disease, but there are a few people who are lucky enough to have high HDL levels. Individuals who are born with a genetic tendency towards high levels of HDL have the lowest incidence of heart disease studied as a group. A number of factors are known to result in an increase in HDL, which will be discussed later in this chapter.

The most successful program for reducing risk to heart disease is one that reduces total blood cholesterol while increasing HDL so that the ratio of total cholesterol in the blood to HDL decreases. Studies have indicated that a person with a total cholesterol–to–HDL ratio of 5 to 1 (for example a total blood cholesterol of 250 and an HDL cholesterol of 50) have the average risk to heart disease; people who have a 3 to 1 ratio of total cholesterol to HDL (for example a total blood cholesterol of 180 and an HDL cholesterol of 60) have one-half the national average risk. As the blood cholesterol–to–HDL ratio increases above 8 to 1, your risk is more than double the national average. Ask your doctor for your cholesterol and HDL values to get some indication of your risk.

For those of you who have heard that alcohol increases the HDL level, it does seem that moderate alcohol consumption results in an increase in HDL. Alcohol intake above the equivalent of two mixed drinks per day, however, does not result in any additional benefit to HDL and is associated with increased risk to liver damage and certain cancers.

Diet and HDL Cholesterol

It is known that individuals who live in Japan and eat a traditional Japanese diet have a much lower death rate from heart disease than people living in the United States. It was found that Japanese men had HDL levels that were about 20 percent higher and total blood cholesterols that were 30 percent lower than levels in American males of the same age, indicating a greatly reduced risk to heart disease. When Japanese men consumed American diets, however, their HDL levels went down and their total cholesterol went up, indicating that the effects were not genetic, but were, to a great extent, related to lifestyle and diet.[8] The Japanese diets that promote HDL increases are lower in total fat, higher in fiber, and richer in vitamins and minerals.

A symptom associated with low HDL levels in males between 16 and 27 years of age appears to be severe cystic acne. Investigations show that severe and persistent cystic acne must, therefore, be considered one of the indications of low levels of HDL and increased risk to heart disease in later life.[9]

Other Risk Factors

Two additional factors known to significantly increase the risk to heart disease are cigarette smoking and elevated blood pressure. Cigarette smoking may contribute to increasing heart disease by delivering to the bloodstream substances that can initiate the atherosclerosis-producing process (hardening of the arteries) or it may cause a reduction in oxygen concentrations of the blood and an increase of carbon monoxide levels, which may also set the stage for heart disease. Individuals who are smokers have been found to have an elevated white blood cell count, an early warning marker to the potential of heart attack in smokers.[10]

Finally, elevated blood pressure has been known to be a major risk factor to heart disease. Individuals whose diastolic blood pressure (the second of the two numbers, for example, the 90 in 140/90) is greater than 90 are found to have a much greater risk to heart disease, stroke, and kidney damage. It was found that by reducing the blood pressure of the individuals in this group, there was a reduction of 17 percent in the death rate from heart disease as compared to an untreated group of individuals with elevated blood pressure.[11] And we have to remember that blood pressure values in the neighborhood of 140/90 are only borderline elevations in blood pressure; much higher values seriously compound the problem.

Based upon this information, the Nutraerobics Program focuses on five factors in attempting to decrease the risk to heart disease: reduction of the blood cholesterol–to–HDL ratio, reduction of blood pressure, reducing smoking, optimizing weight-to-height ratio, and improving exercise tolerance.

Treatment of Existing Heart Problems

Work by many surgeons indicates that it is the rule, not the exception, that people over 30 have some plaque (the material that collects in the arteries and shuts off proper blood flow) in the arteries feeding nourishment to their hearts. If this is so, what can Nutraerobics do to help "dissolve" existing plaque to improve blood flow to the heart in people who already have problems from the wear and tear of their lifestyles on their heart function? Will lifestyle modification help us restore normal blood flow?

Since the early 1970s, scientists have known that hardening of the arteries and heart disease can be reversed in monkeys, animals very similar to humans. Now more recent studies indicate that regression of existing plaque can occur in humans as well. Researchers at the University of Southern California Medical School studied twenty-five patients who had plaque in the arteries of their legs. After thirteen months on a diet modification program, nine of the twenty-five patients showed regression of the pre-existing blockage. Cardiologists at the University of Alabama Medical School reversed atherosclerosis in five of the twenty-five patients by having them modify their diets and quit smoking. Scientists at the University of Minnesota saw a regression of atherosclerosis in three out of twenty-two patients who underwent an operation that lowers blood cholesterol levels by removing part of the intestine.[12]

These case studies indicate one important fact. Mild dietary or lifestyle alteration is not enough if you have existing heart disease. An aggressive program is necessary to lead to the reversal of existing atherosclerotic plaque. The standard dietary approach used by many doctors to manage patients with heart problems is that proposed by the American Heart Association. This program as outlined in the Heart Association Guide is said to be "satisfactory in prevention, but not for reversing atherosclerosis in people who have advanced disease." In more aggressive dietary programs, such as the Nutraerobics Program, the approach is more comprehensive and requires a more detailed evaluation of your biotype. Diet, activity, and stress all need evaluation.

Exercise as Therapy

People who have more vigorous occupations and lifestyles have been shown to have a lower incidence of heart disease. Analysis of heart disease prevalence in Iowa farmers indicated that they had a much lower heart disease death rate than the population at large, and although they consumed more total calories and cholesterol, they drank less alcohol, got more exercise, used fewer tobacco products, and had higher HDL levels.[13]

Monkeys that were fed a high-fat diet and were properly conditioned by exercise were found to have significantly higher HDL levels, lower total blood cholesterol, and substantially reduced overall hardening of the arteries than nonexercised animals. This suggests that moderate exercise may prevent or retard coronary heart disease.[14] A similar study was recently reported on humans, again showing conclusively the importance of a vigorous exercise program in reducing the risk of coronary heart disease.[15]

It was found that men who engaged in vigorous sports to keep fit had an incidence of heart disease less than half that of their colleagues of the same age who reported no vigorous exercise. The investigators conclude from their study that exercise is a natural defense activator of the body, exerting a protective effect on the aging heart against heart attack.

Taking any preventive measure to the extreme, however, does not guarantee complete freedom from disease. At one time exercise was considered so successful, that if you could complete a 26-mile marathon race, you were thought to have "immunity" to heart disease. This has subsequently been proven incorrect in that heart disease has been found in marathon runners. Still, it is clear that improved exercise tolerance, which does not necessitate pushing yourself to extremes like a marathon, will greatly improve overall heart function and may even help in reducing existing atherosclerotic plaque by raising HDL levels.[16]

Diet as Therapy

Let's now look at the type of diet that would be helpful in leading to the regression of existing plaque. It has been suggested that the simplest dietary approach for improving heart function and minimizing the risk to heart disease is to reduce by half the intake of all foods high in saturated fats and vegetable oils from the levels now in the average diet. This could be achieved by implementing the following diet modifications:[17]

Food	Reduction (per day) from average
whole milk and cream	replace with low-fat milk
cheese	from ½ to ¼ ounces (replace with low-fat)
butter	from ⅔ to ¼ ounce
margarine	from ½ to ¼ ounce
cooking fats and oils	from ½ to ¼ ounce
meat and meat products (excluding poultry without skin, fish)	from 5 to 2 ounces
baked goods with shortening	from 10 to 5 ounces
salad dressings, condiments	reduce by 50 percent
deep-fried foods	reduce by 50 percent

These groups contribute 90 percent of the saturated fats in the average diet. Using low-fat cheeses, two-percent milk, cutting out butter and margarine and cooking in fats, reducing red meat consumption and replacing it with chicken (without the skin) and fish, and eliminating animal fats for cooking or baking should be easy to implement and will reduce total calories as fat from the present 43 percent to between 20 and 25 percent. Replacing many processed foods with whole-grain cereals and bread products is also an important part of the fat-reduction program.

There is a question about how vigorously sugars need to be controlled in the diet. It has been pointed out that sugar and fat work together to aggravate the risk to heart disease and elevated blood cholesterol. Cutting sugar consumption by 50 percent of the present average level seems desirable, so that total sugars do not exceed 10 to 15 percent of the calories. You can do this fairly easily by becoming a label reader. Avoid foods and beverages that begin their list of ingredients with sugar, corn sweeteners, fructose, sucrose, or glucose. Just implementing this part of the program has been found to produce a 20 to 30 percent reduction in blood cholesterol all by itself.[18]

The positive effects of this dietary plan are cumulative in reducing your risk to heart disease and can be summarized as follows:

1. Eat less fat

2. Eat less sugar

3. Eat more high-fiber foods

4. Stop eating deep-fried foods

5. Reduce cheese, ice cream, whole milk

Studies have found that this type of program is readily tolerated and leads to dramatic reductions in blood cholesterol, particularly when saturated animal fat is kept low in the diet.[19]

Eggs and Heart Disease

In spite of all the controversy, how does restricting eggs in the diet fit into our blood cholesterol–lowering program? One recent study concluded that "there was no relationship between egg intake and coronary heart disease incidence."[20] It is true that an egg yolk has about 300 milligrams of cholesterol, but this amount is quite small when compared to the 1000 to 2000 milligrams of cholesterol your body manufactures each day from other sources. It is true that if large numbers of egg yolks (more than two each day) are eaten, blood cholesterol will increase (when a half cup of whole eggs was added to the diet each day there was a 9 percent increase in blood cholesterol[21]), but for most people who have elevated blood cholesterol, the level of egg consumption is only to a small degree related to blood cholesterol.

It may not be the egg that is the hazard, but the way it is cooked. The cholesterol in the egg can be chemically converted by cooking at high temperature, such as frying, to a substance that may initiate the atherosclerotic process. Investigators have found that feeding animals pure cholesterol does not lead to increased heart disease, but feeding them heat-damaged cholesterol (oxidized forms of cholesterol) does. This would indicate that soft-boiling or poaching eggs is much more desirable than frying or high-temperature cooking of egg yolk products.

If you love eggs, eat them frequently, and do have a blood cholesterol problem, you might consider using only one yolk for every two or three eggs. This way you still get the nutritional benefit of the egg but only a half to a third of the cholesterol.

Scaring people away from egg consumption may in the long run be very detrimental to the overall nutritional status of the country. The egg is a complete protein and is high in vitamins and minerals. It is one of the least expensive proteins available, costing about 65 to 90 cents per pound of protein. It is soft and can be prepared and eaten many ways. In short, the egg may be the margin of nutritional difference for some people, particularly aged individuals, between protein adequacy and inadequacy. Many older people cannot afford, prepare, or chew meat protein, and the egg may for them be very important in establishing proper nutritional status. Let's not throw the baby out with the bathwater in condemnation of the egg.

Meat Consumption and Cholesterol

What about other foods of concern with regard to elevated blood cholesterol? Recently, excessive meat consumption has been found to be a contributor to increased blood cholesterol. Researchers found that when a half pound of beef was added to the diet of vegetarians, it resulted in a near 20-percent increase in their blood cholesterol levels.[22] Vegetable protein has been shown to reduce blood cholesterol significantly when taken in the diet in place of the same number of calories of meat protein.[23]

Balancing the essential amino acids in vegetable protein by using two parts grains to one part legumes will provide a quality protein comparable to that of meat at about one-third to one-half of the cost with a much lower cholesterol-stimulating effect.[24] Vegetable protein has two major beneficial roles in reducing blood cholesterol: first, vegetable protein contains substances called plant sterols that block the absorption of cholesterol from the intestines into the blood; and second, vegetable protein has a lower ratio of the amino acids lysine to arginine than does meat protein and this ratio appears to be very important in signaling to the liver how much cholesterol it should manufacture. When lysine is present in high levels compared to arginine, as it is in meat protein, the liver synthesizes more cholesterol than when lysine is in lower levels related to arginine, as in vegetable protein. Individuals who supplement their diets with lysine (1000 to 3000 miligrams daily) to treat herpes infections have slight increases in their blood cholesterol as a result of this therapy. Interestingly, it is also found that eating shellfish, which are known to be high in cholesterol, may actually lead to lower blood cholesterol levels. This is a result of the fact that shellfish also contain sterols that effectively reduce cholesterol absorption from the intestine.[25]

Summarizing these observations indicates that a dietary program to lower cholesterol should be low in animal fat and moderate in lean animal protein with restriction of eggs to no more than two per day; it should include more vegetable-based proteins, particularly wheat, corn, soybeans, brown rice, oats, or rye. Visible forms of oil and fat in the diet should be avoided and oil-rich condiments such as mayonnaise, spreads, salad dressings, and sauces should be restricted.

Fiber and Cholesterol

What about the impact of dietary fiber upon blood cholesterol? Dr. Denis Burkitt, who has been a public health service physician in South Africa for over thirty years, was one of the first individuals to recognize the important protective effect of increased dietary fiber for digestive disorders and elevated blood cholesterol.

Recently, a ten-year study was completed looking at dietary fiber and its relationship to coronary heart disease, cancer, and other degenerative diseases.[26] In this study, it was found that mortality for coronary heart disease was about four times higher for men who had the lowest intake of dietary fiber than for those who consumed large quantities of dietary fiber. Rates of death from cancer were also found to be three times higher for the low-fiber consumers than the higher-fiber consumers. The investigators conclude that a diet containing at least 37 grams of dietary fiber per day is a protective diet against heart disease, cancer, and other diseases of Western society.

Dietary fiber is the undigestible cellulose, hemicellulose, and lignins with associated nutrients found in unrefined plant materials. Increased dietary fiber is generally found in a diet higher in unrefined vegetable protein. By switching from predominately animal protein to more vegetable-based proteins, there will be greater intake of dietary fiber.

The best dietary fiber supplement available for both lowering blood cholesterol and improving the management of blood sugar (glucose) seems to be oat bran fiber.[27] Oat bran fiber is now available commercially and 3 to 4 tablespoons used as a supplement each day in the diet can provide 15 to 20 grams of nutritional dietary fiber. It can be stirred into juice, added to cereals, baked into baked goods, or put into other liquid beverages.

When 100 grams (7 tablespoons) of oat bran was included in the diet per day, blood cholesterol was shown to be reduced 13 percent. Oat bran is generally more palatable, better tolerated, and less gas-producing than wheat bran.

One thing that improved fiber content of the diet does is increase the rate at which food moves through the digestive tract so that it has less time to undergo putrefaction in the intestines. It has been known for some time that when constipation develops or when there is prolonged bowel transit time, the blood cholesterol becomes elevated.[28]

Vegetable gums also have a positive impact upon reducing blood cholesterol. A number of natural gums found in unprocessed fruits and vegetables such as guar gum have been shown to both help manage blood sugar levels in the diabetic and reduce blood cholesterol. Recently 9 grams a day of guar gum supplement given in capsule form, which is similar to a commercially available gum called glucomannan, was found to lower blood cholesterol by 17 percent after four weeks of daily supplementation.[29]

One other interesting dietary agent shown to reduce blood cholesterol and improve blood cell dynamics is oil of garlic. Deodorized oil of garlic has been found to contain an active agent that actually encourages the reduction of blood cholesterol and blood triglycerides.[30] Garlic oil was given to sixty-eight patients with coronary heart disease at the level of about 15 milligrams a day, which corresponds to about 3 raw garlic cloves daily, and blood cholesterol was seen to drop about 15 to 20 percent over ten months of supplementation.

Taken as a whole, these results indicate that increased fibers from unrefined fruits and vegetables and starchy grains and legumes all have a beneficial effect on lowering blood cholesterol and decreasing the risk to coronary heart disease. Some nutritionists maintain that almost all vegetable and cereal products have a beneficial effect on lowering blood cholesterol. This diet approach is called the Lente diet and uses more grains, beans, legumes, peas, and vegetables.[31]

What Type of Cooking Oil?

There is strong evidence indicating that the unsaturated vegetable oils (which are liquid at room temperature) are highly preferable to the saturated fats from animal products (which are solid at room temperature). The saturated fats seem to encourage higher blood cholesterol levels than do unsaturated oils.

In addition unsaturated liquid oils are more effective than lightly hydrogenated oils in lowering blood cholesterol.[32] This suggests that corn, safflower, sunflower seed, peanut, sesame seed, and olive oils would be preferable to highly processed, partially hydrogenated oils or spreads. Extensive hydrogenation of vegetable oils has been shown to leave in such products as margarine by-products of the hydrogenation process that may actually promote increased blood cholesterol levels, even though the margarines themselves have no cholesterol in them.[33] This suggests that a small amount of butter would be preferable to margarine if a solid spread must be used, but the use of all solid fats as such should be limited, certainly not frequently used in cooking, while on a blood cholesterol–lowering program.

Oils should not be exposed to high temperatures for long periods of time because they undergo a chemical modification that may encourage the rancidity process. The high-temperature conversion of fats, oils, and cholesterol to chemical by-products during the frying process can make them very much higher in their coronary heart disease–producing abilities.[34] The key message when using oils or oil-rich foods is cook them as short a period a time as possible at lower temperatures to prevent chemical conversion of these oil materials to substances that could initiate increased blood cholesterol levels or damage of the arteries leading to heart disease.[35]

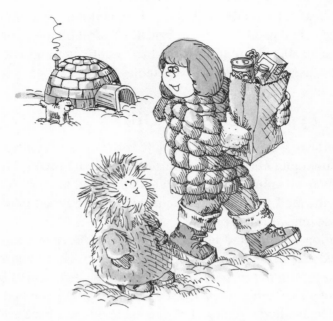

"HI MOM, WHAT'S FOR DINNER?"
"OMEGA-3-EICOSAPENTAENOIC ACID".
"OH BOY!"

Eskimos and Heart Disease

Does this necessarily mean that all oils in the diet are hazardous and should be avoided? Recently, it was found that Greenland Eskimos consume a very high fat diet yet are known to have a very low incidence of heart disease. You might think that this is because the Eskimo is protected against the ill effects of a high fat diet by genetic differences that have occurred over many thousands of years of eating that diet; however, when Greenland Eskimos move to eastern Canada, it is found that within just a few years they have the same high incidence of heart disease as their fellow Canadians.

It seems that in Greenland the Eskimos consumed in their diet oil derived from cold-water mammals and fish. Chemical analysis of this oil demonstrated that it is very high in a unique type of fatty substance called omega-3-eicosapentaenoic acid (EPA).[36] This fatty substance is used in our bodies to manufacture a hormone-like substance called prostacyclin, which prohibits blood cells called platelets from sticking together. This reduces the risk of coronary thrombosis (a blood clot in the heart), producing a heart attack or stroke.

Based upon this information, a study was done in which individuals with elevated blood cholesterol and increased risk to heart disease were placed on a fish-based diet containing 2 to 3 grams per day of the omega-3-EPA oil substance. After eleven weeks, blood cholesterol was found to be reduced and HDL cholesterol was increased, indicating a reduced risk to heart disease in the subjects.[37]

Recently, a commercial concentrate of this fish oil rich in omega-3-EPA has become available under the trade name MaxEPA. The effect on blood cholesterol of taking this oil concentrate was studied in thirteen patients who had heart disease. No other change in diet, medication, or smoking habit was permitted in these individuals. The level of MaxEPA used as a supplement provided 3.5 grams of omega-3-EPA each day, which is equivalent to about 10 grams of MaxEPA daily. After five weeks investigators found that the omega-3-EPA-supplemented diet reduced the risk of heart disease in all patients studied.[38]

It has also been reported that MaxEPA supplementation at the level of 10 grams per day leads to reduced blood pressure and reduced tendency toward sticky platelets which might initiate a blood clot and heart attack. This indicates that a MaxEPA-supplemented program may be extremely important in the therapeutic management of a patient who has elevated blood cholesterol and increased risk to coronary thrombosis.[39]

Minerals and Heart Disease

The first mineral in the diet that usually comes to mind with reference to blood pressure is sodium. It has been estimated that

Americans consume between 10 and 12 grams of salt daily and since salt is about 40 percent sodium, this is equal to between 4 and 5 grams of sodium a day. Of the 10 to 12 grams of salt, approximately 3 grams occur naturally in foods, and the remainder comes from table salt and salt-containing processed foods, even though it is well known that we can get adequate sodium in our diet from unprocessed foods without using the salt shaker or consuming heavily salt-laden foods.

The relationship of sodium to elevated blood pressure is complex. Current information indicates that approximately 20 percent of the population appears to be genetically predisposed to hypertension and may be salt-sensitive. When these individuals are exposed to the average salt intake in the American diet, they may demonstrate elevated blood pressure.[40]

In March, 1981, a five-point program was announced that features a cooperative effort by the FDA and the food industry toward better sodium labeling. The goals of this program are the voluntary reduction of salt in processed foods, expanded consumer education programs on the impact of salt on blood pressure, and continued monitoring of sodium consumption in the average American diet. The objective of this program is to reduce salt consumption by 80 percent in the average person's diet, as spelled out by the U.S. Dietary Goals of the United States Senate in 1976.[41]

The dietary recommendations already given in this chapter, by the nature of their composition, decrease sodium and increase potassium intake, which is beneficial for managing blood pressure. Use of the salt shaker should be limited and foods with salt or sodium high on the list of ingredients should be omitted from the diet in a blood pressure management program.

In one study of two groups with about the same level of sodium and potassium intake, it was found that those with elevated blood pressure had a much lower level of calcium intake per day than those with normal blood pressure. Inadequate calcium intake may be a previously unrecognized factor in the development of elevated blood pressure; calcium intake between 1000 and 1200 milligrams a day may be recommended for the hypertensive individual.[42]

Closely related to calcium is the trace element magnesium, which has also been found to be very important in the prevention of a number of heart disorders. Magnesium is important for the contraction of all muscles in the body, and the early warning signs of a magnesium deficiency can be muscle cramping or twitching and a general sense of nervous irritability.[43] Magnesium intake at the level of 300 to 600 milligrams a day is important to balance calcium intake and promote proper muscle contraction and heart function.[44]

Trace Elements and Heart Disease

One antagonist to calcium and magnesium that can aggravate high blood pressure and heart problems is the toxic trace element cadmium. Recently, it has been found that low-level environmental exposure to cadmium can induce adverse changes in the cardiovascular tissues of animals, and the investigators conclude that the sensitivity of the cardiovascular tissue to low doses of cadmium supports the hypothesis that ingested or inhaled environmental cadmium may contribute to essential hypertension in humans and be a particular problem in the individual who has a low intake of calcium, magnesium, and zinc.[45] Cadmium is found to be high in cigarette smoke, refined foods, and some water supplies.

Zinc is a known antagonist of cadmium and should be consumed in the diet at levels between 15 and 20 milligrams per day. Excessive zinc, however, can suppress copper levels and a copper deficiency can also produce increased risk to coronary heart disease. There must, therefore, be proper balance between zinc and copper.[46] The ratio of zinc to copper should be approximately 10 parts zinc to one part copper, which means that individuals on a blood cholesterol–lowering regimen should be consuming about 20 milligrams of zinc and 2 milligram of copper per day. Excessively high zinc intake (above 100 mg daily) has also been found to reduce HDL cholesterol and may actually contribute to increased risk to coronary heart disease in the sensitive individual.[47]

One other trace element shown to be extremely important in reducing total cholesterol and increasing HDL is chromium. It was found that after supplementing adult men with 200 micrograms of chromium each day, there was a significant increase in HDL cholesterol and a decrease in total blood cholesterol, indicating a reduced risk to coronary heart disease.[48] These results corroborate a previous study done on rabbits, which indicated that chromium supplementation could lead to the regression of existing atherosclerotic plaque in animals that had been fed a high-fat, high-cholesterol diet.

Vitamins, Accessory Nutrients, and Heart Disease

Also important in the management of elevated blood cholesterol and increased risk to heart disease are vitamins and accessory nutrients. Vitamin B-6 has been found very important in the proper metabolism of an amino acid called homocysteine. The inappropriate metabolism of this substance can lead to atherosclerosis, and a chronic B-6 inadequacy has been identified by a number of investigators as being a risk factor to atherosclerotic disease.[49] Intakes of vitamin B-6 at levels of 10 to 20 milligrams per day are suggested as useful in individuals at risk to heart disease.

Another vitamin that has received considerable attention, for its ability to reduce blood cholesterol, is ascorbic acid—vitamin C. Recently, the effect of vitamin C supplementation on blood cholesterol levels in eighty individuals eating egg yolks was examined.[50] It was found that vitamin C supplementation at the level of 2000 milligrams per day did not lead to a uniform response in blood cholesterol, and in many individuals it had no effect whatsoever. This seems consistent with other results that demonstrated that a daily supplemented dose of 2000 milligrams of vitamin C produced the greatest reduction of blood cholesterol in those individuals who had the highest initial blood cholesterol levels. People with near optimal blood cholesterol had no reduction in blood cholesterol after vitamin C supplementation. This would indicate that those who need the reduction the most respond the best to vitamin C therapy.[51]

For a long time, the purported usefulness of vitamin E as protection against heart disease was more anecdote than medical fact. Recently, however, there is accumulating evidence indicating how vitamin E could have a beneficial impact on the prevention of heart disease. Vitamin E has been found to prevent the conversion of a fatty acid in the blood, called arachidonic acid, to a hormone that can stimulate blood platelets to stick together, initiating a heart attack or otherwise contributing to heart disease.[52]

In one human study vitamin E at the level of 600 units per day supplementation was found to lead to a 12 percent increase in HDL cholesterol levels, which is associated with a decreased risk to heart disease, although this study has been questioned by other investigators.[53]

The naturally occurring amino acid carnitine, when supplemented at the level of 400 milligrams three times daily, had a significant impact on reducing blood triglycerides, a form of blood fat associated with increased risk to artery disease.[54] Carnitine has the ability to decrease triglycerides in the blood by increasing the proper metabolism of fats to energy. Using selected carnitine supplementation in people who have long-term elevated blood triglycerides may cause a significant improvement of their metabolism of fats and the reduction of triglycerides.

The need for carnitine in the individual with elevated blood triglycerides may vary considerably; some people may be responsive to as little as 500 milligrams a day.

Two types of carnitine are available: natural L-carnitine and synthetic DL-carnitine. It has been shown that the synthetic DL-carnitine in long-term supplemented doses may produce an adverse set of neuro-

Table 4

**Summary of Aspects
of Nutraerobics Heart Disease Management Program**

Diet	No more than 20% fats
	Remaining fats predominately as unsaturated oils
	Rich in vegetable protein
	Lower in meats
	Lower in sugars
	High in fiber
Exercise	Daily minimum 10–15 minutes of aerobic exercise
Omega-3 oils	5–10 grams MaxEPA supplementation
Fiber	3–5 tablespoons oat bran fiber
Minerals	Lower sodium and salt
	Higher potassium
	300–600 mg magnesium
	800–1200 mg calcium
	20–30 mg zinc
	200 mcg chromium
Vitamins	10–20 mg vitamin B-6
	500–2000 mg vitamin C
	200–600 I.U. vitamin E
	500–3000 mg niacin (optional)
Accessory nutrients	300–1200 mg L-carnitine (optional, for elevated triglycerides)
Lifestyle	Learn how to relax
	Regular vacations
	Stop smoking
	Prudent use of alcohol
	Avoid exposure to toxic minerals and chemicals where possible
	Lose weight if necessary

logical symptoms in some individuals whereas the natural L-carnitine will not.[55] It is, therefore, very important to use the natural source when supplementing with carnitine.

Other substances suggested helpful in the prevention and treatment of coronary artery plaque are mucopolysaccharides or glycosaminoglycans. These substances are called chondroitin sulfate and are generally derived from either the cartilage of sharks or the trachea of beef cattle. Studies have indicated that these complex substances when given in oral supplementation levels of 300 to 1000 milligrams a day have not only growth-stimulating effects but also promote wound healing.[56] These substances seem to have a beneficial effect on the function of the artery wall; they may help prevent calcification of the artery and changes in the artery wall associated with atherosclerosis. This work is still highly speculative at this point and is in need of more clinical proof, but a limited number of human trials have suggested improvement in artery function in patients supplemented with chondroitin sulfate.

Summary Review

In looking over this whole chapter, you probably now understand why we stated that the American Heart Association's dietary approach toward the prevention and management of heart disease may not be broad-based or aggressive enough. Many more dietary and other factors have now been identified as being useful in a successful therapeutic program to minimize risk if your biotype indicates a predisposition to heart disease.

A summary of this information appears in Table 4. This program is for those individuals whose biotype indicates a need for an aggressive approach toward cardiovascular disease prevention or treatment. Based upon the evidence in this chapter, it should be possible for you to reduce your risk to heart disease if you are in a high risk category by as much as 50 percent. Good luck with the implementation of the program.

For those of you whose biotype indicates a high risk to cancer, the next chapter deals specifically with reducing your risk to malignant diseases through specific attention to your biotype uniqueness.

Notes

1. R. I. Levy and J. Moskowitz, "Cardiovascular Research: Decades of Progress, a Decade of Promise," *Science, 217,* 121(1982).

2. L. P. Biese, "Heart II: Risk Evaluation Revisited," *Interface Age* (September 1981):66.

3. R. I. Levy, "Cardiovascular Disease Mortality," in *Annual Review of Public Health,* vol. 2 (Palo Alto, CA: Annual Reviews, Inc., 1981).

4. G. Kolata, "Heart Study Produces a Surprise Result," *Science, 218,* 31(1982).

5. "Trials of Coronary Heart Disease Prevention," *Lancet* (9 October 1982):803.

6. W. B. Kannel and T. Gordon, "The Search for an Optimum Serum Cholesterol," *Lancet* (14 August 1982):374.

7. R. S. Lees, "High Density Lipoproteins and the Risk of Atherosclerosis," *New England Journal of Medicine, 306,* 1546(1982).

8. H. Weshima and Y. Komachi, "High-Density Lipoprotein Cholesterol Levels in Japan," *Journal of the American Medical Association, 247,* 1985(1982).

9. C. Vergani and G. F. Altomare, "Low Levels of HDL in Severe Cystic Acne," *New England Journal of Medicine, 307,* 1151(1982).

10. J. B. Zalokar and J. R. Claude, "Leukocyte Count, Smoking, and Myocardial Infarction," *New England Journal of Medicine, 304,* 465(1981).

11. N. Shulman et al., "The Effect of Treatment on Mortality in 'Mild' Hypertension," *New England Journal of Medicine, 307,* 976(1982).

12. B. Liebman, "Can a Low-fat Diet Clear Clogged Arteries?" *Nutrition Action* (May 1982):3.

13. P. R. Pomrehn and L. F. Burmeister, "Ischemic Heart Disease Mortality in Iowa Farmers," *Journal of the American Medical Association, 248,* 1073(1982).

14. D. M. Kramsch and W. B. Hood, "Reduction of Coronary Atherosclerosis by Moderate Conditioning Exercise in Monkeys," *New England Journal of Medicine, 305,* 1483(1981).

15. J. N. Morris and S. P. W. Chave, "Vigorous Exercise in Leisure-time Protection Against Coronary Heart Disease," *Lancet* (6 December 1980):1207.

16. J. B. Handler and P. M. Shea, "Symptomatic Coronary Artery Disease in a Marathon Runner," *Journal of the American Medical Association, 248,* 717(1982).

17. J. W. Marr and J. N. Morris, "Changing the National Diet to Reduce Coronary Heart Disease," *Lancet* (23 January 1982):217.

18. B. Lewis and A. V. Swan, "Towards an Improved Lipid-Lowering Diet: Additive Effects of Changes in Nutrient Intake," *Lancet* (12 December 1981):1310.

19. C. Ehnholm and P. Puska, "Effect of Diet on Serum Lipoproteins in a Population with a High Risk of Coronary Heart Disease," *New England Journal of Medicine, 307,* 850(1982).

20. T. R. Dawber and J. Pool, "Eggs, Serum Cholesterol, and Coronary Heart Disease," *American Journal of Clinical Nutrition, 36,* 617(1982).

21. S. L. Roberts and W. E. Connor, "Does Egg Feeding Affect Plasma Cholesterol in Humans?" *American Journal of Clinical Nutrition, 34,* 2092(1981).

22. F. M. Sacks and E. H. Kass, "Effect of Ingestion of Meat on Plasma Cholesterol of Vegetarians," *Journal of the American Medical Association, 246,* 640(1981).

23. W. A. Check, "Switch to Soy Protein for Boring but Healthful Diet," *Journal of the American Medical Association, 247,* 3045(1982).

24. F. H. Mattson and J. R. Crouse, "Optimizing the Effect of Plant Sterols on Cholesterol Absorption in Man," *American Journal of Clinical Nutrition, 35,* 697(1982).

25. W. E. Connor and L. L. Gallo, "Lymphatic Absorption of Shellfish Sterols and Their Effects on Cholesterol Absorption," *American Journal of Clinical Nutrition, 34,* 507(1981).

26. D. Kromhout and E. B. Bosschieter, "Dietary Fibre and 10-year Mortality from Coronary Heart Disease, Cancer, and All Causes," *Lancet* (4 September 1982):518.

27. R. W. Kirby and J. W. Anderson, "Oat-bran Intake Selectively Lowers Serum Low-density Lipoprotein Cholesterol in Hypercholesterolemic Men," *American Journal of Clinical Nutrition, 34,* 824(1981).

28. P. Samuel, "Treatment of Hypercholesterolemia with Neomycin—A Time for Reappraisal," *New England Journal of Medicine, 301,* 595(1979).

29. A. R. Khan and M. A. Qadeer, "Effect of Guar Gum on Blood Lipids," *American Journal of Clinical Nutrition, 34,* 2446(1981).

30. A. Bordia, "Effect of Garlic on Blood Lipids in Patients with Coronary Heart Disease," *American Journal of Clinical Nutrition, 34,* 2100(1981).

31. G. E. Fraser and H. Blackburn, "The Effect of Various Vegetable Supplements on Serum Cholesterol," *American Journal of Clinical Nutrition, 34,* 1272(1981).

32. D. C. Laine and I. D. Frantz, "Lightly Hydrogenated Soy Oil Versus Other Vegetable Oils as a Lipid-Lowering Agent," *American Journal of Clinical Nutrition, 35,* 683(1982).

33. F. A. Kummerow, "Trans-Fatty Acids in Margarines, Shortenings, and Cooking Fats," *Artery, 4,* 360(1978).

34. H. Imai and M. Kanisawa, "Angiotoxicity of Oxygenated Sterols and Possible Precursors," *Science, 207,* 651(1980).

35. M. S. Brown and J. L. Goldstein, "Cholesterol Ester Formation in Cultured Human Fibroblasts: Stimulation by Oxygenated Sterols," *Journal of Biological Chem., 250,* 4025(1975).

36. J. Dyerberg and H. O. Bang, "Eicosapentanoic Acid and Prevention of Atherosclerosis," *Lancet* (15 July 1978):117.

37. M. Thorngern and A. Gustafson, "Effects of 11-week Increase in Dietary EPA," *Lancet* (28 November 1981):1190.

38. C. R. M. Hay and R. Saynor, "Effect of Fish Oil on Platelet Kinetics in Patients with Ischemic Heart Disease," *Lancet* (5 June 1982):1269.

39. J. Dyerberg and E. B. Schmidt, "n-3 Polyunsaturated Fatty Acids and Ischemic Heart Disease," *Lancet* (11 September 1982):614.

40. M. A. Weber and J. H. Laragh, *Hypertension: Current Therapy* (New York: Saunders, 1978).

41. USDA, *Nutrition and Your Health: Dietary Guidelines for Americans* (Washington, DC: U.S. Government Printing Office, 1980).

42. D. A. McCarron, C. D. Morris, and C. Cole, "Dietary Calcium and Human Hypertension," *Science, 217,* 267(1982).

43. "Clinical Signs of Magnesium Deficiency," *Nutrition Reviews, 37,* 6(1979).

44. B. M. Altura and B. T. Altura, "Magnesium and Contraction of Smooth Muscle: Relationship to Vascular Disease," *Federation Proceedings, 40,* 2672(1981).

45. S. Kopp and E. F. Derry, "Cardiovascular Actions of Cadmium at Environmental Exposure Levels," *Science, 217,* 837(1982).

46. L. M. Klevay and R. A. Jacobs, "The Ratio of Zinc to Copper of Cholesterol-Lowering Diets," in *Trace Substances in Environmental Health,* D.D. Hemphill, ed., *9,* 131(1975).

47. P. L. Hooper and G. E. Johnson, "Zinc Lowers HDL Cholesterol," *Journal of the American Medical Association, 244,* 1960(1980); J.H. Freeland-Graves and R.

Young, "Effect of Zinc Supplementation on Plasma HDL Cholesterol," *American Journal of Clinical Nutrition, 35,* 988(1982).

48. R. Riales and M-J. Albrink, "Effect of Chromium Chloride Supplementation on Glucose Tolerance and Serum Lipids Including HDL of Adult Men," *American Journal of Clinical Nutrition, 34,* 2670(1981).

49. K. S. McCully and R. B. Wilson, "Homocysteine Theory of Artherosclerosis," *Atherosclerosis, 22,* 2(1975).

50. I. M. Buzzard and J. Bowering, "Effect of Eggs and Ascorbic Acid on Cholesterol Levels in Healthy Young Men," *American Journal of Clinical Nutrition, 36,* 94(1982).

51. E. Ginter, "Pretreatment Serum-Cholesterol and Response to Vitamin C," *Lancet* (3 November 1979):117.

52. D. H. Hwang and J. Donovan, "In Vivo Effects of Vitamin E on Arachidonic Acid Metabolism in Rat Platelets," *Journal of Nutrition, 112,* 1233(1982).

53. W. J. Hermann and J. Faucett, "Effect of Tocopherol on HDL Cholesterol," *American Journal of Clinical Pathology, 72,* 848(1979).

54. P. F. Bougneres and R. Assan, "Hypolipidenic Effect of Carnitine in Uremic Patients," *Lancet* (30 June 1979):1401.

55. G. Bazzato and M. Ciman, "Myasthenia-like Syndrome After DL—But Not L-carnitine," *Lancet* (30 May 1981):1209.

56. L. M. Morrison and D. A. Schjeide, "Growth Stimulating Effects of Acid Mucopolysaccharides," *Proceedings of the Society for Experimental Biology and Medicine, 118,* 770(1965).

8

Cancer and Your Biotype

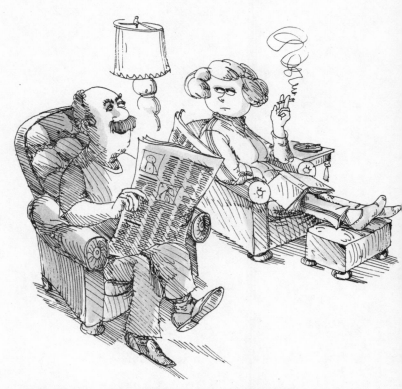

LISTEN TO THIS, "BY 1990 THE RATE OF LUNG CANCER DEATH IN WOMEN WILL BE THE SAME AS MEN."
YOU'VE COME A LONG WAY, BABY.

1. Do you smoke?

1	2	3	4
No	Less than 1 pack per day	1–2 packs per day	More than 2 packs per day

2. Do you eat smoked meats: bacon, ham, hot dogs?

1	2	4
No	Occasionally	Yes, frequently

3. Do you have a high-fat diet?

1	2	3	4
No	I use some butter and deep-fried food	About like the average person	Yes, fatty foods such as cheese and meat and sauces are my favorites

4. Do you dislike orange- or red-colored vegetables and fruits?

1	2	4
No	Somewhat	Yes

5. Do you eat processed foods frequently?

1	2	4
No	Sometimes	Yes

6. Do you have a family history of cancer?

1	2	4
No	It has been in my family	Yes

7. Do you expose yourself to the sun?

1	2	4
No	Periodically	Frequently

8. Have you been exposed frequently to X-rays or radiation?

1	4
No	Yes

If your score exceeds 20 you may be at increased risk to cancer and you should concentrate on this chapter.

"Cancer is not inevitable." So begins a 1982 National Research
Council panel recommendation dealing with the spectrum of problems
related to cancer in the United States. The report goes on to say, "It
is highly likely that the United States will eventually have the option
of adopting a diet that reduces incidence of cancer by approximately
one-third, and it is now well known that what we eat does affect our
chances of getting cancer, especially particular kinds of cancer. This
is good news, because it means by controlling what we eat we may
prevent such diet-sensitive cancers."[1] We do not know the precise
extent to which diet and lifestyle modification will be able to reduce
the incidence of specific cancers, but the evidence is quite clear that by
employing the strategy outlined in this section of the Nutraerobics
Program, a cancer-sensitive individual may be able to significantly
reduce his or her risk to the major cancers of the lung, breast, prostate,
colon, stomach, intestine, and skin.

For more than a decade, the words "diet" and "cancer" mentioned in the same sentence conjured up images of food additives. Any
ingredient that could not be pronounced was suspect as a potential
carcinogen (a substance that can produce cancer). Over the past years,
the FDA has banned more than twenty-five food additives proved toxic
to humans or animals, because the Delaney amendment specifies that
any substance proved a cancer-producing agent in animal or human
trials must be banned from the food supply system.

Most recently, however, food additives have been less implicated
in diet-related cancers than certain natural materials in the foods themselves, such as fat. In a classic series of experiments in 1942, Dr. Albert
Tannenbaum found that dietary fat promoted cancer in animals and
wrote, "The definite increase in the incidence of spontaneous breast
tumors in animals brought about by a fat-enriched diet is significant,
and this effect is the most striking result seen in our studies with
various types of tumors."[2]

This research opened up a whole new field of investigation called
epidemiology, which is concerned with the statistical relationship between lifestyle habits and the incidence of disease. Work in this area

has identified that human cancers may be 70 to 80 percent related to environmental factors, and that diet is possibly one of the major contributing factors. Because environment and nutrition are to a great extent under our control, by modifying our diet and improving our lifestyle to be coincident with our particular genetic susceptibilities and biotype, we can greatly reduce the incidence of the major types of cancer.

Cancers of Affluence

In part, the major cancers we have today—those of the lung, breast, colon, prostate, ovary, uterus, pancreas, and esophagus—are all related to our affluence and excessive lifestyle. Not all individuals have equal sensitivity to this lifestyle; smoking in one may not be nearly the hazard to lung cancer it is in another. Taking into account specific biological sensitivities and relating them to the known risk factors of these cancers can allow an individual to design a lifestyle that helps minimize the risk to cancer.

To do this, we need to see what the major risk factors to the ultimate development of these various types of cancers are. Recently, two British epidemiologists compiled a massive amount of data in a paper on the causes of cancer.[3] This report lists the highest risk factors to cancer as shown in Table 5. It can be seen that almost two-thirds of all cancer deaths can be related to tobacco use and diet. Occupational risks, pollution, alcohol consumption, and reproductive and sexual behaviors constitute an additional 16 percent of the risk factors to cancer, and all of these represent parts of a person's lifestyle and environment that are controllable.

Cancer and the Environment

We are learning that there are substances in the environment that are potentially carcinogenic, but we have also learned that there are processes within our bodies that allow us defense against those sub-

Table 5

Highest Risk Factors to Cancer

Factor	Percent of all cancer deaths
Tobacco	30
Alcohol	3
Diet	35
Food additives	less than 1
Reproductive and sexual behavior	7
Pollution	2
Occupation	4
Medicines	1
Industrial products	less than 1
Infection	10 (?)
Geophysical factors	3

Source: Chemistry and Engineering News, 17 August 1981, p. 23.

stances when we are operating at high efficiency. Environmental agents such as asbestos, polynuclear aromatic hydrocarbons (which come from incomplete combustion of oil and gas products), and chlorinated hydrocarbons (which can come from pesticides, herbicides, or from chlorination of organically polluted water) are all known substances that increase the risk to cancer.

Some people have developed such a paranoia about cancer that they assume all unnatural substances must be carcinogens. This is certainly not the case. In a detailed study done at the National Cancer Institute to screen literally thousands of substances for potential carcinogenicity, or cancer-producing ability, it was found that only 30 percent of the substances had any suspicion of being carcinogens. Even when exposed to a substance that may trigger a cell into the uncontrolled growth we call a malignancy, our body has the ability to defend itself through what is called the immune surveillance system.

The surveillance system is working twenty-four hours a day to protect us against transformed cells in our bodies that could be the origin of a cancer. The key factors are the rate of exposure to substances that may initiate a cancer and the relative defense that our body possesses against those subtances. When our defense is greater than the effects of exposure, we are cancer free. Fortunately, for most of us that system works wonderfully 99.999 percent of the time.

Recommendations to Reduce Cancers

There are a number of things that can be done to reduce your relative risk to cancer if you have a family susceptibility or personal suggestion of risk in your biotype. The National Research Council recommends the following eight dietary changes:[4]

1. The proportion of calories in the diet provided by fats should be reduced from the present 40 percent to no more than 25 percent. Of all the dietary components studied, the evidence was most strong for a relationship between excessive fat intake and occurrence of cancers of the colon, breast, and prostate.

A recent study showed a very strong correlation between mortality from breast and colon cancer and the per capita consumption of meat and fat in different countries of the world.[5] It was suggested from this study that dietary influences in pre-adult life may be important in determining the relative risk in adult life to a number of the common cancers. It was postulated almost fifty years ago that most cancers seen in adult life had their origin some fifteen to twenty years previously, and that it took that length of time for the cancer to become a diagnosed, palpable tumor. If this is so, then the dietary habits we have as younger individuals may have a direct bearing on our ultimate development of cancer in mid to late life.

Although all forms of fat are suspected to be cancer promoters, some types of fat are more potent than others. In experiments where animals were fed only polyunsaturated oils, they developed more tumors than animals fed the same levels of saturated fat. This may be the result of the fact that unsaturated oils in the absence of proper biological antioxidants such as vitamin E are converted in the body to potential carcinogenic substances. If polyunsaturated vegetable oils are eaten as the major fats in the diet, then adequate levels of vitamin E should be taken to prevent conversion of the oils to carcinogenic substances either in the cooking process or in the body.

Fat-rich foods such as seeds, nuts, or oils that have a bitter taste should not be consumed, because this indicates that they have already undergone some chemical conversion to substances that may potentially be cancer producing. For instance, wheat germ which is sweet when fresh becomes bitter upon standing at room temperature, the result of the buildup of rancid by-products from the breakdown of unsaturated oils in the wheat germ.

2. **The daily diet should include whole-grain cereals, fruits, and vegetables, especially those high in vitamin C and beta-carotene.** These foods include citrus fruits, dark green and deep yellow vegetables, and members of the cabbage family. The effect of vitamin C, beta-carotene, and the trace element selenium which are found in these foods will be discussed in greater detail later in this chapter.

3. **The consumption of salt-cured, salt-pickled, and smoked foods should be minimized, because they are associated with increased incidence of cancers of the stomach and esophagus.** In the United States, these foods include sausages, smoked fish, ham, bacon, and hot dogs.

4. **Excessive consumption of alcohol should be avoided, particularly in combination with cigarette smoking.** Such consumption has been associated with an increased risk to cancer of the upper intestinal tract and lungs.

5. **The level of dietary fiber should be increased, utilizing foods that are high in cellulose, lignin, gums, and pectins to protect against cancer of the colon and rectum.**

6.   **Foods rich in vitamin E and members of the B-vitamin family should be increased to prevent processes that could lead to carcinogen production.** These include whole grain and legume products, as well as lean meats and dairy products.

7.   **Foods rich in extraneous chemicals and additives should be minimized in the diet.** Some 3,000 food additives are used intentionally, and an estimated 12,000 are used inadvertently during processing and packaging.

8.   **Foods rich in trace elements such as zinc, magnesium, chromium, selenium, and iodide should be eaten in adequate quantities for the proper integrity of the immune system.** These include brewer's yeast, lean meats, whole grains, green vegetables, and kelp.

In its conclusion the report emphasizes that "the weight of evidence suggests that what we eat during our lifetimes strongly influences the probability of developing certain kinds of cancer, but that it is not now possible, and may never be possible, to specify a single diet that protects all people against all forms of cancer."[6] The program in this chapter, however, is an attempt to define what specific dietary and lifestyle modifications may be required for **you,** based upon your biotype, to minimize your risk of cancer.

Treatment of Cancer

How are diagnosed cancers treated? Advances in surgery and radiation therapy have been such that curative treatment can be delivered to many patients whose tumors have not spread beyond the local and regional areas. Of the 785,000 new patients with cancer (excluding the highly curable forms of skin cancer) annually in the United States, 30 percent fall into this category. For the 550,000 patients whose disease has spread beyond the local or regional area, treatment involves what is called systemic therapy, that is, treating the whole body; some systemic therapies are chemotherapy, hormone therapy, immunotherapy, and radiation therapy.

Chemotherapy is the most widely used treatment today for cancers that have metastasized (spread to other regions of the body from the original site). This procedure may be used in conjunction with surgery or radiation as a "preventive" technique to make sure that all the cancer cells, wherever they may be, are killed. Because of the frequency with which this therapy is used in cancer patients, it is important to know something about its effectiveness and side effects.

Chemotherapy uses chemical agents introduced into the body to kill cancer cells; it was born out of observations made in 1943 that a type of war gas was capable of producing tumor regression in patients with lymphoma (lymph node cancer). Later, in 1955, it was found that substances that blocked folic acid (one of the B-complex vitamins) could produce temporary remission in childhood leukemia and a cure in patients with a kind of cancer called choriocarcinoma. These observations gave birth to the National Cancer Chemotherapy Program. The substances used to kill cancer cells are themselves lethal to all cells, but treatment rests on the fact that they usually kill the more rapidly growing cancer cells faster than they kill normal cells.

Some chemotherapeutic drugs are antimetabolites; that is, they block the metabolism of the cells. Other, inhibitor drugs actually prevent certain enzymes from working in rapidly growing cells. Still other chemotherapeutic agents are derived from heavy metals such as platinum, plant extracts such as vincristine and vinblastine, or the fermentation products of bacteria or fungi (this last group prevents DNA from dividing in rapidly growing tissues).

All of these substances to a degree use the shotgun approach. The hope is that the malignant cells will be harder hit than the normal cells because they are growing faster. Unfortunately, in many cancers the difference between the cancer cell and the normal cell is very small, and the possibility of general toxicity very high; there are almost always toxic adverse side effects. The normal tissues most affected by these toxicity reactions are the rapidly dividing tissues such as bone marrow, the gastrointestinal tract, and hair follicles.

Chemotherapy leads to a decrease in white blood cell count, hair loss, nausea, and vomiting, as well as the potential suppression of ovarian function and reduced sperm synthesis. With a few of the drugs there is actual heart toxicity. A more ominous late toxic manifestation has been the development of secondary tumors, particularly what is called acute myelogenous leukemia, which is actually the result of anticancer agents that are carcinogens as well.

There are, in the face of all these hazards, a number of human cancers that have been very successfully treated with chemotherapy. These include acute lymphocytic leukemia, Hodgkins disease, diffuse histocytic lymphoma, testicular cancer, gestational choriocarcinoma, Wilm's tumor, Ewing's tumor, embryonal rhabdomyosarcoma, and Burkitt's lymphoma. In addition, chemotherapy is probably curative for small-cell lung cancer, acute myelogenous leukemia, and may be helpful for improving the remission of breast cancer and osteogenic sarcoma. As the result of the successful application of surgical techniques followed by radiation and/or chemotherapy, there has been a decline in the United States between 1966 and 1976 of 66 percent for Wilm's tumor, 39 percent for Hodgkins disease, 38 percent for childhood leukemia, 24 percent for non-Hodgkins lymphoma, 23 percent for bone tumors in children, 19 percent for premenopausal breast cancer, and 34 percent for testicular cancer.

There are, however, major tumor types for which chemotherapy, radiation, and surgery have not been overly successful. These include certain types of lung, colon, prostate, and breast cancer. These cancers are those of major public importance and constitute over 60 percent of the total cancer deaths.[7]

Alternative Cancer Therapies

Because of the failure of standard cancer therapies and the unique social stigma associated with the disease cancer, many people have sought alternative treatments, including such things as laetrile, enzyme therapy, vegetarian diets, meganutrient therapy, and other unproven methods. One of the most popular of these alternative methods has been the use of laetrile, which is a derivative of amygdalin, a substance known as a cyanogenic glycoside, which is found in apricot and peach pits.

A clinical trial was done recently in which 178 patients with cancer were treated with amygdalin plus a metabolic therapy program consisting of specified diet, enzymes, and vitamins. The great majority of these patients were in good general condition before treatment and had opted for the alternative therapy. One-third of them had not received any previous chemotherapy. The investigators concluded that there were no substantive benefits observed in terms of cure, improvement, stabilization of cancer, improvement of symptoms, or extension of lifespan. They also suggested that patients exposed to oral amygdalin be instructed about the danger of cyanide poisoning—when taken orally, amygdalin can release cyanide into the bloodstream.[8]

There were undoubtedly procedural errors in this study, but the overall conclusion is one that seems confirmed around the country from other clinical failures with laetrile therapy. One doctor writes, "Laetrile has now had its day in court. The evidence beyond reasonable doubt is that it doesn't benefit patients with advanced cancer, and there is no reason to believe that it would be any more effective in the earlier stages of the disease."[9] He concludes that the time has come to close the books on laetrile and get on with our efforts to understand the riddle of cancer and to improve its prevention and treatment.

Evaluating the Treatment Options

What would be a prudent approach toward the management of an existing cancer? First of all, we need to carefully evaluate the type of cancer. If it is one of the types highly amenable to chemotherapy, then going with traditional therapy would certainly be in your best interests. If, however, it is one of the tumor types that has had marginal to limited success by traditional therapy, then possibly utilizing small amounts of radiation and chemotherapy with limited surgery that would not be disfiguring, and then a strong lifestyle enhancement program to activate the immune system and bolster your body's native abilities to defend itself against cancer would be warranted.

Don't be afraid to ask the difficult questions concerning the cancer. What are the prognoses given standard therapy? What are the side effects? And how do the side effects compare to the possible benefits of the program? What quality of life can people expect to experience if they are successfully managed by the program? Do they have to look forward to a significant debilitation or a high probability of a second tumor?

Cancer is obviously a very personal disease, and decisions about its treatment can truly only be made by the person who has to undergo the treatment. It may not be too long from now when we have selective immunotherapy methods that will attack cancer cells based upon the unique "personality" of the cancer cell without attacking the healthy cells themselves. Such trials are under way, but now we only have the body's own natural defense mechanisms to win the battle for us. The road to cancer treatment should be an option available for patients to decide, each in his or her own way. This decision should be based on informed consent after the best information possible free of threatening, judgmental, or alarmist statements on the part of the medical support team. The final conclusion about a treatment technique should be consistent with the patient's belief system.

Cause of Cancer

What actually causes cancer? And how can knowing the cause be used in putting together a good preventive program, one designed to optimize your body's ability to defend itself against cancer?

The contemporary view is that many cancers are the result of a carcinogenic process whereby the biological clock called the gene, which is in each cell, is altered by a physical or chemical agent so that it loses its ability to control itself and reverts back to an embryonic cell type. This cell continues to grow as a fertilized egg grows in the womb; however, it is undifferentiated and grows invasively, crowding out normal cells.[10]

An obvious example of this association between a chemical agent and the production of cancer is the one-third of the total cancers in the United States that are related to the use of cigarettes and other tobacco products. There is now incontrovertible evidence that cigarette smoking is a causative factor in the major type of cancer today—lung cancer. Not twenty years ago women were said to be immune from lung cancer due to some unknown protective effect. Over the past ten years, however, the incidence of lung cancer in women has rapidly risen, so that it has been projected that by 1990 the rate of lung cancer death in women will be equal to the high rate in men. It was not that women were protected by an unknown immune factor, it was that they were protected by the social stigma against smoking, which has been lifted in the last twenty years. Although the total percentage of the population that is smoking has gone down, there has been a continued increase in smoking by teenage girls.

Chemicals strongly suspected of being carcinogenic in humans include those encountered in occupational settings such as certain coloring agents, asbestos, benzene, vinyl chloride, and medicinal agents such as inhaled arsenic, diethylstilbestrol, and anabolic steroids. Lastly, there are environmental chemicals such as polynuclear aromatic hydrocarbons.

The latent period between exposure to a carcinogen and the ultimate expression of a cancer is fairly long and necessitates conversion of the initial substance into the ultimate carcinogen in the body. This process can be stopped by appropriate body function at a number of stages before it actually produces the agent able to initiate a cancer growth.

One of the agents that seems to promote the conversion of substances in our body to carcinogens are the biochemical workhorses found within liver cells called cytochromes. One of the most important of these cytochromes in carcinogen production is called cytochrome P-450.[11] Cytochrome P-450 is found in different levels in the livers of different individuals. Alcohol consumption increases the level of cyto-

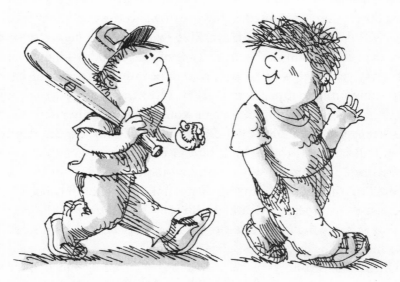

IS IT TRUE THAT WATCHING TOO MUCH LATE
NIGHT TELEVISION IS CARSONOGENIC?

chrome P-450, and this may be why alcoholics have increased risk to certain cancers. Individuals who have higher levels of this enzyme within their body, as determined by their environment and genetics, may be at higher risk to conversion of various environmental substances inhaled or ingested into the ultimate cancer-producing material. The same argument holds for the enzyme aromatic hydrocarbon hydroxylase, which converts combustion products into carcinogens in our body.

This is a direct example of biochemical individuality and shows why some people can be cigarette smokers and have no problem with lung cancer, while others develop the disease from just a small amount of exposure to certain substances in cigarettes. The message is once again clear. People must balance their exposure to carcinogens based upon their genetic susceptibility factors.

Lung Cancer Prevention

One kind of small-cell cancer of the lung is often called oat-cell cancer. It is one of the most common and most deadly cancers, killing nearly all patients within two years.

Recently, considerable progress has been made in understanding how a normal lung cell is transformed into an oat-type cancer cell.[12] Once a normal lung cell has been transformed by carcinogens into a malignant oat cell, this malignant cell turns spontaneously into other types of lung cancer after a number of months. From this research may come better ways of treating oat-cell carcinoma, but at present it leads us to an appreciation of how important it is that the immune defense system of the individual recognize the oat-cell type as a foreign cell and kill it before it has a chance to multiply and transform its function.

For some time people have been utilizing supplemental doses of vitamin A as an immunoprotective agent against lung cancer, in that preliminary work seemed to suggest that vitamin A could activate the immune system to prevent chemical carcinogenesis. Recently, however, the study of lung cancer incidence in one company's employees over a nineteen-year period seemed to indicate that lung cancer was lower in those individuals who consumed high levels of dietary beta-carotene rather than vitamin A.[13]

In fact, the original theory proposed that it is beta-carotene, the pigment found in orange and red vegetables and fruit, and not vitamin A, found in eggs and dairy products and some meats, that reduces the risk of cancer in humans. Vitamin A can be highly toxic if taken in large quantities, leading to liver damage, whereas beta-carotene is not toxic, although it does serve as the material from which vitamin A is made as it is needed in the body. The only adverse side effects of high levels of beta-carotene are a yellowing of the skin (hypercarotenemia) and a slight lowering in white blood cell count.[14]

Several excellent studies have recently confirmed the important role of beta-carotene in preventing chemical carcinogenesis and particularly lung cancer in humans.[15] The level of beta-carotene consumed in the diets of individuals with a lower incidence of lung cancer is 10,000 to 30,000 units per day. This group had 0.4 percent incidence of lung cancer, whereas in those individuals eating low beta-carotene diets (between 100 and 3,000 units per day) the incidence was 3 percent, or a sixfold higher risk to lung cancer.[16]

An interesting related finding is that a higher incidence of cancer has been found in individuals who have low levels of blood cholesterol, meaning below 170 milligrams percent.[17] It has been suggested that low blood cholesterol correlates with low level of vitamin A in the blood, and the low level of vitamin A indicates a low intake of beta-carotene, which may be why individuals with low levels of blood cholesterol have higher incidences of cancer.[18] This does not mean that low blood cholesterol causes cancer; rather, it is the effect. It is obvious that vitamin A adequacy is important for immune defense, but that adequacy can be achieved at levels of intake between 5,000 and 20,000 units per day. Amounts above this may produce symptoms of vitamin A excess, which include hair loss, headaches, skin problems, and liver changes.

Nutrients and Cancer Defense

Recent work indicates that immune activation and defense against lung cancer may be extended also to adequacy of vitamins E and C. Reports show that vitamin E and vitamin C levels in newly diagnosed lung cancer victims were less than half those in noncancer individuals. There may be a possible interrelationship between Vitamins A, C, E, and beta-carotene and the relative risk to lung cancer, a relationship that needs to be studied in greater detail.[19]

The message that comes out of these studies on lung cancer and nutrition is that a number of factors in the diet may give rise to improved immunity and defense against chemical carcinogenesis. It is interesting to note that the shark is an animal that never gets cancer. Although the shark is an extremely primitive animal, it can be fed high levels of known carcinogenic substances, such as aflatoxin B-1 (which

comes from moldy grain and is one of the most powerful liver carcinogens known), with no ill effect.[20] The resistance of the shark to cancer
may be related to the uniqueness of its immune system. If we can find
better, more selective ways of activating specialized immune cells in
our body, including the so called "killer cells" that are lethal to cancer
cells, we will increase our resistance to and therapeutic success with
cancer manyfold. The effectiveness of our immune system is therefore
indirectly controlled by our nutrition and our lifestyle.[21]

Recently, immune system proteins such as interferon and other
glycoproteins have been shown to have powerful suppressing effects on
cancer cells.[22] That lower calorie intake and reduced body mass can
increase the activity of interferon may be one of the reasons why cancer
risk seems lower in people who are underweight than in those who are
overweight.[23] Enhanced immune function seems to be derived from a
slightly lower-calorie, lower-protein intake with increased levels of
zinc, copper, vitamin C and vitamin E, as well as selenium.

For the white blood cells involved in immune defense to work
correctly, they must be properly nourished so that they can manufacture the levels of energy necessary for hand-to-hand combat with
human cancer cells.[24] It is important to note that the nutrients needed
by the immune system do not come in high quantities in highly processed convenience foods. Many Americans depending on them may not
even be meeting their RDA levels, much less the specific levels required
for adequate immune defense.

Trace Elements and Cancer

The elements zinc, selenium, and manganese are extremely important in the immune system. A zinc deficiency can lead to a low level
of functioning of the thymus gland, which is a small gland located at
the base of the neck responsible for activating white blood cells to
become active defensive agents called T-lymphocytes. Loss of thymus
function is associated with increased aging and disorders of the immune system.[25]

Studies have demonstrated that human cancer incidence is associated to some degree with the level of selenium in the soil of various regions in the United States.[26] Those areas that have low soil selenium have higher incidence of cancer than areas of higher soil selenium. Tumors in mice can be increased by a decrease in the selenium content of the diet, or decreased by increasing the selenium content of the diet.[27] Cancer mortality in humans correlates with lower levels of dietary selenium intake.[28] Two hundred micrograms of selenium daily as organic selenium from high-selenium yeast is recommended for immune activation and protection against cancer-producing processes.[29]

Manganese, like selenium, may not be gotten in adequate quantities in many individuals' dietary intakes.[30] Manganese has been found to activate superoxide dismutase, an enzyme produced by blood cells that is extremely important in the activity of the immune system.[31] Manganese is also important in the activation of a substance that protects against carcinogenesis called coenzyme Q.[32] The level of manganese intake required to activate these substances may be between 5 and 20 milligrams a day.

Vitamin and Mineral Therapy

The use of various nutrients in therapeutic doses to activate the immune system and to reduce the incidence of cancer and the use of these nutrients in the treatment of certain forms of cancer has traditionally been an area of nutrition called quackery by the medical profession. Recently, the National Cancer Institute, however, launched a series of investigations to evaluate the effect of vitamin and mineral therapy in cancer.[33] This program, a first by the NCI, will focus primarily on prevention of cancer through nutritional supplementation. A number of foods have been suggested to reduce the risk of cancer, such as brussels sprouts, cabbage, certain fruits, and black tea, which contain high levels of selenium and manganese. The NCI is going to be looking at what it is in these foods and others that contributes to the lowering of cancer incidence.

One biochemist doing work in cancer research writes, "I think physicians eventually will discover that there are nutritional ways of preventing cancer at a very early age by assuring an optimal concentration of certain vitamins to force all cells exposed to carcinogens in the direction of normal differentiation." This, of course, is the approach advocated by the Nutraerobics Program. Not all people need broad-based nutritional supplementation, but for those individuals at risk to cancer due to genetic propensity or lifestyle, alteration of diet and lifestyle may be extremely important in reducing that risk.

Vitamins and Cancer

Dr. Linus Pauling, a two-time Nobel laureate, has been a champion of the importance of nutrition and, specifically, vitamin C in reducing the incidence of cancer and even in potential treatment of certain cancers. From his work has come the report from laboratories around the world that 2000 to 3000 milligrams of vitamin C daily can stimulate the immune system.[34] Pauling's work has also pointed out that high-level vitamin-C therapy was useful in the prolongation in life of diagnosed cancer victims[35], although these findings have not received total agreement within the medical community.[36] Recent work does indicate that vitamin C is utilized and excreted much more rapidly in smokers than in nonsmokers and, therefore, smokers may be more prone to vitamin-C depletion and a suppressed immune system which leads to high risk to various forms of cancer.[37]

Vitamins C and E when used together can improve the management of some tumors by inhibiting cancer growth, enhancing the effects of chemotherapy, perhaps reducing the side effects of chemotherapy, and even stimulating host immune functions. Preliminary studies in cancer patients who are administered 400 units of vitamin E and 500 milligrams of vitamin C daily show improved chemotherapeutic treatment of colon cancer. Vitamin E in supplemented doses also reduces the adverse side effects of heart toxicity in cancer patients treated with the chemotherapeutic drug adriamycin.[38]

One vitamin that should be used cautiously in supplemented doses in certain chemotherapeutic programs is the B-complex vitamin folic acid. Some of the chemotherapeutic agents work as anti–folic acid agents, which means that supplementation with this B vitamin when these medications are being used can actually reduce the effectiveness of the therapy.[39] But, in general, individuals with cancer have been shown to have a much more rapid excretion of many of the water-soluble B vitamins, and evidence suggests that increased levels of the majority of the B-vitamins are helpful in maintaining appetite and improving body defenses in the cancer patient.[40]

Breast Cancer and Nutraerobics

Alcohol consumption may constitute an increased risk factor to the incidence of breast cancer in women.[41] Women who are both smokers and alcoholic beverage consumers have an even higher incidence of cancer, indicating that there may be an adverse multiplier factor in effect when both these habits are involved simultaneously. The results of this study indicated that women who drank beer, wine, or distilled alcohol had one and a half to two times the rate of cancer of those women who never drank. The estimated increase in the rate was greatest for those who had drunk most frequently during the year preceding the cancer diagnosis.

One of the explanations as to why alcohol consumption may increase the risk to breast cancer has to do with alcohol's adverse effect upon the liver. The liver metabolizes a woman's estrogens (female hormones) so that they can be excreted. The inability to properly metabolize estrogens can lead to the buildup of certain estrogenic substances within the body that can overly stimulate receptors in the breast, ovary, or uterine wall and initiate a cancer process. Women who have high levels of the two hormones estrone and estradiol are known to have increased incidence of breast and ovarian cancer.[42]

Many of the first-generation oral contraceptives produced imbalances in these estrogens and it was found that there was a disproportionately large number of endometrial (uterine) cancers in women taking these medications.[43] These products have subsequently been taken off the market and replaced by what are called combination-hormone oral contraceptives which balance the hormones and prevent the risk to cancer.[44]

Evidence now suggests that if a reduction in the luteal-phase (prior to ovulation) estrogen production can be achieved in women, a 20 percent reduction in the risk to breast cancer is possible; this reduction can occur if the rate of metabolism of the estrogens is increased in the liver.[45] Increased liver activity can be achieved by the proper level of the B-complex vitamins, vitamin C, and the trace elements zinc, copper, manganese, and selenium. Decreased production of estrogen can be achieved by a lower-fat diet, idealizing the weight-to-height ratio, and exposure of the naked eye to sunlight, which stimulates the secretion the hormone melatonin which blocks estrogen overproduction.[46]

In those women who have recurring breast tenderness due to fibrocystic disease, caffeine should be restricted and vitamin E should be supplemented at 400 to 600 units per day, as is discussed in Chapter 9.

Digestive Cancers

One major cancer of the digestive tract is colon cancer. Recently, the chemical structure of a substance manufactured by bacteria that could initiate cancer in the colon was discovered.[47] This substance and others produced by bacterial putrefaction of materials in the digestive tract may increase the risk to cancers of the colon. The best way of preventing the buildup of these substances is to stimulate proper intestinal regularity and prevent constipation. High-meat, high-fat, low-fiber diets encourage longer residence time of fecal material in the bowel and greater potential bacterial putrefaction and carcinogen development.[48] Fiber intake between 20 and 35 grams per day seems to be desirable in improving digestive function and reducing the risk to colon cancer.

Another factor found to reduce the risk to colon cancer comes from the natural antibiotic activity of cultured milk products such as yogurt and kefir that contain lactobacillus acidophilus and lactobacillus bulgaricus.[49] It has been observed that these cultures are capable of producing metabolites that inhibit the growth of a variety of bacteria in the intestines capable of producing carcinogens. Such cultured dairy products may be anticarcinogenic.[50]

Other forms of digestive cancer that have received considerable attention are stomach cancer and its relationship to smoked food consumption, pancreatic cancer and its relationship to coffee consumption, and bladder cancer and its relationship to saccharin. A recent study indicates that the consumption of foods smoked, cured, or pickled with nitrates may increase the risk to stomach cancer. Nitrates or nitrites are converted to carcinogens called nitrosamines in the stomach; however, the formation of nitrosamines can be reduced by taking vitamin C at the same meal.[51] This means that bacon and eggs and orange juice are far superior to bacon and eggs and coffee relative to the potential for nitrosamine formation.

What about coffee and its suggested effect on increased risk to pancreatic cancer? Since the initial report that coffee may cause pancreatic cancer, many studies have been done. The most recent study indicates that a moderate intake of coffee (3 to 8 cups per day) does not statistically increase the risk to pancreatic cancer.[52] We do know that increased coffee consumption will elevate blood pressure and increase the level of the hormone adrenaline in the blood, but this in itself has no direct impact upon increasing the risk of cancer. (If you are going to consume decaffeinated coffee, however, drink one made by the water-extracted process. The solvent-extracted process leaves residues of ethylene dichloride that may in themselves be low-grade carcinogens.)

What about saccharin and bladder cancer? Studies seem to clear saccharin of blame, but it is important to point out again that certain people are more sensitive to synthetic substances than others. The safest policy is to avoid exposure to petrochemically derived substances whenever possible, and when not possible, to use as little of the substance as you can.

Skin Cancer

The same message is applicable to one other known carcinogen— excessive sun exposure. There is no excuse these days for people to overexpose their bodies to the harmful ultraviolet rays of the sun. We now have sunscreens made with derivatives of para-aminobenzoic acid (PABA) that effectively block out the sun's harmful rays. If you plan on being in the sun, use common sense. Do not try to get a tan the first day. Protect your skin against the carcinogenic rays of the sun by using the appropriate grade of sunscreen to meet your skin's need. Light-skinned individuals may need a 15-rated sun block, darker-skinned individuals may get away with an 8-rated one, but no one is immune to the cancer-producing effects of ultraviolet light.

Cancer and Your Drinking Water

The United States Environmental Protection Agency has noted as a significant health problem related to the risk to certain cancers the contamination of our drinking water.[53] The U.S. General Accounting Office issued a statement in 1981 that said, "Unsafe drinking water is causing outbreaks of disease or poisoning in thousands of communities throughout the United States . . . furthermore the blame for increasing outbreaks of water-borne disease is many times the state's failure to enforce safe drinking water standards."[54]

Drinking water can be contaminated with physical agents such as sand or sediment; inorganic toxic chemicals such as lead, mercury, arsenic, cadmium, or radioactive elements; organic chemicals such as PCBs (polychlorinated biphenyls), DDT, chloroform, or carbon tetrachloride; or biological entities such as bacteria or viruses. In many regions of the United States the only water purification method used is to kill bacteria by chlorination. Chlorination, however, can actually contribute to **increased** levels of potentially cancer-causing chlorinated hydrocarbons if the water before chlorination is polluted with organic substances.

Because of these problems, many people have purchased "point-of-use" home water purification units. Many of these are no more than sophisticated-looking expensive toys, however. They may have a filter and activated charcoal, but they do not remove much other than some color- and taste-producing substances. Inorganic and potentially carcinogenic organic substances may still escape untreated into the drinking water. Alternatives such as distillation and reverse osmosis units are improvements, but they still have their problems. Distillation is very expensive because it is energy consumptive and in areas with hard water the unit needs servicing frequently. Reverse osmosis units are able to remove contaminants well, but the membranes are very delicate and need constant inspection, and the volume of water processed by the system is limited.

The best alternative for home water purification seems to be a multiple-stage system that first has a filter to remove sediment, followed by a carbon absorption unit to remove organic materials and chlorinated hydrocarbons, and then an exchange resin to remove toxic inorganic materials and reduce the hardness and residue. This will produce water equivalent in quality to double distillation without the high energy cost and equipment problem because the system can work under normal home water pressure.

In areas of the United States where water is heavily polluted, or aquifers have been contaminated by leaching of pollutants from chemical industries, purification of all cooking and drinking water is essential in reducing the exposure to water-borne carcinogens and toxins. Remember that, between cooking and drinking, water is a large proportion of what you take into your system, so its quality is very important in establishing your overall health.

Table 6

Summary of the Nutraerobics Program for Cancer Risk Reduction

Component	Reduces risk to:
Stop smoking	Lung cancer
Reduced alcohol	Digestive and breast cancer
Reduced fat	Breast, ovarian, and colon cancer
Increased fiber	Colon cancer
Reduced nitrates and other additives	Bladder, stomach, and digestive cancer
Lactobacillus-cultured dairy products	Colon-rectal cancer
Increased vitamin C	All cancers
Increased zinc, copper, selenium, and manganese	All cancers
Reduced estrogen exposure	Breast, uterine, ovarian cancer
Reduced caffeine	Breast and pancreatic cancer
Increased beta-carotene	Lung cancer
Normalized vitamin A	All cancers
Reduced exposure to ultraviolet light and X-rays	Skin cancer

Summary of the Program

If you are confused, it is understandable—there is considerable material in this chapter. Let's use the summary of the Nutraerobics Program approach to reducing cancer risk as shown in Table 6.

The major objective of the Nutraerobics Program is to design a lifestyle that minimizes your exposure to known cancer-producing substances and activates your immune defense system to its maximum extent. When you are thinking good thoughts and positively reinforcing yourself with the way you live, your immune system is unbelievably successful in winning the battle in which weak cancer cells are pitted against the strong lymphocytes. You don't have to lead a strange lifestyle to reduce your cancer risk by a third or more; following Table 6 will do it. Let your knowledge of your biotype be your guide and enjoy life while contributing to the reduction in risk to cancer.

Changes in hormone levels may be associated with dietary and lifestyle changes. This not only may change the risk to cancer, but also to other specific male and female health problems. The next chapter will explore the management of these specific male and female difficulties.

Notes

1. *Diet, Nutrition and Cancer* (Washington, DC: National Academy Press, 1982).

2. P. Hausman, "The Cancers of Affluence," *Nutrition Action,* (December 1981):7.

3. "Massive Data on Cancer Risk Factors Compiled," *Chemical and Engineering News* (17 August 1981):20.

4. *Diet, Nutrition and Cancer.*

5. L. J. Kinlen, "Meat and Fat Consumption and Cancer Mortality," *Lancet* (24 April 1982):946.

6. T. H. Maugh, "Cancer is Not Inevitable," *Science, 217,* 36(1982).

7. E. Frei, "The National Cancer Chemotherapy Program," *Science, 217,* 600(1982).

8. C. G. Moertel et al., "A Clinical Trial of Amygdalin (Laetrile) in the Treatment of

Human Cancer," *New England Journal of Medicine, 306,* 201(1982).

9. A. S. Relman, "Closing the Books on Laetrile," *New England Journal of Medicine, 306,* 236(1982).

10. E. Farber, "Chemical Carcinogenesis," *New England Journal of Medicine, 305,* 1379(1981).

11. L. S. Alexander and H. M. Goff, "Chemicals, Cancer, and Cytochrome P-450," *Journal of Chemical Education, 59,* 179(1982).

12. G. Kolata, "Cell Biology Yields Clues to Lung Cancer," *Science, 218,* 38(1982).

13. R. B. Shekelle and J. Stamler, "Dietary Vitamin A and the Risk of Cancer in the Western Electric Study," *Lancet* (28 November 1981):1185.

14. M. J. Stampfer and C. H. Hennekens, "Carotene, Carrots, and White Blood Cells," *Lancet* (11 September 1982):615.

15. "Dietary Carotene and the Risk of Lung Cancer," *Nutrition Reviews, 40,* 265(1982).

16. G. Wolf, "Is Dietary B-Carotene an Anti-Cancer Agent," *Nutrition Reviews, 40,* 257(1982).

17. "Cholesterol, Cancer and Stroke," *Nutrition and the M.D., 8,* 1(1982).

18. J. D. Kark and C. G. Hames, "Retinol, Carotene, and the Cancer/Cholesterol Connection," *Lancet* (20 June 1981):1371.

19. B. Y. LeGardeur, "Vitamins A, C, and E in Relation to Lung Cancer Incidence," *American Journal of Clinical Nutrition, 35,* 851(1982).

20. C. Luer, "Sharks Fed Carcinogens in Cancer Study," *Clinical Chemistry News* (June 1982):15.

21. J. Murray, "Toward a Nutritional Concept of Host Resistance to Malignancy and Infection," *Perspectives in Biology and Medicine* (Winter 1981):290.

22. E. Gresser, M. T. Thomas, and D. Broute-Boye, "Interferon and Cell Division," *Proceedings of Experimental Biology and Medicine, 137,* 1285(1971).

23. R. A. Good and G. Fernandes, "Nutritional Modulation of Immune Responses," *Federation Proceedings," 39,* 3098(1980).

24. M. F. McCarty, "Optimized Mitochondrial Function as a Nutritional Strategy in Cancer Immunotherapy," *Medical Hypotheses, 7,* 50(1981).

25. M. E. Weksler and G. Goldstein, "Immunological Studies on Aging IV. The Contribution of the Thymus Involution to Immune Deficiencies," *Journal of Experimental Medicine, 148,* 996(1978).

26. R. J. Shamberger and C. E. Willis, "Selenium Distributions and Human Cancer Mortality," *CRC Critical Review Clinical Laboratory Science, 2,* 211(1971).

27. G. N. Schrauzer, "Effects of Selenium and Arsenic on the Genesis of Mammary Tumors in Mice," *Annals of Clinical and Laboratory Science, 4,* 441(1974).

28. G. N. Schrauzer, "Cancer Mortality Correlation Studies III. Statistical Associations with Dietary Selenium Intakes," *Bioinorganic Chemistry, 7,* 23(1977).

29. G. N. Schrauzer, "Selenium and Cancer: A Review," *Bioinorganic Chemistry, 5,* 275(1976).

30. L. S. Hurley, "Manganese and Other Trace Elements," in *Present Knowledge in Nutrition,* 4th ed. (New York: The Nutrition Foundation, 1976), p. 345.

31. S. J. Weiss and A. F. LoBaglio, "Superoxide Generation by Human Monocytes," *American Journal of Hematology, 4,* 1(1978).

32. N. F. Khmara, "Effect of Manganese on Ubiquinone Content in Rats," *UK Biokhim Zh, 40,* 367(1968).

33. P. Gounby, "Research on Vitamin-Cancer Relationship Getting Big Boost," *Journal of the American Medical Association, 247,* 1799(1982).

34. R. Anderson and A. J. van Rensburg, "The Effects of Increasing Weekly Doses of Ascorbate on Certain Cellular and Humoral Immune Functions in Normal Volunteers," *American Journal of Clinical Nutrition, 33,* 71(1980).

35. E. Cameron and L. Pauling, "Supplemental Ascorbate in the Supportive Treatment of Cancer: Prolongation of Survival Times in Terminal Human Cancer," *Proceedings of the National Academy of Sciences, USA, 73,* 3685(1976).

36. E. T. Creagan and S. Frytak, "Failure of High-Dose Vitamin C Therapy to Benefit Patients with Advanced Cancer," *New England Journal of Medicine, 301,* 687(1979).

37. A. B. Kallner and D. H. Hornig, "On the Requirements of Ascorbic Acid in Man: Steady State Turnover in Smokers," *American Journal of Clinical Nutrition, 34,* 1347(1981).

38. C. E. Myers and R. C. Young, "Adriamycin: The Role of Lipid Peroxidation in Cardiac Toxicity and Tumor Response," *Science, 197,* 165(1977).

39. T. K. Basu, "Significance of Vitamins in Cancer," *Oncology, 33,* 183(1976).

40. T. K. Basu and D. C. Williams, "The Thiamine Status of Cancer Patients,"

International Journal of Vitamin and Nutrition Research, 44, 53(1974).

41. L. Rosenberg et al., "Breast Cancer and Alcoholic Beverage Consumption," *Lancet* (30 January 1982):267

42. B. Zumoff, "The Role of Endogenous Estrogen Excess in Human Breast Cancer," *Anticancer Research, 1,* 39(1981).

43. S. G. Silverberg and E. L. Makowski, "Endometrial Carcinoma in Young Women Taking Oral Contraceptive Agents," *Obstetrics and Gynecology, 46,* 503(1975).

44. B. S. Hulka and B. G. Greenberg, "Protection Against Endometrial Carcinoma by Combination-Product Oral Contraceptives," *Journal of the American Medical Associaton, 247,* 475(1982).

45. B. MacMahon and J. Brown, "Age at Menarche, Urine Estrogens, and Breast Cancer Risk," *International Journal of Cancer, 74,* 117(1982).

46. A. J. Levy and S. P. Markey, "Light Suppresses Melatonin Secretion in Humans," *Science, 210,* 1267(1980).

47. D. G. Kingston, "Mutagen Implicated in Human Colon Cancer," *Chemical and Engineering News* (27 September 1982):22.

48. D. Kromhout and C. Coulander, "Dietary Fibre and 10 Year Mortality From Coronary Heart Disease, Cancer and All Causes," *Lancet* (4 September 1982):518.

49. K. M. Shahani and A. Kilara, "Natural Antibiotic Activity of Lactobacillus Acidophilus and Bulgaricus," *Cultured Dairy Products Journal, 11,* 14(1976).

50. Natasha Trenev, private communication, No. Hollywood, California; D. K. Sinha, "Development of Nonfermented Acidophilus

Milk and Testing its Properties," Doctoral Dissertation, University of Nebraska, 1979.

51. L. Kolonel and M. W. Hinds, "Association of Diet and Place of Birth with Stomach Cancer Incidence in Hawaii Japanese and Caucasians," *American Journal of Clinical Nutrition, 39,* 2478(1981).

52. A. Feinstein and R. N. Battista, "Coffee and Pancreatic Cancer," *Journal of the* *American Medical Association, 246,* 957(1981).

53. R. J. Bull, "Health Effects of Drinking Water Disinfectants," *Environmental Science and Technology, 16,* 554(1982).

54. J. D. Miller, "The New Pollution: Ground Water Contamination," *Environment, 24,* 8(1982).

9

Male and Female Problems

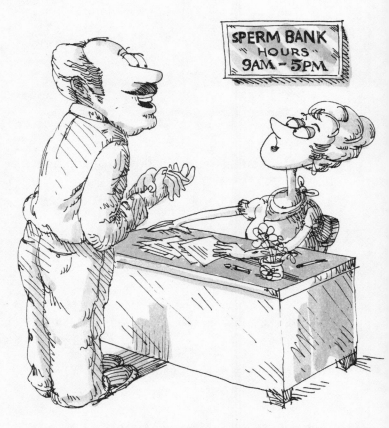

TELL ME, PLEASE, WHAT ARE YOUR CURRENT INTEREST RATES?

For women only:

1. Do you suffer from difficult periods?

1	2	3	4
No	Occasionally	Frequently	Always

2. Do you have breast tenderness or lumps?

1	2	3	4
No	Occasionally	Frequently	Always

3. Do you have premenstrual depression or tension?

1	2	3	4
No	Occasionally	Frequently	Always

4. Do you have excessive facial or body hair?

1	2	4
No	Some	Yes, extensive

5. Are you wrinkling faster than you should, have prematurely gray hair, or stretch marks on your skin?

1	2	4
No	Somewhat	Yes

For men only:

1. Do you suffer from a low sex drive?

1	2	3	4
No	Occasionally	Frequently	Always

2. Do you have a high blood pressure problem?

1	2	4
No	Some	Yes

3. Do you have prostate problems?

1	2	4
No	Moderate	Yes

4. Do you carry excess fat in your chest and upper arms?

1	2	4
No	Some	Yes, extensive

5. Do you smoke or drink alcoholic beverages routinely?

1	2	4
No	Somewhat	Probably more than I should

If your total score exceeds 12 you may have a hormone imbalance, and you should concentrate on this chapter.

Fortunately, to keep life interesting, there are very significant differences between men and women. These differences result in need for modification of the Nutraerobics Program according to sex-related uniquenesses. The diet and lifestyle needed to optimize a woman's physiological function may be different from those for a man, and in this chapter we explore those subtle differences and unique problems related to the specificity of the male and female of the species.

It is hard to believe, but it is now felt that the difference between the sexes is to a great extent determined by differences in the levels of exquisitely small amounts of substances called steroid hormones. These hormones, such as estrogen, progesterone, and testosterone, modulate the development of the fetus and give rise to certain characteristics we associate with males and females. They also have impact upon the functioning of men and women throughout their entire lives.

Hormones are actually produced as a result of a complex series of reactions that starts in the brain. The brain releases certain substances into the bloodstream that travel to the various hormone-secreting organs and stimulate the release of hormones such as testosterone from the testes or estrogen from the ovaries, which then have their effect upon adjacent tissues. The hormones also travel in the bloodstream back to the brain in a feedback process that tells the brain to turn off the secretion of any more releasing substances, a mechanism that regulates the proper levels of hormones.

Stress and Hormone Levels

As with any system in the body, however, there are ways this self-controlling system can be interrupted and cause either excessive or deficient amounts of specific hormones. Because these hormones are released as a result of chemical messages received from the brain, it is possible that features of your lifestyle can have an impact upon the production of hormones, and we know that hormones have a distinct influence on behavior and function. As mentioned earlier, studies have indicated that pregnant women under very high stress may expose the fetus to differing levels of hormones **in utero** and actually alter the development and possibly even the behavior of their offspring.[1] And an interesting experiment was done in Sweden indicating that stress and demanding physiological tasks may have a direct suppressive effect upon certain hormone secretions.[2] Men who enlisted in a special forces branch of the army were placed under very rigorous and demanding requirements for two weeks with virtually no sleep. They were tested during the course of this training, and after a period of ten days it was found that their testosterone levels were actually lower than those of women of a comparable age.

Nutrients and Hormones

The hormones estrogen, progesterone, and testosterone are all derived in your body from cholesterol, which is manufactured in the liver. Since the metabolism of cholesterol is under certain aspects of dietary control, so is the production of these hormones. The receptivity of certain tissues to the action of these hormones may also be regulated by essential nutrients, so once again tailoring nutrition and lifestyle to meet your biotype needs may help normalize hormonal problems previously unrecognized as being related to your lifestyle.

As work continues on the essential nutrients needed to optimize human function, it becomes clear that there are major differences between the needs of men and those of women. The most recent RDA (1980) for females up to the age of 19 years recommends significantly different levels of specific nutrients than that for males of the same age. Young females require a substantially greater iron intake than males of the same age; however, it is difficult to establish the individual requirement for a specific woman, as the need can vary widely.

Women and Iron Deficiency

Iron deficiency is a potential problem from adolescence to menopause and can make women highly susceptible to a variety of anemias (lack of adequate red blood cells or hemoglobin). Anemia may be the result of both inadequate iron intake, due to the consumption of iron-poor foods or dieting, and the increased iron requirement women have because of menstruation and childbearing. (Not all anemias are directly related to iron deficiency, however; some are related to inadequate intakes of folic acid, vitamin B-12, and copper, which we discuss later in this chapter.) Studies done by the USDA have indicated that 40 percent of women have an iron deficiency, based on an RDA of 18 milligrams per day. One of the difficulties in establishing a specific optimal amount for iron in women is that intestinal absorption can vary widely from individual to individual. It is well known that vitamin C enhances the absorption of iron, whereas substances such as tannin in tea and phosphorus in processed foods depress iron absorption.[3]

The requirement for iron is substantially increased during pregnancy; the total increased need for iron during gestation, to compensate for the baby's need, is approximately 750 milligrams. A daily supplement of 30 to 60 milligrams of elemental iron is therefore recommended during pregnancy. If dietary iron is deficient, the fetus tends to deplete the mother's stores of iron, leading to a maternal anemia. The levels of intake of the other nutrients that work with iron to prevent anemias range between 400 and 1000 micrograms of folic acid, 5 to 20 micrograms of vitamin B-12, and 2 to 5 milligrams of copper daily.

A chronic deficiency of iron in women may lead to increased susceptibility to infection. The early warning manifestations of iron deficiency include: cracks at the corners of the nose and mouth, spooning of the fingernails, a painful and red tongue, and intestinal and muscle pain. One interesting symptom associated with iron deficiency is a red or pink color imparted to the urine after an iron-deficient individual consumes a half cup of diced beets. Treatment with iron leads to disappearance of the color in the urine within a week. Some investigators have suggested that the pink or red color in the urine after eating beets is the result of low stomach acid secretion, which leads to malabsorption of the iron. This can be treated either by giving betaine hydrochloride as a stomach acid replacement, or more iron and vitamin C.[4]

Behavioral changes are also very common in chronic iron deficiency, often manifesting themselves as compulsive eating habits: a person may eat one food in large quantities without control or crave ice. The compulsive eating of ice, called phagophagia, can also be found in women who have had blood loss due to unrecognized hemorrhages or bleeding cystic ovaries.

In children, iron deficiency has been characterized as leading to decreased attention span and problems with perception. Children appear solemn and irritable, a condition that seems to be amplified during the first few years of menstruation in adolescent girls.[5]

The times of greatest susceptibility to iron deficiency in women occur as a girl moves into adolescence, when she increases her total iron stores by 25 percent during her growth spurt—yet most teenage diets are deficient in iron. Other times an iron deficiency can show itself in a woman are during childbearing, when she is under heavy exercise demand, or when she has unusually heavy flow during the menses. A vegetarian diet may aggravate the condition because it provides little absorbable iron unless it is high in vitamin C, (more than 250 milligrams of vitamin C per day, taken along with the food). Other women suspected to be at increased risk to iron deficiency include chronic aspirin users, or women whose tests show low hemoglobin and hematocrit levels in their blood with a low mean corpuscular volume (MCV). In these cases an iron supplement of 20 to 40 milligrams per day, in a chelated or complexed form may be needed. Inorganic iron salts such as ferrous fumarate or ferrous sulphate tend to produce intestinal problems at these doses and may not be very useful.[6]

Unless there is an iron deficiency, iron should not be used in excessive quantities because it can accumulate in the body and lead to toxic side effects; accumulation in the joint spaces causes arthritic-like pain. Exceeding 30 to 40 milligrams per day in the nonpregnant woman should be monitored carefully for potential side effects of toxicity if continued for an extended period of time.

Women and Hypothyroidism

Another problem more prevalent in women is hypothyroidism, the condition in which an underactive thyroid gland results in a lowered metabolic rate and general loss of vigor. Clinical hypothyroidism is generally diagnosed by a blood test indicating the levels of various thyroid hormones or the hormone secreted from the brain that stimulates the production these hormones. This test is not very good, however, for identifying a borderline or chronic hypothyroid condition. A better way of detecting borderline hypothyroidism in women is to take the underarm temperature upon waking, but before rising, each morning for a period of two weeks. The average temperature is related to the thyroid gland's activity, and a low body temperature upon waking —below 97.8° F, on the average—suggests borderline hypothyroidism.[7]

Recently, borderline or subclinical hypothyroidism has been associated with infertility in women.[8] In a study of 150 women aged 25 to 34 years who had long-standing infertility due to the inability to ovulate, it was found that a great percentage of them were subclinically hypothyroid when monitored by detailed biochemical testing. Normalizing thyroid function led to improved ovulation and a number of the women became pregnant. The investigators conclude that subclinical hypothyroidism may be of greater importance in infertile women with menstrual disorders than is usually thought, and that standard screening methods used by doctors to evaluate thyroid function are inadequate to pick up this problem.

Subclinical hypothyroidism may be the result of either of two different problems. Either the thyroid gland itself is not secreting enough thyroid hormone, which could be the result of iodine deficiency, or the hormone that is secreted is not being properly activated, so that it does not have the properties necessary to stimulate ovulation. In exploring these two possibilities, investigators found that a zinc deficiency may impair the conversion of the released thyroid hormone to its active substance.[9] Because so many women are on diet programs and because our foods are so poor in zinc, it may be very common for a woman to be chronically zinc deficient and therefore, in this case, subclinically hypothyroid. Other symptoms of a zinc deficiency include poor appetite, eczema, lethargy, and increased susceptibility to infection.

Anorexia Nervosa and Bulimia

Anorexia nervosa, in which an individual virtually starves herself, is recognized as a complex condition related to psychophysiological problems occurring predominately in adolescent girls and characterized by emaciation, fear of gaining weight, and distortions of body image. Recently it has been suggested that anorexia nervosa may also have a direct relationship to a zinc deficiency state, in that a zinc deficiency can depress appetite.[10] In one study, thirty female patients hospitalized for anorexia nervosa were found to have very poor perception for bitter and sour taste; foods were generally perceived as tasteless. The administration of zinc at the level of 30 milligrams per day led to improved taste perception and improved appetite. Whether a zinc deficiency actually causes anorexia nervosa or whether it is associated with the symptoms of this condition is yet undetermined, but zinc supplementation did result in improved appetite.

Bulimia, on the other hand, is binge eating; the term literally means "ox hunger" or a voracious appetite. This syndrome, only recognized since 1980, is characterized by the sudden, impulsive ingestion of a large amount of food in a short period of time; it may not necessarily lead to obesity, because many bulimic individuals purposely vomit to get rid of their meals right after eating. It has been estimated that the ratio of bulimia to anorexia nervosa is four to one. It appears that bulimia is related to a great extent to certain behavior problems. It has been reported that almost half the patients with anorexia nervosa experience episodes of bulimia and that 43 percent of these had eating bouts at least several times a week.[11] Not only hunger but frustration, tension, emptiness, and boredom apparently induce the craving for food. Binging and purging dispel the tension, even though accompanied by a constant fear of not being able to stop eating. Frequent vomiting can lead to irritation of the throat and extensive dental erosion and decay. Bulimia is associated with menstrual disturbances, especially amenorrhea or the lack of menstrual periods.[11] Because of the similarities between anorexia nervosa and bulimia, it has been suggested that zinc supplementation, along with a good high-potency B-complex vitamin supplement and psychological counseling, may be helpful in the management of this condition.

The psychological profile most often seen in the anorexic or bulimic is that of an intellectually gifted, hard-driving individual who sets high (often unachievable) goals and standards. The expectations for personal accomplishment or achievement may be continually increased by these individuals, so that they never reach their goals. The resulting sense of frustration can be displaced into an eating disorder related to fear of physical imperfections. Interestingly, it has recently been found that this same personality profile is found in males who are compulsive runners. This may indicate that compulsive personality disorders exhibit an abnormal fear of fatness.

Premenstrual Tension

Another problem unique to women that has received considerable attention recently is the premenstrual syndrome. In two celebrated legal cases the courts reduced a charge of murder to one of manslaughter on the grounds of diminished responsibility because the defendant was a woman purportedly in the severe throes of premenstrual tension (PMT), a triggering factor in aggression.[12] In the less sensationalized, everyday lives of a large number of women, the premenstrual syndrome can be a very aggravating and frustrating collection of symptoms, including depression, anxiety, and confusion, that a woman may have to look forward to every month until menopause.

A magnesium deficiency has been implicated as a possible factor in some of the symptoms related to premenstrual tension.[13] Many women who have PMT, however, do not show a low blood magnesium level, which has tended to dispute the magnesium-deficiency theory. Recently, however, it was found that although women with PMT may not have low blood magnesium, they may have low magnesium inside the cells, which is where it has its effect. Low cellular magnesium can only be recognized by doing an analysis of a cell such as the red blood cell.[14] Using this type of determination, it was found that women with PMT had significantly lower magnesium content of their red blood cells than women without PMT and suggests that a clinical trial of magnesium at the levels of 200 to 600 milligrams per day two to three days before the onset of the premenstrual syndrome may be helpful. Vitamin B-6 (20–50 mg) and zinc (20–30 mg) have also been used in conjunction with magnesium to help control this problem. The symptoms of PMT can also be aggravated by blood sugar problems, particularly low blood sugar, as discussed in Chapter 5. Lastly, the amino acid tryptophan has been found useful in treating the depression that accompanies PMT in some women.

Oral Contraceptives

The use of oral contraceptives is not without some physiological hazard to women. A number of women have premenstrual tension and depression aggravated by their use. This is sometimes called oral contraceptive–induced depression.

Recently a study was done exploring the factors that affect the relationship of oral contraceptive use to ovarian cancer. One hundred forty-four women under the age of 60 who had had ovarian cancer and 139 women under the age of 60 who were selected from the general population without cancer were screened for their various health habits and oral contraceptive use. In younger women taking oral contraceptives there appeared to be a statistical increase of risk to ovarian cancer compared to women the same age not taking the medication.[15] This study contradicts previous studies that suggested there may be a decreased risk to ovarian cancer in women taking oral contraceptives. The authors point out that the previous studies did not take into account such factors as age at first use, length of use, recentness of use, or the type of formulation. The study went on to indicate that the greatest risk was in women who had not had children, who were under the age of 40, who had initiated the use of oral contraceptives in their middle teens, and who had continued them for many years.

Data also suggest that there may be an increase in ovarian or uterine cysts after prolonged use of oral contraceptives, and these tumors in women under 40 are related to the increased incidence of malignancy. It was found that in older women who have had children, the use of oral contraceptive medication does not increase, but may actually reduce, the risk of ovarian epithelial tumors.[16]

It is also well known that women who are on oral contraceptives have greater need for zinc and vitamin B-6, as well as folic acid, and that the supplementation of these three agents may be very useful in preventing some of the adverse psychological side effects of oral contraceptive medication, including depression and anxiety.[17] Recommended maintenance levels for women on oral contraceptives are 20 milligrams of zinc, 25 milligrams of vitamin B-6, and 800 micrograms of folic acid.[18]

Folic Acid and Cervical Dysplasia

One of the adverse side effects of taking oral contraceptives is a thickening of the wall of the cervix and increased tendency toward bleeding and cyst formation, called cervical dysplasia. In a recent double-blind study of 47 young women with mild or moderate dysplasia of the uterine cervix, which had been diagnosed by Pap smears, the supplementation of their diet with folic acid at 10,000 micrograms per day for three months led to reversal of the condition and a return to normal cervical tissue.[19]

The dose of folic acid used in this study would certainly be considered a supplemental dose, in that normal dietary levels are about 400 micrograms per day. To get the high dose used in this study as a supplement would require many tablets in the United States, as the FDA has limited the amount of folic acid in a nonpregnancy formula to 400 micrograms and in a pregnancy formula to 800 micrograms per tablet. Folic acid is not a toxic vitamin, but if given in supplemental doses to a person who is vitamin B-12 deficient, it can mask the symptoms of a vitamin B-12 deficiency and lead to irreversible nervous system damage. In order to prevent this, a limit was put on the level of folic acid in a supplement below that which would mask the vitamin B-12 deficiency. When initiating any folic acid therapy, therefore, it is important for the patient to be getting the proper amounts of B-12; supplemental B-12 or a vitamin B-12 injection may be necessary.

Dysmenorrhea

Dysmenorrhea—women suffering from this condition have painful, heavy periods—sometimes with serious psychological problems is a significant problem for many women. A new medical treatment utilizes a series of hormone inhibitors called prostaglandin inhibitors to provide relief from menstrual cramps.[20] One of these substances, called flufenamic acid, was demonstrated to provide complete relief of menstrual cramps in sixteen patients studied. Based upon this work, it seems that excessive production of a few of the prostaglandin hormones may be the cause of the pain, cramping, backache, diarrhea, headache, and insomnia associated with dysmenorrhea. One of these prostaglandins, which is called prostaglandin F-2-alpha, is manufactured in the uterine wall and exerts a muscle-contracting effect.

A nutritional approach to the management of dysmenorrhea has become available through the recognition that certain dietary fatty substances can also serve as blocking agents for prostaglandins like F-2-alpha. One of these substances is called MaxEPA, which is a registered trademark for a fish oil concentrate that is rich in a fatty acid called omega-3-eicosapentaenoic acid. This material is used in the body to manufacture a specific prostaglandin able to counteract the activity of the native prostaglandin manufactured by some dysmenorrheic women in excessive quantities. Supplemental doses of MaxEPA from 3 to 10 grams a day, along with vitamin B-6 (20 mg), zinc (20 mg), magnesium (200 mg), calcium (400 to 600 mg), and where necessary the amino acid tryptophan (1–2 g), have led to considerable reduction of menstrual pain and cramping in some women.

It is also known that menstrual activity and difficulty with the menses are related to other aspects of lifestyle, diet, for example. High-fat diets can alter hormone levels and can contribute to increased problems with menstruation.[21] For women who have a considerable problem with dysmenorrhea, a diet consisting of increased complex carbohydrates, moderate protein, and reduced fat would be suggested. Many women have found that switching to a more vegetable-based diet is successful in reducing difficulties with the menses.

Exercise and Menstruation

Exercise can reduce the length of time of the menses and in the extreme cases actually produce menstrual irregularity.[22] It was found that only 41 percent of the women who competed in the Montreal Olympics in 1976 had regular menstruation. Physical exercise in which women are pushing themselves to high levels of aerobic training, including such things as running, gymnastics, and ballet dancing, all have been demonstrated to delay the onset of menarche in adolescent girls and once menstruation begins to reduce the time of the menstrual period each month over nonexercising women of the same age. Even female joggers who do a slow and easy 5 to 30 miles per week have been shown to have significantly fewer menses per year than their less energetic counterparts.[23]

Some investigators suggest that the reduced menstrual activity is the result of improved lean body mass, and that extra body fat stores, found more frequently in the nonexercising woman, can trigger prolonged menstruation. It is important to point out, though, that even women who are amenorrheic and have had no periods may still be ovulating and may become pregnant; therefore, exercise is not a fail-safe form of birth control.

What are the long-term consequences for the woman who may have shortened her period or caused menstrual irregularities by exercising? Obstetrically, the prognosis appears good—women athletes have shorter labors and fewer complications in labor.[24] Exercising women also have less dysmenorrhea and more calcium-dense bones than nonexercising women. So the effects of exercising on menstruation do not appear harmful, except possibly in extreme cases where the woman is pushing herself so far that she is actually undergoing muscle wasting or bone loss as a result of her training schedule.

Appetite and Ovulation

Women often experience appetite changes before and after ovulation. It has recently been found that in the preovulatory phase of the cycle—some seven to ten days before ovulation—there is an increase in metabolic activity requiring approximately 300 to 500 calories more per day; after ovulation there is a lowering of the basal metabolic rate and body temperature and the energy requirements go down 300 to 500 calories per day.[25]

This suggests that increased hunger before ovulation may be a result of the woman's natural compensation for increased energy needs, due to the higher basal metabolic rate. During the preovulatory period a woman would lose weight more quickly while dieting than after ovulation when her basal metabolic rate and her energy expenditure go down. This may explain why women have more cyclical plateaus when undergoing weight loss programs than men. These plateaus may be correlated with the effects of the menstrual cycle on basal metabolic rate. It may also account for why women after menopause —after losing the monthly increased metabolic rate—have more difficulty in maintaining proper weight. Exercise may be of value in the menopausal woman for stabilizing basal metabolic rate and helping in weight management.

Smoking and the Menses

One other interesting relationship between the menses and lifestyle is the recent observation that women who smoke have earlier menopause than those who do not.[26] Recent work indicates that smoking women have substantially lower levels of all three of the major estrogens in the first phase of their menstrual cycle than nonsmoking women of the same age.[27] (The effects of smoking on hormone production appear not to be totally selective with women, in that smoking men are found to have much lower levels of the male hormone testosterone than nonsmoking men.[28]) This lowering of estrogen in women may also increase the risk of bone loss from the skeleton, leading to osteoporosis, as estrogen is a skeletal protective hormone. There is some evidence to suggest that smoking women do have higher risk to osteoporosis than nonsmoking women.[29]

Fibrocystic Disease

In fibrocystic disease of the breasts, or cystic mastitis, a woman has breast tenderness correlated with the menstrual cycle, or ongoing breast tenderness that leads to swelling, discomfort, and noticeable lumps in the breast. The majority of these lumps are not cancerous, but rather areas of localized irritation and inflammation. This condition may continue to progress and worsen until menopause. There is strong clinical support that variation in the estrogen levels is a factor in the development of this painful condition.[30] The breast is a site for stimulation by the estrogenic hormones produced by the ovaries, and overstimulation can lead to breast irritation.

Recently, many attempts have been made to evaluate the relationship between fibrocystic problems of the breast and breast cancer. One study found that women who had fibrocystic disease had some sevenfold higher incidence of breast cancer than women without the cystic condition.[31] The association of fibrocystic disease with a higher incidence of breast cancer does not mean that cancer is caused by lumpy breasts; rather, it shows that there may be some underlying mechanism that ties these two problems together.[32] Given this, a biopsy is not suggested in many fibrocystic cases, in that a biopsy itself doubles the risk of breast cancer. Aggressive hormone therapy may also not be called for because of its adverse side effects.

Is there any other way, then, to reduce breast tenderness in the woman suffering from recurrent fibrocystic condition of the breast? Two very interesting reports have appeared recently that demonstrate the impact that diet and lifestyle may have on reducing breast tenderness. These two approaches are vitamin E supplementation and avoidance of caffeine and related substances called methylxanthines.[33]

Supplemental vitamin E at levels of 400 to 600 units per day has been shown very helpful in the treatment of fibrocystic disease, and diets free of coffee, tea, cola, and chocolate, all of which contain methylxanthines, help significantly to reduce breast tenderness in affected women.[34] This list of substances to be avoided also includes other caffeine-containing soft drinks and over-the-counter caffeine-containing medications. Evidence of improvement was found in 88 percent of the women who supplemented with vitamin E and reduced their consumption of the xanthine compounds. In most patients these changes usually took more than two months to become evident; by six months the improvement was dramatic. Some people have worried about adverse side effects of vitamin E taken at this level, but no adverse side effects of significance in long-term supplementation at doses between 400 and 600 units per day have been identified. Very high levels of vitamin E can be related to hypothyroidism in women, but this generally occurs at doses of more than 1000 units per day.[35]

Other Nutrients and the Female

Another vitamin known to have effects on hormones when used in supplemental doses in women is vitamin B-6. When vitamin B-6 is taken in excess of 300 milligrams per day, it has been found to suppress prolactin in women, which may lead to reduced milk production in the lactating woman.[36] On the positive side, vitamin B-6 supplementation at 100 to 200 milligrams per day has been found to increase growth hormones in exercising women and stimulate muscle mass formation in place of fat stores.

One last nutritional impact upon hormone status of great concern to menopausal women is discussed in the next chapter—the effect of

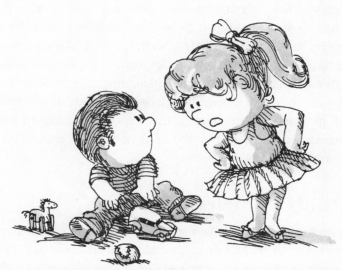

SO WHAT IF WOMEN HAVE THE POTENTIAL FOR HYPOTHYROIDISM, ANOREXIA NERVOSA, BULIMIA, PREMENSTRUAL TENSION, ORAL CONTRACEPTIVE-INDUCED DEPRESSION, OVARIAN CYSTS, CERVICAL DYSPLASIA, DYSMENORRHEA, AND FIBROCYSTIC DISEASES? I STILL ENJOY BEING A GIRL.

meat protein on increasing calcium loss from bone. Two recent studies indicate that excessive dietary protein, particularly from meat, increases the urinary loss of calcium and the potential risk to bone demineralization, especially postmenopausally, after the protective effect of estrogen is lost.[37] When protein consumption exceeds 120 grams per day, there is need to increase calcium intake to accommodate the increased calcium loss. In the absence of increased calcium, a woman will be in a negative calcium balance and have increased risk to the problems of bone loss.

Nutrition for Men

Now, what nutrition and lifestyle modifications pertain specifically to health problems in men?

Vitamin E has a reputation for being a virility vitamin leading to sexual potency. Although this has been demonstrated in rat and mouse studies, it has never been shown to be the case in humans. Vitamin E does, however, have a demonstrated positive effect in the management of one reproductive disorder in males called Peyronies disease. In Peyronies disease a segment of the flexible connective tissue of the penis is replaced with an inelastic scar, which causes distortion upon erection and results in pain.[38] The cause of the scar is not known; however, reports of treatment with 200 to 600 units of vitamin E daily have had 70 to 80 percent success.

Infertility in Males

Male impotency problems have been associated with deficiency states of selenium, zinc, and an amino acid called carnitine. The trace element selenium, found in liver, whole grains grown in soils with adequate selenium, and selenium-rich brewer's yeast, is concentrated in the testes and appears very important in sperm production.[39] Suggested adequate levels are between 100 and 300 micrograms a day as organic selenium. A person consuming a highly processed diet may not be getting adequate selenium and may be at risk not only to inappropriate reproductive function but also to cancer and heart disease, as discussed in Chapters 7 and 8.[40]

Zinc has been found very important in normalizing testosterone production and increasing sperm counts in zinc-deprived males.[41] Levels of zinc intake from 15 to 30 milligram per day are considered important for improving body functions dependent on zinc. In the cases of extreme deprivation, zinc has been used at levels over 100 milligrams per day to improve hormone levels.

It has been suggested that the amino acid carnitine is very important in promoting proper sperm motility.[44] Some men with fertility problems have an adequate number of sperm, but the sperm lack adequate motility, so that infertility results. Men have much higher carnitine levels than women, and carnitine is found to be high in the testes of men.[42]

Carnitine is manufactured in our bodies from the amino acid lysine, and it is known that lysine-depleted animals become infertile due to carnitine insufficiency. The testes seem to be the first tissue to show deficiencies of carnitine or lysine. There is, however, evidence indicating that the carnitine need in some individuals may be greater than the amount they can manufacture in their own bodies, so supplementation becomes essential. Supplements of carnitine from 300 to 800 milligram a day may be helpful; or increasing the level of high-quality dietary protein rich in lysine and methionine, along with vitamin C supplementation, may also stimulate carnitine synthesis in the body.

Many other factors can affect male fertility: mumps at puberty that damages the sperm-producing cells, gonorrhea and other reproductive tract infections that scar the reproductive passages, excessive heat around the scrotum from working near ovens or taking hot baths, drugs like marijuana and alcohol, and exposure to lead and industrial chemicals. Nutrition may play an important role in improving both sperm production and sperm motility in males with nutritionally related problems, but it should be part of a complete program that evaluates these other factors as well.

Wernicke-Korsakoff Syndrome and Osteoarthritis

One problem that may have a relationship to male physiology is an alcohol-induced memory loss condition called the Wernicke-Korsakoff syndrome. Symptoms include mental confusion, disturbances in balance, problems with vision, and short-term memory loss. This syndrome affects men consuming alcohol in large quantities, although the quantity varies from person to person; some men end up with alcohol-induced memory loss at lower levels of alcohol consumption than others.[44] This syndrome is preventable by supplementing with magnesium and vitamin B-1 at levels of 400 to 600 milligram of magnesium and 20 to 200 milligrams of vitamin B-1.

Another problem seen frequently in men is a condition of inflammation of the joints called osteoarthritis. The amino acid L-glutamine and vitamin B-3 in the form of niacinamide have been shown to have a marked anti-inflammatory effect when given orally; they are useful in the management of inflammation associated with arthralgia or arthritis-like pain.[45] Doses range from 500 to 1000 milligrams of L-glutamine three times daily and 100 to 500 milligrams of niacinamide three times daily.

Prostate Problems

One very common problem unique to males is prostatic hypertrophy, or an enlargement of the prostate gland, which can result in pain on urination, a poor urinary flow, and tenderness when sitting. Although the cause of this enlargement can range from low-grade infection to physical irritation, it has been found that symptom relief can be achieved in many men by using vitamin E (400 to 800 units), zinc (20 to 40 mg), flax seed oil, which is rich in linolenic acid (6 to 10 g), and selenium (100 to 300 mcg) daily. This therapy needs to be continued for six to eight weeks to determine if it will be successful. A number of men with prostate problems have found that the problems return when they terminate the program, only to go away again when the supplements are resumed.

Light and Health

Lastly, the other lifestyle alteration that may be necessary for improving hormone balance in men and women and reducing arthritis-like pain is exposure of the unshielded eyes to full-spectrum sunlight. Sunlight may be "an essential nutrient" for many individuals, in that it stimulates the secretion of certain hormones, such as melatonin, which controls estrogen secretion in women.[46]

In a recent study, the effect of full-spectrum sunlight on individuals 40 to 60 years of age who had had the diagnosis of rheumatoid arthritis was examined. The results of the study indicated that expo-sure to wave lengths of light nearer the blue portion of the solar spectrum, which are not found in fluorescent lights or incandescent bulbs to any great extent, reduced pain, and the longer the exposure to the light, the more pain reduction occurred.[47]

This is very important, because we as a society are living more of our life indoors, illuminated by synthetic lighting that may be very poor in the blue portion of the sun's spectrum. This component appears necessary for proper stimulation of the endocrine or hormone system. Although this observation has been delineated in men as being impor-tant, it undoubtedly has impact on women as well. Even when we are out of doors, we commonly use sunglasses or eyeglasses, which block out the blue portion of the spectrum and may be similar in impact to living indoors. Exposure of the uncovered eye to full-spectrum sunlight seems an essential part of a person's defense against sex hormone imbalances. This may explain why some people taking their vacation in Florida, Hawaii, or the Caribbean come home for the first time with the absence of those aches and pains that they went on vacation with. It is another example of the important subtle role that the environment plays in controlling aspects of our function.

In the next chapter we will explore the Nutraerobics bone loss prevention relationships, and detail ways of keeping the calcium in your bones where it should be.

Notes

1. J. D. Yalom and N. Fisk, "Prenatal Exposure to Female Hormones: Effect on Psychosexual Development in Boys," *Archives of General Psychiatry, 28,* 554(1973).

2. "Prenatal Determination of Adult Sexual Behavior," *Lancet* (21 November 1981):1149.

3. M. Winick, *Nutritional Disorders of American Women* (New York: Wiley, 1977).

4. F. A. Oski, "The Nonhematologic Manifestations of Iron Deficiency," *American Journal of Disabilities in Children, 133,* 315(1979).

5. M. Chrisholm, "Tissue Changes Associated with Iron Deficiency," *Clinical Haematology, 2,* 303(1979).

6. J. Williams, "Iron Deficiency Treatment," *Western Journal of Medicine, 134,* 496(1981).

7. B. Barnes, in *Hypothyroidism: The Unsuspected Illness* (New York: Random House, 1974).

8. H. G. Bohnet and F. A. Leidenberger, "Subclinical Hypothyroidism and Infertility," *Lancet* (5 December 1981):1278.

9. J. E. Morley and J. M. Hershman, "Zinc Deficiency, Chronic Starvation and Hypothalamic-Pituitary-Thyroid Function," *American Journal of Clinical Nutrition, 33,* 1767(1980).

10. R. C. Casper and J. M. Davis, "An Evaluation of Trace Metals, Vitamins and Taste Function in Anorexia Nervosa," *American Journal Clinical Nutrition, 33,* 1801(1980).

11. R. C. Casper, "Bulimia and Diet," *Archives of General Psychiatry, 37,* 1030(1980).

12. P. T. D'Orban, "Premenstrual Syndrome: A Disease of the Mind," *Lancet* (19 December 1981):1415.

13. A. Nicholas, "Treatment of the Premenstrual Syndrome with Magnesium," in J. Durlach, ed., *First International Symposium on Magnesium Deficiency in Human Pathology* (Paris: Springer-Verlag, 1973), p. 261.

14. G. E. Abraham and M. M. Lubran, "Serum and Red Cell Magnesium in Patients with Premenstrual Tension," *American Journal of Clinical Nutrition, 34,* 2364(1981).

15. D. W. Cramer and R. C. Knapp, "Factors Affecting the Association of Oral Contraceptives and Ovarian Cancer," *New England Journal of Medicine, 307,* 1047(1982).

16. J. L. Bennington and S. L. Haber, "Incidence and Relative Frequency of Benign and Malignant Ovarian Neophasms," *Obstetrics and Gynecology, 32,* 627(1968).

17. B. T. Nobbs, "Pyridoxal Phosphate Status in Clinical Depression," *Lancet* (9 March 1974):405.

18. D. P. Rose and P. W. Adams, "EGOT Activities and Effect of Vitamin B-6 Supplementation in Women Using Oral Contraceptives," *American Journal of Clinical Nutrition, 26,* 48(1973).

19. C. E. Butterworth and C. L. Krumdieck, "Improvement in Cervical Dysplasia Associated with Folic Acid Therapy in Users of Oral Contraceptives," *American Journal of Clinical Nutrition, 35,* 73(1982).

20. J. R. Dingfelder, "Prostaglandin Inhibitors," *New England Journal of Medicine, 307,* 746(1982).

21. P. Hill and E. L. Wynder, "Diet, Lifestyle and Menstrual Activity," *American Journal of Clinical Nutrition, 33,* 1192(1980).

22. "Running, Jumping, and Amenorrhea," *Lancet* (18 September 1982):638.

23. E. Dale and A. L. Wilhite, "Menstrual Dysfunction in Distance Runners," *Obstetrics and Gynecology," 54,* 47(1979).

24. G. J. Erdelyi, "Gynecological Survey of Female Athletes," *Journal of Sports Medicine and Physical Fitness," 2,* 174(1962); R. W. Rebar, "Reproductive Function in Women Athletes," *Journal of American Medicine Association, 246,* 14(1981).

25. S. J. Solomon and D. H. Calloway, "Menstrual Cycle and Basal Metabolic Rate

in Women," *American Journal of Clinical Nutrition, 36,* 611(1982).

26. H. Jick, J. Porter, and A. S. Morrison, "Relation Between Smoking and Age of Natural Menopause," *Lancet* (14 April 1977):1345.

27. B. MacMahon, P. Cole, and J. Brown, "Cigarette Smoking and Urinary Estrogens," *New England Journal of Medicine, 307,* 1062(1982).

28. Surgeon General of the United States, *The Health Consequences of Smoking: A Report of the Surgeon General,* (Washington, DC: U.S. Dept. of Health and and Human Services, 1980), p. 235.

29. H. H. Hussey, "Osteoporosis Among Women Who Smoke Cigarettes," *Journal of American Medical Association, 235,* 1367(1976).

30. P. M. Vogel and K. S. McCarty, "The Correlation of Histologic Changes in the Human Breast with the Menstrual Cycle," *American Journal of Pathology, 104,* 23(1981).

31. M. M. Black and A. J. Asire, "Association of Atypical Characteristics of Benign Breast Lesions with Subsequent Risk of Breast Cancer," *Cancer, 29,* 338(1972).

32. S. M. Love and W. Silen, "Fibrocystic Disease of the Breast," *New England Journal of Medicine, 307,* 1010(1982).

33. R. S. London and P. J. Goldstein, "Medical Management of Mammary Dysplasia," *Obstetrics and Gynecology, 59,* 519(1982).

34. A. Brooks, "Methylxanthines and Their Effect on Fibrocystic Disease of the Breast," *Journal of Reproductive Medicine, 26,* 279(1981).

35. P. M. Farrell and J. G. Bieri, "Megavitamin E Supplementation in Man," *American Journal of Clinical Nutrition, 28,* 1381(1975).

36. C. Moretti and F. Fraroli, "Pyridoxine (B-6) Suppresses the Rise in Prolactin and Increases Growth Hormone Induced by Exercise," *Lancet* (12 August 1982):444.

37. A. Licata, "Acute Effects of Increased Meat Protein on Urinary Electrolytes and Serum Parathyroid Hormone," *American Journal of Clinical Nutrition, 34,* 1779(1981); J. Lutz and H. M. Linkswiter, "Calcium Metabolism in Postmenopausal and Osteoporotic Women Consuming Two Levels of Dietary Protein," *American Journal of Clinical Nutrition, 34,* 2178(1981).

38. C. J. Devine, "Peyronie's Disease," *Journal of American Medical Association, 244,* 392(1980).

39. D. Behne and W. Elger, "Selenium in the Testes of the Rat," *Journal of Nutrition, 112,* 1682(1982).

40. G. Schrauzer, "Selenium in Medicine," *Bioinorganic Chemistry, 6,* 114 (1979).

41. H. H. Sandstead and S. J. Darby, "Human Zinc Deficiency: Endocrine Manifestations and Response to Treatment," *American Journal of Clinical Nutrition, 20,* 422(19697); L. D. Antonious, "Zinc and Sexual Dysfunction," *Lancet* (8 November 1980):1034.

42. G. Cederblad, "Carnitine Levels in the Testes," *Clinica Chim. Acta 67,* 207(1977).

43. P. R. Borum and H. P. Broquist, "Carnitine," *Journal of Nutrition, 107,* 1209(1977).

44. M. Victor and G. H. Collins, *The Wernicke-Korsakoff Syndrome* (Philadelphia: F. A. Davis, 1971).

45. P. Jain and N. K. Khanna, "Evaluation of Anti-inflammatory and Analgesic Properties of L-glutamine," *Agents and Actions, 11,* 3(1981).

46. J. Ott, *Light and Health* (New York: Bantam, 1977).

47. S. F. McDonald, "Effect of Visible Lightwaves on Arthritis Pain," *International Journal for Biosocial Research, 3,* 49(1982).

10

Bone Loss and Calcium
Where It Shouldn't Be

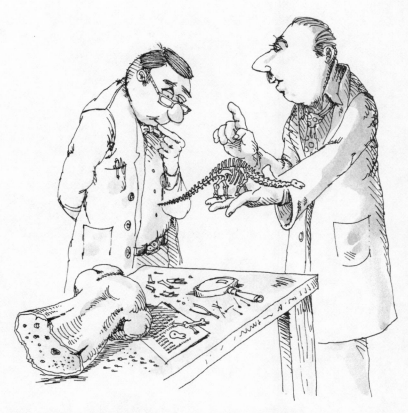

EITHER WE HAVE DISCOVERED A NEW SPECIES OF DINOSAUR, OR THAT'S THE MOST EXTREME EXAMPLE OF BONE LOSS I'VE EVER SEEN.

1. Do you have arthritis, osteoporosis, or kidney stones?

1	2	3	4
No	Occasionally	Frequently	All the time

2. Do you suffer from the loss of teeth due to gum disease (periodontal problems)?

1	2	3	4
No	Small Amount	It's a problem	Extensive tooth loss

3. Are you a postmenopausal female who is eating the standard American diet?

1	4
No	Yes

4. Are your teeth difficult to keep clean due to a lot of calculus formation?

1	2	3	4
No	Occasionally	Frequently	All the time

5. Do you suffer from leg cramps or recurring muscle cramps?

1	2	3	4
No	Occasionally	Frequently	All the time

If your total score exceeds 11 you may have a problem with calcium status and bone loss and you should concentrate on Chapter 10.

You probably consider your skeleton one of the least interesting and least important parts of your body. You assume that those bones are going to be there to hold you up throughout your life and that rather nonliving part of your body is of minor concern. It may come as a surprise to learn that in older age the majority of our health problems are related directly or indirectly to the calcium that is deposited in those bones. Disease conditions such as osteoporosis, which is loss of calcium from bones and easy fracture, periodontal disease, which causes tooth loss due to calcium loss from bones in the jaw, and increased deposition of calcium in muscle tissue and other organs, which leads to a series of diseases called sclerosis, are all associated with aging.

You have a distinct risk of these problems, if your lifestyle includes one or more of the following: smoking, excess alcohol, extreme emotional stress, physical inactivity, little or no consumption of milk or other dairy products, heavy reliance on processed foods, high meat consumption, low citrus fruit consumption, and high intake of empty-calorie foods. These are all characteristics associated with increased risk to bone loss from your skeleton, and increased risk to deposition of this lost calcium in soft tissues like muscles and organs. Loss of bone is an inevitable process of aging, yet the rate at which it is lost is highly dependent upon the individual and his or her own lifestyle. To understand how to prevent bone loss we need to know something about what controls the deposition of calcium in bone and its maintenance throughout one's lifetime.

Control of Calcium

Bone is actually an active tissue like the rest of your body; although it generally turns over a little more slowly than other tissues, it is constantly being broken down and replenished. When calcium is reabsorbed, or removed from bone by the body, new calcium must be deposited in order for your skeleton to remain in a constant state of balance. The control of this process of bone breakdown and bone reformation is one of the most complex areas of human biochemistry.

Bone consists of a complex mineral called hydroxyapatite which is made up of calcium and phosphorus. Your body cannot manufacture calcium and phosphorus; they can only be gotten through the diet. Calcium is poorly absorbed from the diet and needs to be transported into the blood from the intestinal tract by way of specific calcium-binding proteins that are stimulated by vitamin D. Vitamin D can either be gotten directly from the diet or manufactured in the skin when exposed to natural sunlight. Once calcium is in the bloodstream, its deposition in bone is controlled by a hormone released by the thyroid gland called calcitonin. Another hormone, secreted by the parathyroid gland and called parathyroid hormone, controls calcium resorption from bones. When these processes are in balance, your skeleton is neither growing nor diminishing in magnitude and your bone density is constant. When resorption exceeds deposition, however, you are in a net bone loss situation and over time will slowly, progressively, have weaker bones which are more susceptible to spontaneous fracture.[1]

Bone Loss and Aging

Symptoms that may indicate the risk to bone loss are recurring nocturnal leg cramps, heavy plaque or calculus formation around the teeth, recession of the gum line around the teeth, tendency toward kidney stone formation, and osteoarthritic changes in the joints that lead to pain and tenderness. As people get older they tend to lose the ability to manufacture the hormones that stimulate bone reformation and they have higher levels of the hormones that stimulate bone calcium resorption.

Therefore, as one gets older it is more and more important to pay attention to the lifestyle and dietary factors that contribute to improved bone calcium balance. Some of the things that contribute to bone loss in the older individual are: physical inactivity, removal of milk from the diet, decreased exposure to natural sunlight, increased dependency upon highly processed foods which are low in calcium and high in phosphorus, and the attendant hormonal changes associated with aging. Sadly, conditions like osteoarthritis or osteoporosis are common in the older segment of our population, although for many these conditions could be avoided by appropriate modification of diet and lifestyle.

Bone loss occurs particularly in the menopausal woman, who no longer has the additional protective effect of the female hormone estrogen. When estrogen levels decline after menopause, a woman can experience rapid bone loss, the rate dependent upon her health and dietary status at that time. If her bones are already in a weakened state, this bone loss may lead to the clinical signs of osteoporosis at a fairly early age. However, if her bones have high calcium density and the rate of loss can be retarded, then the problem of bone loss may not ever be seen during her lifetime.

Calcium and Your Teeth

Dentists may be one of the first health practitioners to recognize the signs of bone loss because one of the first places in the body where it is seen clinically is in the jaw. Bone loss from the jaw produces pockets around the teeth, allowing bacterial infection and periodontal disease to proceed and ultimately lead to the loss of teeth. Periodontal disease is the major cause of the loss of teeth in the adult and is also the most prevalent degenerative disease in Western society. Some investigators feel that periodontal disease may be an early warning sign to more severe problems of calcium loss, including osteoporosis.[2]

Vitamin D and Your Bones

Vitamin D is converted in the body to a hormone called 1,25 dihydroxivitamin D which is the active substance in the promotion of calcium absorption from the intestines. Proper exposure to sunlight or dietary vitamin D provides enough of the initial substance in the body, but this vitamin D must be converted by our kidneys and livers to the hormonal form for calcium to be properly managed. If your blood is too acidic, it inactivates the conversion of vitamin D to its hormonal form and can prevent proper calcium absorption.[3] Health conditions that can make the blood too acid include diabetes, fasting, or the temporary anaerobic metabolism that occurs when the body is severely strained or overworked (when you want to or have to, you can make your muscles continue to perform even though the bloodstream can't possibly deliver enough oxygen to them at the time; it is this principle that allows you to build up the aerobic condition of whatever portion of your body you're exercising by pushing yourself a little further each time). To decrease blood acidity, the diet should be made higher in alkaline residue foods such as dairy products, vegetables, fruits, and soft grains such as corn, brown rice, or millet, and lower in acid residue foods such as meats, confectionary goods, fats, and highly processed foods.

It has been shown that vitamin D can be manufactured in the skin if you expose 30 percent of your body to the sunlight for half an hour,[4] although this value varies with the latitude and altitude at which you live. If you live in a northern latitude or a cold climate you are not getting as much sunlight as if you lived closer to the equator. Vitamin D supplementation may be required in these cases to promote adequacy, but it should be recalled that excessive vitamin D can lead to toxic side effects promoting calcification of muscles and other organs. The suggested range of dose for vitamin D in the adult is between 400 and 1000 units per day. It is impossible to get a toxic amount of vitamin D by exposing yourself to too much sunlight because the body can regulate the manufacture of vitamin D in your skin.

Calcium and Phosphorus Relationship

The levels of calcium and phosphorus in the diet play a significant role in controlling bone status. As the diet becomes higher in phosphorus and lower in calcium, it encourages bone breakdown and calcium loss from bones. The reason for this is that phosphorus stimulates the secretion of parathyroid hormone which increases calcium resorption, whereas dietary calcium increases the secretion of calcitonin which causes bone reformation.[5]

Recently, it was found that monkeys maintained on a low-calcium, high-phosphorus diet lost skeletal mass continually while on that diet.[6] The loss of skeletal mass does not become symptomatic until the bone loses more than 30 percent of its calcium. This is why many bone problems seem to come on suddenly when the problem has in fact been slowly progressing for years. Interestingly, the dietary calcium-to-phosphorus ratio found to produce these bone loss conditions in monkeys was identical to that seen in the average American diet—about one part calcium for every two parts of phosphorus. When the ratio was one part calcium to one part phosphorus, the bone loss was prevented.

In human studies, it was found that people on a high-phosphorus, low-calcium diet from the consumption of foods rich in phosphate food additives displayed high levels of parathyroid hormone and clinical features suggesting increased bone loss.[7] The authors of the study conclude that the use of phosphate food additives should be carefully controlled in our food supply because they have a stimulating effect on adult bone calcium resorption and lead to net calcium loss. This means you should become a label reader. If you already are, you have noticed in the list of ingredients in foods such things as pyrophosphate, polyphosphate, sodium phosphate, potassium phosphate, or phosphoric acid. These are all phosphate additives that increase the dietary intake of phosphorus with no calcium to balance them. The other major sources of dietary phosphorus not balanced with calcium in the standard American diet include excessive meats, particularly red meat (which has one part of calcium to every thirty parts of phosphorus), and soft drinks (which use phosphorus to reduce acidity that would otherwise actually dissolve teeth). The total amount of phosphorus consumed in diet from all these sources each day is about 1500 to 1700 milligrams which, if compared to only about 800 milligrams of calcium intake every day, causes a distinct calcium imbalance and encourages bone loss.

Protein and Bone Status

A number of medical investigators have recently found that consumption of high levels of dietary protein in excess of 120 grams per day may stimulate bone calcium resorption and encourage long-term bone loss.[8] This may be a particular problem in individuals who are eating protein-rich foods in hopes of managing blood sugar problems. It is quite easy when concentrating on protein-rich foods such as meats at each meal to exceed 120 grams of dietary protein.

The solution to the problem of bone loss appears to be reducing total dietary phosphorus intake by limiting the consumption of meats, reducing soft drink consumption, not depending upon highly processed phosphorus-rich foods, and not exceeding dietary protein limits of about 100 to 120 grams a day, along with increasing calcium and magnesium consumption by eating more dairy products, preferably cultured dairy products (yogurt, kefir, buttermilk), fruits, vegetables, and grains, and where necessary supplementing with calcium.

Calcium Allowance

Increased calcium intake may be important in children who have poor bone growth, in pregnant women who are on a low calcium dietary intake, and in older-age individuals who are susceptible to bone loss problems.[9] Symptoms such as leg cramps at night, loss of bone around the teeth with pocket formation in the gums, sore and swollen joints, and spastic colon may all be indications of relative calcium deficiency.

A number of investigators suggest that the recommended 800 milligrams per day for calcium is actually too low and that a better target value would be 1200 milligrams per day to keep people in proper calcium balance.[10] Even at the level of 800 milligrams per day of calcium, more than 40 percent of the population has been found to be deficient using present dietary intakes as norms. It is very difficult to get 1200 milligrams of calcium in the absence of supplementation if an individual is not consuming dairy products routinely.

Calcium supplementation can best be achieved by using calcium lactate, calcium gluconate, dolomite, or a chelated form of calcium (sometimes labeled a proteinate complex of calcium). Substances such as bone meal may not be as desirable as a source of calcium due to potential lead contamination. Levels of calcium supplementation should be in the range of 400 to 800 milligrams per day so that the total dietary plus supplemental intake is about 1200 milligrams. Magnesium should also be consumed at levels of between 400 and 600 milligrams per day as the total dietary plus any supplementary intake.

With these recommended intakes, the ratio of calcium to phosphorus in the diet will be about one part calcium to one and one-half parts phosphorus, a much better ratio than the present one part calcium to two parts phosphorus.

Oral Health Effects
of Calcium–Phosphorus Imbalance

What type of health problems might we associate with the present trend toward lower-calcium, higher-phosphorus diets? The most common and possibly the most interesting is periodontal disease, which traditionally has been viewed as an oral hygiene problem rather than as a problem of lifestyle or nutrition. This condition used to be known as pyorrhea, but due to the stigma associated with the term, it now goes by the more fashionable name periodontal disease.

A number of factors contribute to the development of periodontal disease. The major theories cite calculus formation or poor oral hygiene that cause infection of the gums or factors within individuals bodies that dispose them to bone loss, which then sets the stage for bacteria to grow between the teeth and the gums leading to loosening of the teeth in the jaw. As the disease progresses, the gum swells and creates a ledge where bacterial plaque and calculus collect. Toxic products of the action of the bacteria result in chronic infection and the gums are irritated further. Finally, pockets form between the teeth and the gum, the gum line recedes, and eventually teeth are lost.

This process, from its initial stages to the final loss of a tooth, requires many years and one professional concludes that there is no disease that seems to be triggered by more factors than human periodontal disease.[11] Conditions that increase the risk to this disease include plaque and calculus formation, faulty dental restoration work, poor tooth alignment, and physiological factors such as a depressed immune system status, poor nutritional status, or hormonal imbalances. A number of researchers now feel that oral hygiene may be the least important variable in the termination of the progression of human periodontal disease and that nutritional and physiological factors play a much more important role.[12]

Prevention of Tooth Loss

Lifestyle and dietary factors shown to directly influence the tendency toward bone loss in the jaw predisposing one toward periodontal disease include the low-calcium, high-phosphorus diet, excessive consumption of alcohol, cigarette smoking, low vitamin-C intake, and zinc depletion. Another associated factor is poor alignment of the jaw. Proper alignment of the two jaws is necessary to put stress on the jaw bones to stimulate bone reformation. It is now well recognized that when individuals do not have proper physical stress on their skeletons, their bones lose calcium content. A malocclusion (where the jaws do not bring the teeth into proper contact with one another) may cause localized loss of bone in particular areas and necessitate the attention of a dentist to realign the jaws properly.[13]

Conditions that trigger the need for increased calcium intake may also predispose one toward periodontal disease. These include pregnancy, lactation, and trauma-induced stress.

It can be said, almost as a point of reference, that all men and women over the age of 50 who are consuming the standard American diet should be on calcium and probably magnesium supplementation to achieve adequacy and that they should look carefully at factors such as cigarette smoking, alcohol consumption, oral hygiene, and diet as factors that may contribute to bone demineralization leading to periodontal disease or, in the more serious cases, osteoarthritis or osteoporosis.

Osteoarthritis and Calcium

What is osteoarthritis and how does the loss of calcium from bone lead to problems associated with it? When calcium is lost from bone it may be deposited in the joint spaces or in muscle; these small calcium deposits irritate the sensitive tissues in joints, which in turn leads to inflammation, pain and stiffness, and long-term changes in the joints themselves. The irony of this situation is that low calcium intake can lead to the calcification of soft tissue. Many people think the deposition of calcium in the soft tissue means calcium excess; however, the problem is not too much but rather too little, or at least too little calcium as compared to too much phosphorus.

Other Nutrients in Bone Formation

Let's go beyond calcium, magnesium, phosphorus, and dietary protein and look at the role other nutrients play in bone formation. It is known that the hydroxyapatite mineral deposits found in your bones actually form on a matrix of protein called collagen. Collagen is manufactured by your bone cells and requires adequate levels of vitamin C for its construction. Deficiency states of vitamin C can lead to alterations in the collagen and result in imperfect bone mineralization.

Vitamin C also aids in the formation of connective tissue that helps prevent the penetration of bacteria from your oral cavity into the soft gum tissues of your mouth, which could then lead to increased risk to periodontal disease. It has been suggested that vitamin C in excess of the Recommended Dietary Allowance may be required both to optimize the synthesis of collagen in bone formation and to provide proper resistance to bacterial invasion in the gums.[14]

A recent study indicated that vitamin-C supplementation was extremely useful in helping prevent periodontal disease in an animal model.[15] Vitamin C has also been found very helpful in reducing inflammatory response that occurs when there is a localized tissue irritation.[16] For people with considerable irritation of the gums and the start of pocket formation around the teeth, folic acid (at 400 to 1000 mcg a day) and vitamin B-6 (at 20 to 50 mg a day) supplementation has been found useful along with flossing the contents of a 100-unit vitamin E capsule up in between the teeth. Lastly, zinc (at 20 to 30 mg a day) and copper (at 2 to 5 mg a day) have been found very helpful in reducing the active process of tissue inflammation and bone loss. Zinc has also been found helpful in preventing cavities in children who are very prone to cavity formation.

Zinc and Cavity Prevention

In a recent study, two groups of animals were fed a high-sugar diet, one of which was also supplemented with zinc. It was found that the rate of cavity formation of the zinc-supplemented animals, even though they received a high amount of sugar, was extremely low compared to that in the group without zinc supplementation. The conclusion drawn was that zinc activates the immune response to prevent the growth of bacteria in the mouth that leads to cavities.

For cavities to be formed, three things seem to be necessary. First, there must be bacteria in the mouth—no problem, they are always present. Second, there must be something for the bacteria to live on—generally simple sugars, certainly more than adequate in the American diet. Third, there must be a reduced immune defense in the mouth against the growth of the bacteria—which can be caused by inadequate zinc and vitamin C. It is also interesting to note that unrefined cereal grains have been found to contain substances called lectins that actually prohibit the bacteria from sticking to the teeth and getting a foothold where they can grow and cause cavities.[17]

Osteoporosis and Calcium Therapy

In putting this all together, it is important for the diet to be high in unrefined cereal grains, adequate in zinc, copper, and vitamin C, low in sugar, not excessive in dietary protein, and properly balanced in calcium, magnesium, and phosphorus to promote proper bone formation and control calcium in the body. It has been found that even in women who have diagnosed osteoporosis, supplementation of vitamin D and calcium can be extremely helpful in promoting improved bone density.[18]

In a recent report, postmenopausal women showing bone thinning who were given vitamin D by injection, oral daily doses of 800 milligrams of calcium as calcium glutamate, and 8 grams a day of a refined veal bone powder extract were found to have increased bone density after eighteen months of supplementation.[19]

Milk Intolerance and Toxic Minerals

Although everyone ages and loses some bone, less than a third of the aging population actually develop osteoporosis. Apart from the dietary and lifestyle factors we have discussed, these individuals may also have an underlying allergic response to milk or an excess body burden of the toxic minerals lead, cadmium, and aluminum, both of which can contribute to bone loss.[20]

A form of milk intolerance called lactose intolerance, which afflicts 31 percent of adult Caucasians, 45 percent of Orientals, and 65 percent of blacks, can lead to bone loss.[21] People with lactose intolerance should either eliminate milk from the diet or substitute cultured dairy products such as buttermilk or yogurt, which have reduced lactose content. Sometimes lactose intolerance is not obvious because the classic symptoms of diarrhea or gas are absent, although long-term, slow, but progressive bone loss may be present. If you have a history of milk sensitivity, you might suspect lactose intolerance as contributing to bone loss.

The toxic minerals lead, cadmium, and aluminum can accumulate in the body. For some time it has been known that lead coming from inhaled dust or automobile exhaust, or from canned foods, can contribute to bone calcium displacement. Also, it has been known that cadmium can contribute to bone loss and in extreme cases lead to a condition called "itai-itai" disease, which has weakened bone and gross skeletal abnormalities associated with it.

It is only recently that aluminum, which for a long time was thought to be a safe and nontoxic element, is now implicated as having an adverse effect upon the skeleton. Aluminum accumulation in the body is associated with the overproduction of parathyroid hormone, the hormone that stimulates bone breakdown and calcium resorption.[22] The accumulation of aluminum may be a result of continual consumption of aluminum-containing antacid materials for the treatment of excess stomach acid.[23] Individuals who have extensive aluminum deposition with extremely high levels of calcium loss have been treated successfully with calcitonin hormone therapy, which tries to balance the excessive production of parathyroid hormone.[24]

The best defense against aluminum accumulation from low-level exposure such as antacids or cooking acid or alkaline foods in aluminum cookware is adequate calcium, magnesium, and vitamin D intake. It was recently found that cooking tomato sauce in a 6-inch diameter pot caused approximately 25 milligrams of aluminum to leach from the pot into the tomato sauce. The investigators point out that whether this is clinically important or not remains to be seen, but it could constitute a long-term, slow buildup of aluminum in people who use aluminum cookware frequently.[25]

Fluoride and Bone Integrity

What about fluoride? Does fluoride supplementation in fact improve oral health and bone density in infants, children, or adults?

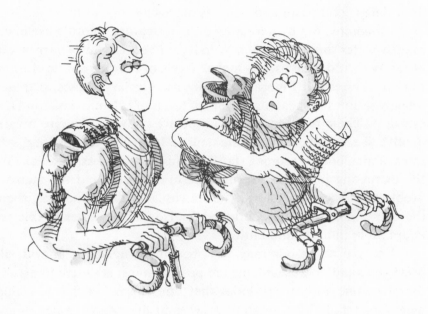

DO YOU THINK SHE FLUNKED ME BECAUSE I ANSWERED
THAT THE FIRST RECORDED INCIDENT OF BONE LOSS
WAS ADAM'S RIB?

Fluoride therapy began as a means of preventing cavities in the middle 1940s based upon the lower incidence of cavities in communities whose water supplies were adjusted upward in fluoride to one part per million, compared with similar cities with no fluoride supplementation. Over the thirty-five years that fluoride has been used, however, there has been increasing evidence that the prevalence of cavities is declining in communities with unfluoridated water as well as in those with fluoridated water. This phenomenon may be related to an increase of fluoride in the food chain, in that many commercial food processors now use fluoridated water, or the fact that people are brushing with fluoridated toothpaste and dentists are using topical fluoride.

As pointed out by a number of investigators, fluoride use in community water supplies is not hazard free. There is a fairly narrow range of safety for fluoride use, as higher levels of fluoride can lead to mottling of the teeth.[26] Fluoride is being used in large doses to treat osteoporosis in women, along with high levels of calcium, vitamin D, and estrogen. These high doses of fluoride are known to lead to a variety of adverse side effects, including nausea, low-energy states, and symptoms of metabolic poisoning (fatigue, muscle weakness, nausea). Given the increasing prevalence of fluoride in our diets and the increasing problems of excessive fluoride in individuals, called fluorosis, there is the question of whether continued fluoridation of water at this point is desirable in all communities.

Because our foods may now be much higher in fluoride than previously and because infants are possibly most sensitive to excessive fluorides, one author concludes that "the dosage of fluoride supplements for infants in communities without fluoridated water needs to be reassessed in the light of evidence regarding the fluoride content of formulas and baby foods."[27]

An Integrated Approach to Bone Integrity

Remember that certain individuals have greater calcium need than others, particularly women, but that excessive calcium for any individual can create problems of its own. Vitamin D supplementation should be approached with caution, and calcium should be properly balanced with magnesium, so that the total dietary calcium, including any supplement, is 1200 milligrams per day, balanced with 1600 to 1800 milligrams of phosphorus each day from the diet. Magnesium intake should be about half the level of calcium in the diet, and vitamin C, folic acid, vitamin B-6, and zinc should all be within sufficient dietary levels to meet your specific needs for optimal function according to your biotype. If the variables discussed in this chapter are taken into account adequately, a considerable reduction in risk to calcium metabolism problems of later life may result, both increasing bone integrity and decreasing the risk to soft-tissue calcification and sclerosis.

Exercise for Bone Integrity

Does exercise play any role in stimulating the skeleton to reform new bone? Studies done on astronauts indicate that when they are immobilized for a period of time, they lose calcium very rapidly from bone. A similar phenomenon is seen in hospitalized or bed-ridden elderly patients, who may lose bone very quickly due to the lack of skeletal stimulation. It is absolutely essential that people put muscular stress on the skeleton to stimulate new bone to be formed. Any type of stress on the skeleton that uses gravity as a stressor will help stimulate new bone—a routine walking program, stationary exercises, even vigorous yardwork and housework. A sedentary lifestyle encourages bone loss, even in the face of the application of proper nutrition and the other variables discussed in this chapter. There is no guarantee that by applying all of the concepts of this chapter that you will be free of bone demineralization or soft-tissue calcification throughout your life, but you will have greatly loaded the dice in favor of decreased risk to major calcium problems such as periodontal disease, osteoporosis, and osteoarthritis.

Dr. Weston Price and Bone Status

Weston Price was a dentist who some seventy years ago observed that when cultures that had eaten a primitive diet for centuries suddenly switched to a Westernized diet, their oral health degenerated quickly and their skeletal and bone structure was altered in succeeding generations. This observation, made from travels around the world by

Dr. Price and his wife and documented in his book **Nutrition and Physical Degeneration,**[28] has only recently been confirmed in a detailed animal study. Investigators found that when monkeys were raised on natural (hard) diets or highly processed (soft) diets, the natural diets resulted in proper oral development and excellent bone and tooth structures. The soft, highly processed diets, however, resulted in rotated and displaced teeth, crowded molars, and narrower dental arches.

Isn't it telling that over the past forty years we have seen greater and greater need for orthodontic work on our youngsters, due to tooth crowding and changes in the jaw? This increased need for braces is not just due to increased sensitivity to the cosmetic appearance of the teeth. If, in fact, the observations from animal studies prove applicable to humans, it suggests wide-ranging implications concerning anatomical structure and functional capacity as they relate to diet and lifestyle.[29]

Proper skeletal development and calcium maintenance starts in the womb and follows people throughout their lives, based upon the way they treat themselves. Diseases stemming from calcium metabolism problems may be strongly related to the important role that lifestyle and nutrition, in relation to an individual's biotype, play in controlling the maintenance of the skeleton in mid to late life.

A set of vertical disease symptoms that many times goes along with bone loss is joint and muscle pain, or what some people term arthritis or arthralgia. Interestingly, these symptoms are often related to an allergy to certain foods or to poor digestion and assimilation of nutrients from the diet. Optimal health is gained by not only eating good food, exercising, and practicing a supportive lifestyle, but also by digesting, assimilating, and utilizing the nutrients in the diet as well as excreting the waste products properly. In the next chapter we will discuss the important role that allergy and maldigestion have in causing headaches, intestinal problems, and the pains of "arthritis."

Notes

1. H. Spencer and D. Osis, "Factors Contributing to Calcium Loss in Aging," *American Journal of Clinical Nutrition, 36,* 776(1982).

2. L. Lutwak, L. Krook, and P. A. Hendrickson, "Calcium Deficiency and Human Periodontal Disease," *Israel Journal of Medical Science, 7,* 504(1971).

3. L. Schneider and M. Haussler, "Experimental Diabetes Reduces Circulating 1,25-dihydroxy vitamin D-3," *Science, 196,* 1452(1977).

4. M. S. Deugun and C. Cohen, "Vitamin D Nutrition in Relation to Season and Occupation," *American Journal of Clinical Nutrition, 34,* 1501(1981).

5. R. G. Henika, "Food and Nutrition Research," *Nutrition News, 41,* 3(1978).

6. M. Anderson et al., "Long-term Effect of a Low Calcium:Phosphate Ratio on Skeleton of Monkeys," *Journal of Nutrition, 107,* 834(1977).

7. R. Raines-Bell and H. Draper, "Physiological Responses of Human Adults to Foods Containing Phosphate Additives," *Journal of Nutrition, 107,* 42(1977).

8. S. Margen and D. H. Calloway, "Studies in the Mechanism of Calciuria Induced by Protein Feeding," *Federation Proceedings, 29,* 566(1970).

9. P. Marie and F. H. Glorieux, "Histological Osteomalacia Due to Dietary Calcium Deficiency in Children," *New England Journal of Medicine, 307,* 584(1982).

10. A. Albanese, *Bone Loss: Detection and Therapy* (New York: Alan R. Liss, 1977).

11. M. C. Alfano, "Controversies, Perspectives, and Clinical Implications of Nutrition in Periodontal Disease," *Dental Clinics of North America, 20,* 519(1976).

12. P. H. Hendrickson, "Periodontal Disease and Calcium Deficiency," *Acta Odontologica Scandinavica, 26,* Supplement 50, 1968.

13. K. E. Wickal and P. Brussee, "Effects of a Calcium and Vitamin D Supplement on Alveolar Ridge Resorption," *Journal of Prosthetic Dentistry, 41,* 4(1979).

14. J. C. Gallagher and B. L. Riggs, "Nutrition and Bone Disease," *New England Journal of Medicine, 298,* 193(1978).

15. G. Kolata, "Vitamin C Prevents Periodontal Disease in an Animal Model," *Science, 209,* 1113(1981).

16. S. C. Sharma and W. M. Wilson, "Cellular Interaction of Ascorbic Acid with Histamine, Prostaglandins in the Immediate Hypersensitivity Reaction," *International Journal of Vitamin and Nutrition Research, 50,* 163(1980).

17. R. J. Gibbons and I. Dankers, "Inhibition of Lectin-Binding to Saliva-Treated Hydroxyapatite," *American Journal of Clinical Nutrition, 36,* 276(1982).

18. C. J. Lee and G. H. Johnson, "Effects of Supplementation with Calcium on Bone Density in Elderly Females with Osteoporosis," *American Journal of Clinical Nutrition, 34,* 819(1981).

19. O. Epstein and S. Sherlock, "Vitamin D, Hydroxyapatite, and Calcium Gluconate Treatment of Cortical Bone Thinning," *American Journal of Clinical Nutrition, 36,* 426(1982).

20. M. Kleerkoper and A. M. Parfitt, "Nutritional, Endocrine and Demographic Aspects of Osteoporosis," *Orthopedic Clinics of North America, 12,* 547(1981).

21. "Lactose Intolerance and Bone Loss," *Nutrition Reviews, 39,* 119(1981).

22. G. H. Mayor and P. K. Ku, "Aluminum Absorption and Effect of Parathyroid Hormone," *Science, 197,* 1187(1977).

23. H. Spencer and D. Osis, "Effect of Small Doses of Aluminum-Containing Antacids on Calcium and Phosphorus Metabolism," *American Journal of Clinical Nutrition, 36,* 32(1982).

24. S. Ott and D. J. Sherrard, "The Prevalence of Bone Aluminum Deposition in Renal Osteodystrophy and Its Relation to Calcitriol Therapy," *New England Journal of Medicine, 307,* 709(1982).

25. G. A. Trapp, "Aluminum Pots as a Source of Dietary Aluminum," *New England Journal of Medicine, 304,* 172(1981).

26. D. H. Leverett, "Fluorides and the Changing Prevalence of Dental Caries," *Science, 217,* 26(1982).

27. Ibid.

28. W. Price, *Nutrition and Physical Degeneration* (Santa Monica, CA: The Price-Pottenger Nutrition Foundation, 1975).

29. R. S. Corruccini and R. M. Beecher, "Occlusal Variation Related to Soft Diet in a Nonhuman Primate," *Science, 218,* 74(1982).

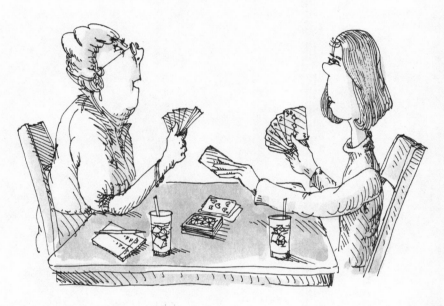

11

The Link Between Arthritis, Headache, and Intestinal Problems

CAN YOU BELIEVE IT?
I'M ALLERGIC TO MY IMMUNE SYSTEM.

1. Do you have a depressed appetite?

1	2	3	4
No	Occasionally	Frequently	All the time

2. Do you have an abnormal craving for sweets?

1	2	3	4
No	Occasionally	Frequently	All the time

3. Do you have rough skin?

1	2	3	4
No	Occasionally	Frequently	All the time

4. Do you suffer from stomach or intestinal pain?

1	2	3	4
No	Occasionally	Frequently	All the time

5. Do you suffer from symptoms of morning stiffness, joint pain or stiffness?

1	2	3	4
No	Occasionally	Frequently	All the time

If your score exceeds thirteen, you may have a problem with maldigestion or allergy and you should concentrate on Chapter 11.

This chapter deals with the immune system, its important ability to protect you from disease, and what happens when it goes haywire, recognizes you as foreign, and actually attacks your own body.

Your Immune System

The immune system is the defensive team of your body which protects you twenty-four hours a day against infectious diseases, chemicals in the environment, drugs, foreign substances, and even your own body's cells, if they have been transformed into malignant cells. This defensive system has its origin in the white and red blood cells and in the lymphatic system, which is composed of the lymph glands and the bloodstream. Circulating through this system and stored in the various lymph glands are specialized blood cells called lymphocytes, which are given the responsibility for protecting against all sorts of hazards and disease-producing substances. Lymphocytes are divided into two types: T-lymphocytes (which are activated in the thymus gland, located at the base of your neck, near the throat) and B-lymphocytes.

The T-lymphocytes have the responsibility for doing hand-to-hand combat with invading foreign bacteria or viruses or your own transformed cells. Some scientists call this system the *surveillance system,* indicating that the T-lymphocytes guard the territory of your body all day long, making sure there is no invasion by troops of the opposition. The T-lymphocytes recognize a foreign cell by their sense of touch, known as membrane receptivity. Once a T-lymphocyte recognizes a foreigner, it attacks that substance by engulfing it and secreting chemicals that kill it, a process called *phagocytosis.* Some of the substances used to kill the foreign cells include superoxide (a very chemically reactive form of oxygen) and hydrogen peroxide and singlet oxygen (other vigorous oxidizing agents). These materials are lethal to foreign cells; therefore, when T-lymphocytes are working correctly, they are tremendously effective defensive forces. Most of the foreign substances that enter your body are relatively weak and ill-prepared to deal with these strong and very active T-lymphocytes.

Although you are exposed each day to countless potentially disease-producing bacteria and viruses, you rarely become ill, because your T-lymphocytes are able to work actively 99.999 percent of the time. It is only when the T-lymphocytes are reduced in activity, or when you are exposed to too much of the foreign invader, or exposed to some new invader your body's defensive system is not used to that you become ill. Your nutritional and general health status can directly affect the condition of your T-lymphocytes and, therefore, either activate or inactivate your body's defensive system.

The second important type of defensive cell is the B-lymphocyte, which, instead of engaging in hand-to-hand combat, sends into your bloodstream chemical missiles called antibodies, which seek out foreign substances and destroy them. Different B-lymphocytes manufacture specific antibodies for specific foreign substances that you may have been exposed to in your life—these are the things you have an immunity against. Vaccination works precisely because of this very powerful memory built into the B-lymphocyte that allows it to recognize substances it has previously been exposed to. It quickly secretes the antibodies necessary to glue these foreign substances together and take them to the liver where they can be detoxified and ultimately excreted before they cause you harm.

When the T- and B-lymphocytes are working properly you have a powerful defensive team engaged in a twenty-four-hour search and destroy mission in your body to protect you from any foreign invaders. When, however, this sytem is either deactivated or overly sensitized, it can lead to harm.

Problems with the Immune System

Obviously, when the system is understaffed or sluggish, you are more susceptible to many disease-producing organisms and even to cancer.[1] What about when the immune system is too activated?

An overactive immune system is termed **hypersensitive** and can be related to the presence of an allergy or a condition of autoimmunity —"being allergic to yourself." An overactive B- or T-lymphocyte system can, therefore, do you just as much harm as an underactive system. Of the symptoms at the beginning of this chapter, some are associated with reduced immunity and others with hypersensitivity.

Problems of the digestive tract, such as irritable bowel, and symptoms of arthritis are associated with a hypersensitive immune system; poor wound healing and a tendency to "get every bug that comes along" are more associated with an underactive immune system. What the Nutraerobics Program strives for is an optimal state of health—where your immune system is neither underactive nor overactive.

Let's start with how we can activate an underactive immune system for the individual who is at greater risk to infection, flu, and possibly even cancer. It has been recently pointed out that many nutrients have positive effects on activating the immune system.[2] Previously, medical doctors thought that only fairly significant nutrient deficiency states led to immune suppression; however, there is now concern that current suboptimal nutrition may cause chronic immune system impairment. The degree that suboptimal nutrition influences your immune system, of course, depends upon your biochemical individuality.

Water-Soluble Vitamins and Immunity

A number of water-soluble and fat-soluble vitamins as well as minerals and protein have a direct effect in activating the immune system in people who have chronic impaired immunity due to borderline nutritional deficiency. A deficiency of vitamin B-6 is known to depress B- and T-lymphocyte function and seems to accompany deficiencies of vitamin B-12 and folic acid. The ranges of these nutrients proven useful in activating the immune system in individuals who have apparent deficiency are 10 to 50 milligrams of B-6, 10 to 50 micrograms of B-12, and 400 to 1000 micrograms of folic acid.

Of the water-soluble vitamins, the one with the greatest effect upon the immune system, however, is vitamin C. Vitamin C has been shown to play a very important role in activating T-lymphocytes and the vitamin-C content of white blood cells can become depleted during violent infections, pregnancy, and in older persons.[3] Recently, vitamin-

C supplementation at levels of 1000 to 3000 milligrams per day has been found to activate T-lymphocytes in normal subjects and may be considered a reasonable range of intake as a supplemental dose. The Recommended Dietary Allowance of between 40 and 60 milligrams per day is far below this level for optimal immune defense.[4]

A B-complex vitamin that activates the immune process is pantothenic acid. A pantothenic acid deficiency has been shown to lead to depressed B-lymphocyte response and is also indicated to be related to intestinal conditions such as ulcerative colitis and even Crohn's disease.[5] These intestinal tract disorders can result in severe ulceration of the intestine and the need for surgical intervention; the use of pantothenic acid as calcium pantothenate at levels between 200 and 1000 milligrams a day has been suggested as useful in the management of these conditions.

Fat-Soluble Vitamins and Immunity

In the fat-soluble vitamin area, there has been considerable interest in vitamin A and its supposed ability to activate the immune system. A vitamin A deficiency in animals has been shown to depress both B- and T-lymphocyte function, which suggests that supplemental doses of vitamin A may activate the human immune system. Vitamin A, however, can be toxic at levels above 25,000 units per day. Toxicity symptoms of vitamin A include hair loss, headaches, dryness of the mucous membranes, skin problems, and digestive disorders, as well as increased liver damage.

Some people take supplemental vitamin A to reduce the risk to lung cancer from smoking. Recently, however, evidence indicates that the most powerful protective agent against lung cancer is not vitamin A but rather a close relative called beta-carotene.[6] Beta-carotene is the pigment found in orange and red vegetables and fruits and has been shown in human studies to be a potential protective agent against smoking-induced lung cancer at levels of intake of about 10,000 to 30,000 units per day. One of the benefits of using beta-carotene rather than vitamin A is that there appears to be no direct toxicity from carotene other than a slight yellowing of the skin in some people, which is not a toxic reaction.

Vitamin E is another fat-soluble vitamin that has been shown to have effects upon the immune system. A vitamin-E deficiency can depress immune function and general resistance to disease. On the other hand, doses of vitamin E in excess of 1000 units per day have been shown to suppress the immune system.[7] Given these observations, it would appear that the best range of supplemental vitamin E for promotion of immune defense is between 100 and 600 units a day. The observation that vitamin E in doses in excess of 1000 units a day inhibits aspects of the immune system may account for why vitamin E has found some useful application in the management of symptoms of autoimmune diseases such as scleroderma, myesthenia gravis, rheumatoid arthritis, and systemic lupus erythematosus (SLE).[8] These are conditions characterized by an overactive immune system; in these cases the actual suppression of immune hypersensitivity might be achieved by high doses of vitamin E.

Minerals and Immunity

Trace minerals also play a very important role in activating the immune system. Iron deficiency, the nutritional deficiency that has been targeted by the USDA as the most prevalent in American society, is known to lead to immune suppression. As is the case with many of the trace elements, however, if a little is good, a whole lot more is not necessarily better. Excessive iron can also lead to immune suppression. The optimal daily dose of iron for most individuals is between 15 and 30 milligrams per day.

Zinc is another element that we are going to talk much about in this chapter, because of its powerful effect on the immune system. A zinc deficiency in the chronic state can lead to impaired wound healing, growth and developmental retardation in children, eczemic skin problems, and poor hair growth. Zinc-deficient individuals show an improvement of not only their immune function but these other problem areas when body zinc stores are replenished. The level of zinc required for proper maintenance of immune function is between 15 and 30 milligrams per day.

Selenium and magnesium have also been shown to be important as activators of the immune process. A modest deficiency of selenium along with a vitamin-E deficiency can greatly increase the risk to infection, and may also increase the risk to cancer.[9] The level of selenium required can vary between 100 and 300 micrograms a day, and organic selenium from high-selenium brewer's yeast is better than inorganic selenium such as selenite or selenate.

Finally, magnesium depletion may lead to unusual sensitivity of the skin to rash and a decreased function of the thymus gland, the gland that activates T-lymphocyte function. Magnesium intake should ideally be 400 to 600 milligrams daily for proper immune system status.

Protein and Fats in Immunity

Another class of nutrients important in stabilizing immune function is dietary protein. Deficiencies of any of the essential amino acids, which are complete in high-quality dietary protein but not in imbalanced proteins, such as certain vegetable proteins or heat-rendered animal protein, can result in impairment of immunity system and increase the risk to disease. Long-term protein deficiency states or amino acid imbalance, which have been associated with individuals on poorly controlled weight loss diets for an extended period of time, vegetarians with inappropriate daily protein intake, or individuals who cannot digest and assimilate protein correctly, can lead to great risk of infection. Some of the first signs of this difficulty are hair loss and skin disorders.

Possibly the most exciting new work relating nutrition to improved immunity is the work on dietary oils and their impact on immune function. It was found that people who have been on high saturated-animal-fat diets, or diets rich in partially hydrogenated vegetable oils, or people who have basically cut almost all of the fat out of their diets for a long period of time may have a suppressed immune system due to an essential fatty acid deficiency. It is now recognized that one of the white blood cell types involved in immunity, called the mast cell, secretes prostaglandins and leukotrienes, substances necessary for the inflammatory response (your body's method of dealing with localized infection and repairing cell damage). Their release from the mast cell is dependent upon dietary essential fatty acids coming from vegetable oils such as safflower, sunflower seed, and fish oils derived from cold-water fish.[10]

Putting this all together, a good program for activating the immune system is to balance high-quality dietary protein at levels between 70 and 100 grams per day, administer zinc, vitamin B-12, folic acid, vitamin C, and vitamin E along with polyunsaturated vegetable oils, while decreasing the level of saturated fat intake.

Immunity and Allergy

But what if your problem is one of an overactive immune system and you are suffering from symptoms that resemble allergies, or maybe even in the extreme case arthritis-like symptoms with morning stiffness and pain, reduced joint range mobility, and a need to take anti-inflammatories like aspirin?

Let's look at allergies. It is now recognized that certain tissue reactions, particularly those in connective tissue, lymphatic tissue, intestinal mucosal tissue, and skin, may be related to an unsuspected or unknown allergy. **Allergy** comes from the Greek words **allos,** meaning "other," and **ergon,** meaning "work," and basically means that your immune system is doing other work; that is, it is working on things it doesn't need to; it has gone faulty. When your immune system is working normally, mast cells initiate the inflammatory response to eliminate true noxious agents and damaged tissue; in an allergy or hypersensitivity the mast cells initiate that same inflammatory response against an otherwise benign substance, which is then termed an allergen. Inflammation-producing substances secreted by the mast cells cause changes in smooth muscles, blood vessels, mucous glands, and sensory nerve endings, producing the swelling, tenderness, and pain associated with allergy. If this reaction occurs in the brain, it is called a cerebral allergy and can lead to headaches and behavioral problems.[11]

We are now gaining a better understanding of the prevalence and complexity in the allergic response of one class of allergens—those found in food. In descending order of prevalence the most common food allergens are wheat, milk, corn, soy, yeast, chocolate, tea and coffee, beef, citrus fruits, shellfish, eggs, and potatoes. No food is free of allergic potential, but these are the most common. The symptoms of allergy can be quite complex, including not only the classic examples of diarrhea, hives on the skin, and intestinal complaints including pain and bloating, but also the more complex and difficult to define indications such as a sense of tiredness, inability to concentrate, increased risk to intestinal diseases, skin disorders including eczema, and even, in some isolated examples, vision changes.

One way of checking for a suspected food allergy is to eliminate the foods that have the highest probability of being allergy-producing from the diet for a period of three to five days. After the elimination period, reintroduce the foods one at a time. A food should be reintroduced in reasonable quantities and then the symptoms watched for for a period of three to five hours after the consumption. The most common symptoms indicating the presence of allergy are not only intestinal complaints, headaches, and skin rashes, but also rapid heartbeat, sleepiness, shortness of breath, muscle pain or weakness, and a feeling of mental confusion. Once the allergy-producing food has been identified, a diet can be developed whereby the offending food is either rotated in the diet every third or fourth day or eliminated entirely. A number of excellent books now discuss how to implement a diversified food rotation diet.[12]

Migraine Headache and Allergy

One of the most troublesome symptoms associated with long-term unrecognized allergy is migraine headache. Migraines affect about 20 percent of the population, the majority affected being women. Food

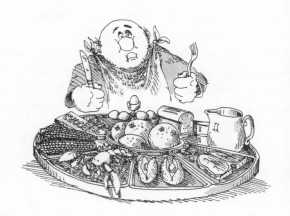

YOU MEAN A DIVERSIFIED FOOD ROTATION DIET ISN'T WHEAT, MILK, CORN, SOY, YEAST, CHOCOLATE, TEA, COFFEE, BEEF, CITRUS FRUITS, SHELLFISH, EGGS, AND POTATOES ON A LAZY SUSAN?

allergy has now been demonstrated in follow-up studies to be involved in possibly as many as two-thirds of the cases of individuals suffering from this condition.[13] In a recent study, sixteen migraine patients were found to be free of headaches after eliminating the offending food from the diet.[14]

Although food allergy may not be the cause of migraine in all patients, it could be a cause in some—it may indicate increased exposure of the individual to immune activating substances that produce brain biochemical effects. Some investigators have concluded there is no convincing evidence that allergic reactions to foods are responsible for migraine attacks and that any evidence in support of this claim is just circumstantial.[15] However, clinical studies have indicated considerable improvement in migraine headache patients when the food allergens can be identified and eliminated.

In a very recent study, it was found that patients who do suffer from diet-related migraine have a genetically determined lower level in their bodies of a specific enzyme important in the detoxification of certain substances from food; if these substances are not detoxified, they can produce adverse effects upon brain function.[16] These substances from food are chemically related to tyramine, which is found in chocolate, cheese, bananas, coffee, and tea.

As was pointed out in Chapter 5, it has also been found that there are substances in certain dietary proteins, particularly in wheat and milk, that may be responsible for increasing the level of certain neurotransmitter active substances, exorphins, in the blood that result from the incomplete breakdown of dietary protein.

Arthritis and Allergy

Now, what is the relationship of these observations to arthritis-like symptoms? It is well known that the overactivation of the mast cell releases inflammation-producing substances that can produce pain and swelling in localized tissue. This overactivation can come as a consequence of the buildup of immune complexes, which are actually the rubble and debris of the overactivated immune system. These immune complexes develop from incompletely digested proteins that are absorbed into the blood, or from other allergy-producing materials.[17] By reducing the number of these immune complexes through food allergen elimination, the offending substances can then be eliminated from the blood, thereby reducing the hypersensitive reaction of the mast cell. The mast cell is capable of increasing localized tissue destruction when it is overly stimulated and this may be the link between arthritis and allergy.

How then do we go about reducing the potential absorption of these immune activating substances from the intestines? First, reduce or eliminate the food allergens from the diet. Second, increase intestinal regularity and prevent constipation. Constipation can lead to the buildup of these immune sensitizing substances in the intestines, resulting in the slow release of these substances into the blood. To correct this, a higher-fiber diet should be employed to improve intestinal regularity. One of the best fibers now being used to increase intestinal function and decrease the exposure of the body to these food allergic substances is oat bran fiber. Two to three tablespoonfuls of oat bran fiber each day, stirred into juice, added to cereals, or cooked into bread, can provide 15 to 20 grams of dietary fiber. This amount is now suggested as useful for normalizing intestinal function and reducing not only the risk to allergic substances being absorbed into the blood but also other intestinal tract processes that could result in increasing risk to colon cancer or diverticular disease.[18] Third, improved protein digestion is important for those who are poor protein digesters. Oral pancreatic enzyme supplements taken with each meal have been shown to help some people with food allergy. (These products may be known as pancreatin tablets).

Immunity and Arthritis

Also of considerable concern is the balance of zinc and copper. As was previously mentioned, zinc is extremely important in activating the immune system but it must be in balance with the trace element copper. There is now strong evidence to suggest that certain of the rheumatoid arthritis–like diseases may be related to the imbalance between zinc and copper. Some workers have indicated that arthritic-like pain can be treated by administering zinc; other investigators have indicated that copper plays a significant role in reducing the same type of symptoms. These results may appear conflicting because zinc and copper are antagonists in the body; when zinc levels go up, copper generally goes down, and vice versa.

Large supplemental doses of zinc can have the actual pharmaco-logical effect of tending to spur T-lymphocytes to activity far in excess of what would be considered normal. In some people this activation may produce an adverse reaction and lead to a depletion of copper, which is necessary for proper immune status. Given this, it would appear that the specific balance of zinc and copper is highly individual-ized and both trace elements should be examined closely for their role in optimizing immune defense.

If an individual has poor wound healing, a poor sense of taste and smell, hair loss, and lowered immune defense, it may signal the need for zinc in therapeutic doses of from 15 to 30 milligrams a day.[19] If, however, there is arthritic-like pain, including stiff knuckles, swollen knees, and trouble getting out of bed in the morning, it may indicate a need to look at the potential requirement for copper, particularly if this comes in conjunction with bone loss and a generalized tendency towards allergy.

The level of zinc that has been used varies from 15 to 40 milligrams per day and has been proven beneficial in these copper-sensitive individuals. In twenty-four patients who had symptoms of rheumatoid arthritis, the use of zinc supplements of from 50 to 150 milligrams a day were helpful in reducing the symptoms of arthritis.[20] Other studies seem to indicate that copper given in therapeutic doses is the missing link. Particular success has been obtained with a substance called copper aspirinate, a compound of copper and aspirin (copper salicyclate).

It is clear that these studies, taken together, indicate that the balance between copper and zinc is extremely important in regulating the immune system and preventing the symptoms of hypersensitivity. The program needs to be individualized, based upon your own particular biochemistry and recognizing that what zinc may not do, copper may, and vice versa.

A problem with zinc and copper balance may be particularly aggravated if there is also an overload of iron. Iron can accumulate in certain joints of the body, initiate the arthritic-like response, and hypersensitize the immune system. Again, we have a case where a nutrient may be deficient in some, but in excess in others; this excess can produce adverse symptoms. Certainly this is the case with iron, which in many individuals is deficient, but in others an excess from supplementation or iron-rich water supplies overactivates the immune response.[21]

Acquired Immunodeficiency Syndrome (AIDS)

The Acquired Immunodeficiency Syndrome is characterized by a severe defect in immunity that predisposes an individual to infection or certain cancers, such as the unusual Kaposi's Sarcoma. This condition has attracted considerable attention due to its rapid increase and unknown cause.[22] The predominant theory as to its cause is that it is virally transmitted, with an incubation period of longer than one year for exposed adults. The defect in the immune system caused by this infection results in improper function of the T-lymphocyte cell.[23] This defect may be related to the fact that AIDS victims have low levels of the hormone thymosin (secreted by the thymus gland), which normally activates and regulates the T-lymphocyte.[24] It has recently been found that individuals with AIDS have altered ratios of two types of T-lymphocytes: helper and suppressor cells. Whereas in normal individuals there is a predominance of helper cells, in the AIDS patient the suppressor cells are in excess, shutting down the immune response.[25] This reversal in helper/suppressor cell numbers may reflect the alteration in thymosin output by the thymus gland and account for the report that some types of immunodeficiencies have been successfully treated with synthetic analogues of thymosin.[26] Although this approach to the treatment of AIDS is still experimental, it opens the door for new treatments based on activation of the thymus gland. Such treatments include the use of vitamin C in large quantities, and the amino acid arginine. Vitamin C has been administered orally up to levels just before diarrhea is produced and continued throughout the treatment (20 grams or more per day). Arginine is suggested to have thymotropic effects when given in supplementary doses (3 to 5 grams per day).[27] It is important to recognize that a disorder that impairs immunity has a resultant direct impact on cancer and on opportunistic infections that can be life-threatening, a sequence consistent with the model of disease outlined in the Nutraerobics approach. Considerably more work on what causes AIDS, and why certain individuals are more susceptible to it than others, must be done; but the evidence today points us toward a viral agent that inactivates the immune system by involvement with the thymus gland, and opens the door for potential therapy using thymosin, vitamin C, arginine, and other thymus-activating substances.

Stress and Immunity

Is nutritional status the only feature controlling your body's immune system? No, your stress level, as evaluated in your biotype in Chapter 2, is an important factor as well. Your body and mind are in direct relationship with one another and the way you perceive your world can have a dramatic impact upon your immune system. It was found that the rate of cancer in animals could be varied tremendously by the stress under which the animals were placed. Highly stressed animals had a depressed immune system and a much greater incidence of cancer than the animals housed in low-stress conditions.[28]

It is also known that the onset of rheumatoid arthritis, ulcers, or ulcerative bowel disease in many patients occurs simultaneously with a major stressor in their lives. Physiological stress can come from pregnancy, a family problem, an emotional disturbance, or a major physical trauma. These examples illustrate the important role that the mind has in modulating the immune system. If, in fact, your biotype indicates you are under high distress, stress may be one of the first places you want to concentrate on in improving your resistance to disease.

Stress reduction techniques such as exercise, biofeedback, and imagery might all be important parts of a program for activating your immune system. Scientists call this the neuroendocrinology of the immune system, indicating that your central nervous system and your perception of the world about you have an impact upon your T- and B-lymphocytes and your ultimate protection against the disease process. The old adage "To think good thoughts is to think healthy" seems to be true as we now view the important impact of mental outlook and immunity.

If you have more than 300 points on the Stress Indicator test in Chapter 2, there is strong evidence suggesting that your lifestyle is adversely affecting your defense mechanisms. Concentrating on the factors that made your score high and trying to reduce the stress load in your life and improve your nutritional status will help to promote proper immune defense.

This may be as simple as finding some time for yourself each day, learning how to relax, and finding a way to enjoy leisure time. If you are a person who does not know how to take a vacation, has no hobbies or recreational outlets other than your work, you may be a highly distressed individual who is in the active throes of immune suppression and increased risk to diseases of either the hypersensitized or immune-suppressed type.

By analyzing your biotype and designing your lifestyle to accommodate your specific uniquenesses, you should be able to improve your immune status immensely. In evaluating your nutritional needs in concert with your level of stress, recall that you march to a different drummer from anyone else, and nutrition and stress may have an impact upon your immune system different from others who seem to be leading a similar lifestyle.

Many people ask, "When is the best time to introduce this Nutra-erobics Program?" The answer is simple—the sooner the better. The next two chapters will discuss the impact of the program during pregnancy, infancy, and childhood. Optimal health should start at conception and continue through fetal development into childhood. Many later-age problems have their origin in these initial stages; the following chapter has information on how to prevent these problems.

Notes

1. "Immune Disorders," *Journal of the American Medical Association,* November 26, 1982.

2. W. R. Beisel et al., "Single Nutrient Effects on Immunologic Functions," *Journal of the American Medical Association, 245,* 53(1981).

3. W. R. Thomas and P. G. Holt, "Vitamin C and Immunity," *Clinical and Experimental Immunology, 32,* 370(1978).

4. R. Anderson and A. J. van Rensberg, "The Effects of Increasing Weekly Doses of Ascorbate on Cellular and Immune Function in Normal Volunteers," *American Journal of Clinical Nutrition, 33,* 71(1980).

5. R. E. Hodges and R. E. Bleiler, "Factors Affecting Human Antibody Responses. III: Responses in Pantothenic Acid Deficient Men," *American Journal of Clinical Nutrition, 11,* 85(1962).

6. G. Wolf, "Is Dietary Carotene an Anti-cancer Agent?" *Nutrition Reviews, 40,* 257(1982).

7. C. F. Nockels, "Protective Effects of Supplemental Vitamin E Against Infection," *Federation Proceedings, 38,* 2134(1979).

8. S. Ayres and R. Mihan, "Is Vitamin E Involved in the Autoimmune Mechanism?" *Cutis, 21,* 321(1978).

9. G. N. Schrauzer, "Selenium and Cancer: A Review," *Bioinorganic Chemistry, 5,* 275(1976); R. J. Shamberger and R. E. Willis, "Selenium in the Diet and Cancer," *Cleveland Clinic Quarterly, 39,* 119(1972).

10. N. A. Nelson, R. C. Kelly, and R. A. Johnson, "Prostaglandins and the Arachidonic Acid Cascade," *Chemical and Engineering News* (16 August 1982):80.

11. P. D. Buisseret, "Allergy," *Scientific American* (June 1982):86.

12. M. Mandell, *The 5-Day Allergy Relief Diet* (New York: Bantam, 1980).

13. J. Monro and J. Brostoff, "Food Allergy in Migraine," *Lancet* (5 July 1980):1014.

14. E. C. Grant, "Food Allergies and Migraine," *Lancet* (5 May 1979):966.

15. D. Stevenson, "Food Allergies and Migraine," *Lancet* (14 July 1979):103.

16. R. Pleatfield and J. Littlewood, "Platelet Phenosulfotransferase Deficiency in Dietary Migraine," *Lancet* (1 May 1982):983.

17. W. Hemmings, *Food Antigens and the Gut* (London: Lancaster Press, 1979).

18. A. Ryding and B. Odegaard, "Prophylactic Effect of Dietary Fibre in Duodenal Ulcer Disease," *Lancet* (2 October 1982):736.

19. "Oral Zinc and Immunoregulation," *Nutrition Reviews, 40,* 12(1982).

20. J. Sorenson, "Therapeutic Uses of Copper," in *Copper in the Environment, Part II* (New York: Wiley, 1979).

21. D. R. Blake and J. M. C. Gutteridge, "Importance of Iron in Rheumatoid Disease," *Lancet* (21 November 1981):1142.

22. A. S. Fauci, "The Acquired Immune Deficiency Syndrome," *Journal of the American Medical Association, 249,* 2375(1983).

23. R. Hirschhorn, "Metabolic Defects and Immunodeficiency Disorders," *New England Journal of Medicine, 308,* 714(1983).

24. M. Dardenne, and B. Safai, "Low Serum Thymic Hormone Levels in Patients with Acquired Immunodeficiency Syndrome," *New England Journal of Medicine, 309,* 48(1983).

25. A. Rubenstein and M. Hollander, "Acquired Immunodeficiency with Reversed T_4/T_8 Ratios in Infants Born to Promiscuous and Drug-Addicted Mothers," *Journal of the American Medical Association, 249,* 2350(1983).

26. F. Aiuti and G. Goldstein, "Thymopoietin Pentapeptide Treatment of Primary Immunodeficiencies," *Lancet* (12 March 1983):551.

27. A. Barbul and E. Seifter, "Wound Healing and Thymotropic Effects of Arginine: A Pituitary Mechanism of Action," *American Journal of Clinical Nutrition, 37,* 786(1983).

28. V. Riley, "Mouse Mammary Tumors: Alteration of Incidence as an Apparent Function of Stress," *Science, 189,* 465(1975).

12

Protecting the Unborn

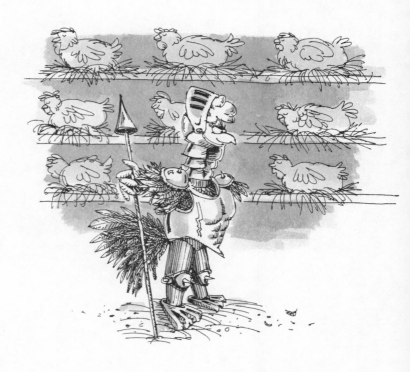

For parents:

1. Does your child have frequent respiratory infections, flu, or colds?

1	2	3	4
No	Occasionally	Frequently	Always

2. Does your child have learning disabilities or behavior problems?

1	2	3	4
No	Occasionally	Frequently	Always

3. Does your child have a problem with bed-wetting?

1	2	3	4
No	Occasionally	Frequently	Always

4. Is your child small for his or her age?

1	3	4
No	Somewhat	Yes, definitely

5. Does your child have an underweight or overweight problem?

1	4
No	Yes

If your score exceeded 12, then your child has metabolic problems controllable by dietary revision and you should concentrate on this chapter and the next.

For expectant or future parents:

1. Do you expect to breastfeed your infant?

1	2	4
Yes	Possibly at first	No

2. Do you plan to supplement with vitamins or minerals during the pregnancy?

1	2	4
Yes, modestly	Possibly	No or yes, with high levels

3. Is the expectant mother over 40 years of age?

1	4
No	Yes

4. Does the prospective mother drink milk or consume dairy products routinely?

1	2	3	4
Yes	Sometimes	Rarely	Never

5. Does the prospective mother have episodes of low blood sugar or hypoglycemia?

1	2	3	4
No	Sometimes	Frequently	Yes, severe

6. Does the expectant mother smoke or drink alcohol?

1	2	3	4
No	Sometimes	Frequently	All the time

If your score exceeded 12, then you have metabolic uniquenesses controllable by dietary revision and you should concentrate on this chapter and the next.

It was only forty years ago that a physician made the startling observation that suboptimal nutrition during pregnancy in the cats he was using in his work led to developmental abnormalities in their offspring, and that these abnormalities increased in severity with each succeeding generation that was raised on the suboptimal diet. This problem became so acute that by the third generation the cats were unable to have any successful live births.[1]

One cannot account for this startling rate of degeneration on the basis of genetic changes alone because it takes literally thousands of years to produce a profound inheritable genetic change that can be traced from generation to generation. The situation this physician observed occurred so quickly that the poor diet must have been the direct cause of the abnormal development of the fetuses. This proposition has considerable implications, for it has generally been believed that if nutrition is truly deficient, a stillbirth or fetal death will occur; otherwise, if there is a state of marginal malnutrition, it is the mother who suffers, for the fetus takes all it needs first. Birth defects have not been thought of as the result of malnutrition.

Suboptimal Nutrition and Pregnancy

Recently, the idea that suboptimal nutrition may play a role in the success of a pregnancy has been rekindled. It has been found that by controlling the level of various nutrients in the diet of a pregnant animal for even a short period of time during the early phases of pregnancy, there can be a considerable variation in the percent of fetuses ultimately born with malformations.[2]

The most important observation from this work is that many of the alterations in fetal development occur very soon after conception. In humans, it is known that the eyes are almost completely developed by the forty-third to fifty-fifth day after conception. The first three to eight weeks of the pregnancy may be one of the most critical periods of time in determining the ultimate development of the fetus, yet at this time many women may not even know they are pregnant. This means that the state of health of the mother, and possibly of the father, prior to conception may have a considerable bearing on the success of the development of the fetus, not to mention the maternal health status throughout all of the pregnancy.

Factors Affecting Fetal Development

It has often been thought that the woman bears the burden of responsibility for birth defects since the egg resides in her body and the fetus develops there. This myth must be put to rest, for there is now evidence indicating that the health of the sperm may also have a direct bearing upon the development of the fetus.

Sperm samples from forty-three cigarette smokers were found to have a signicantly greater percentage of abnormal sperm forms than samples from forty-three nonsmokers. In the light of this and other work showing increased chromosomal damage in the sperm of cigarette smokers, it has been suggested that the sperm abnormalities in cigarette smokers may reflect genetic damage to these cells as a consequence of exposure to smoke products and may ultimately contribute to increased risk to various birth defects.[3] It is also known that sperm that is older as a consequence of abstinence, or possibly a product of an older-age male, has a greater number of sperm abnormalities than younger-age sperm.

There are many other factors that may contribute to fetal abnormalities. Both men and women are exposed to many agents of unknown potential hazard in the environment through food, air, water, and direct skin contact.

One agent hotly contested as a potential birth defect–producing substance is caffeine. Studies recently published have indicated that the effect of caffeine on pregnant animals seems to be that of increased risk to cleft palate, delayed skeletal development, an increased percentage of abortions, and a moderate degree of fetal growth retardation.[4]

One doctor points out three case histories of women who drank twelve to twenty cups of coffee a day and smoked cigarettes, who gave birth to infants with significant birth defects and concludes that, "Moderately high levels of caffeine or coffee intake may be teratogenic (birth defect producing), but we have not established a safe level of consumption. It would seem prudent for pregnant women and those planning to have a baby to limit their caffeine intake."[5] Most current evidence seems to indicate that prudent intake of coffee at levels of two to three cups a day does not increase the risk to fetal abnormalities but that higher levels of coffee intake may, in fact, increase the risk, particularly in conjunction with cigarette smoking.

It is also known that excessive alcohol consumption during the early phase of pregnancy and throughout the gestation period can encourage fetal abnormalities. An acute case is known as the fetal alcohol syndrome, in which the infant may be born with significant impairment of brain function and the nervous sytem.

Even exposure to environmental chemicals during pregnancy, such as solvents, cleaning materials, oven cleaners, insecticides, pesticides, and paint fumes, may increase the risk at certain stages of pregnancy to fetal development abnormalities. Pregnancy is a critical period and every precaution should be taken to design the environment, both preconception and during pregnancy, to protect the developing fetus from exposure to toxic substances and afford the fetus optimal opportunity for development through proper nutrition.

Diet and Problem Pregnancy

It has been almost forty years since it was found that there is a strong correlation between the quality of diet of a pregnant woman and the health of her offspring.[6] Studies reported in 1982 indicate that there is a risk of nutritional deficiency in the newborn, even in uneventful pregnancies in an economically favored population.[7] These investigators conclude that nutritional surveillance during pregnancy must remain an important and pivotal part of preventive health care and that the pregnancy period is the optimal time to initiate a Living Life

Insurance Program that will follow that new individual throughout his or her entire life.

Proper nutrition throughout pregnancy can help avoid some of the major complications of pregnancy such as eclampsia or toxemia.[8] One doctor was able to reduce the pregnancy toxemia rate in an urban hospital by a factor of five by instituting nutrition education classes for pregnant women and getting them to eat high-quality foods, such as whole-grain breads, dairy products, eggs, fresh fruits and vegetables, and give up the empty-calorie "junk" and snack foods and sugar-rich beverages they had been previously consuming. He expressed amazement that the success of the program was such a revelation to many of his obstetrical colleagues. It would seem to be common sense that eating well during pregnancy may be as important in determining the quality of the pregnancy as any other single feature in the habits of the mother.

If the observation that suboptimal nutrition leads to poor development *in utero* is correct, and if this problem can be amplified from generation to generation, it is possible that some people may be moving into a second or third generation equivalent to the cats in the study. Adults who were poorly nourished as fetuses may now have increased problems with conception and pregnancy of their own. Infertility of unknown origin is being seen in larger numbers of couples around the country. Might these problems be related to the legacy that these individuals carry with them as it relates to their own poor nutritional and health status begun during their development *in utero?*

Vitamin Supplementation During Pregnancy

Obviously, the answer to that question is very difficult because many factors have an impact upon a person's physiological function, but there is preliminary evidence indicating that improved vitamin and mineral intake during pregnancy can have a significant impact upon improving fetal development. Women who had previously given birth to one or more infants with the fetal abnormality called neural-tube defect, when recruited into a trial of multivitamin supplementation during pregnancy, had a significant reduction in neural-tube defects in infants born after the supplementation.[9] Supplements used in the study were of standard potency, including the Recommended Dietary Allowance levels of the major known vitamins, with added iron, calcium, and phosphorus.

The link between vitamin deficiency and neural-tube defects was recognized in 1965, when it was first realized that a folic acid deficiency might be related to the problem. More recently, significant associations have also been found between the increased risk to neural-tube defects and vitamin-C, vitamin-B-2, and vitamin-A deficiencies during pregnancy.

What are the benefits, then, of nutritional supplements during pregnancy? Optimal fetal growth and development in the mother's uterus depends upon a steady supply of nutrients from the mother to the fetus. The fetus is nourished exclusively by the mother's blood sugar and generates no energy for growth from either protein or fat itself. One of the reasons why many infants born to diabetic mothers have very large birth weights is that the mother has a very high level of sugar in her blood and, therefore, feeds the fetus more, which results in larger birth-weight babies. Fetal malnutrition may result from deficiency of proper levels of blood sugar delivered to the fetus, or inadequate level of the vitamins and minerals necessary for the proper metabolism by the fetus of the blood sugar.

Blood Sugar and Fetal Development

It is well established that women who are diabetic are at higher risk to problems in pregnancy than women who are not diabetic; however, women who may have a tendency toward low blood sugar, or hypoglycemia, may have actually a greater risk to pregnancy complications than women who are diabetic.[10] From a study of over 10,000 pregnant women it was concluded that hypoglycemic women actually had more complications in delivery and children with lower Apgar scores (a measure of infant vitality after birth), and increased perinatal mortality than did diabetic women.

Unfortunately most doctors screen their pregnant patients only for diabetes, not for hypoglycemia. If a woman shows the symptoms of hypoglycemia before pregnancy—shakiness before meals, confusion or emotionally depressed states if a meal is missed, compulsive appetite for sweet foods, and abnormal tiredness or muscle weakness after eating—she should be tested so this low blood sugar condition can be identified and managed properly throughout the pregnancy if it exists.

To help properly manage the level of sugar in the blood, a variety of vitamins and minerals may be necessary in the diet of a mother, based upon her own unique genetic need. This is another good reason for a woman who is planning on having a child to develop her own Nutraerobics biotype so that she can manage her unique requirements during pregnancy for optimal nutrition of the fetus.

Problems of Excessive Nutrients in Pregnancy

What, then, are the risks associated with nutritional supplements during pregnancy? Due to the fact that the fetus cannot protect itself, nor tell the mother what the impact of vitamin supplementation is, it is wise not to supplement with any vitamin or mineral in high levels during pregnancy unless there is a specific demonstrated need.

Vitamin A has an RDA of 5000 units during pregnancy, which represents an increase of 25 percent over the allowance for nonpregnant adult women. The added allowance is required for fetal storage of vitamin A. Dietary sources can readily provide the necessary amount of vitamin A if the mother is on a high-quality diet from animal and vegetable products, so there is usually no need for supplementation. Vitamin A intakes during pregnancy in excess of 50,000 units may lead to increased risk to birth defects according to animal studies. Although confirmatory evidence in human studies is still lacking, excessive vitamin A is not advised during pregnancy.

Vitamin D requirements are usually not increased in pregnancy and, in fact, there is evidence that a markedly excessive intake may actively cause maternal loss of calcium and predispose the fetus to develop severe forms of high blood calcium. The RDA for vitamin D is 400 units per day, which can be obtained, again, through the diet if milk and other dairy products are consumed.

The need for Vitamin E may rise an average of 40 to 50 percent during pregnancy and return to normal levels after delivery. The rise occurs primarily in the second trimester and probably reflects the increased blood fats associated with pregnancy. There is some evidence that increased vitamin E above the 30 units suggested by the RDA may be helpful—levels of 100 to 400 units can be used safely during pregnancy.

Most investigations have shown an increased need for the water-soluble vitamins throughout pregnancy. There may be a number of genetically determined metabolic conditions that require increased levels of B vitamins during pregnancy. Pregnant women who tend to get sore muscles and stiffness during the pregnancy may have greater need for vitamin B-1 to reduce pyruvic and lactic acid buildup, indicators of this B-vitamin deficiency state.

A vitamin B-2 deficiency is characterized in the expectant mother by chapped lips, fissures at the corners of the mouth, dermatitis of the face, and soreness of the hands and feet. Levels of vitamin B-2 between 2 and 20 milligrams per day are suggested. There is no known adverse effect upon the fetus from taking larger amounts of this water-soluble vitamin.

Vitamin B-3 (niacin) in large quantities may produce flushing, which is an unpleasant side effect, but there are no known adverse effects upon the fetus from taking large doses of B-3.

Vitamin B-6 in very large doses has been used to treat the nausea of pregnancy. One of the problems in taking large doses of B-6 in the latter stage of pregnancy is that it seems to depress the hormone prolactin and prevent proper milk flow and production in the woman who is going to breastfeed.[11] Proper quantities of B-6, however, are necessary; a chronic B-6 deficiency during pregnancy might increase the risk to fetal atherosclerosis, or alterations in the arteries feeding the heart, that could lead in later life to heart disease.[12] Levels of B-6 during pregnancy should range from 10 to 100 milligrams per day.

Vitamin B-12 and folic acid are two other water-soluble vitamins that should be taken in greater doses during pregnancy. These two vitamins work together to promote the manufacture of red blood cells in the mother and DNA (the genetic material) production in the fetus. The RDA for vitamin B-12 during pregnancy has been established at 5 micrograms and that of folic acid at 800 micrograms. Higher levels may be used with safety.

Vitamin C is distinctly needed in adequate quantities during pregnancy. It has been recently reported that aborigines in Australia, who are notoriously vitamin C depleted, give birth to infants who develop a syndrome that resembles sudden infant death syndrome, and that by administering vitamin C to the mothers this condition was virtually eliminated.[12] This does not suggest that sudden infant death syndrome is necessarily caused by a vitamin-C deficiency, only that vitamin C has an important effect on the neonatal vitality of the developing fetus. Levels of vitamin C between 500 and 1000 milligrams a day are considered in the ideal range. Very high levels in the thousands of milligrams per day may be excessive because we do not know the long-term side effects of high-level vitamin-C administration during pregnancy.

In conclusion, it can be said that supplementation during pregnancy with vitamins and minerals within a prudent range of the RDAs is possibly beneficial, but that supplementation in the megavitamin range should be avoided, since we do not yet know what the potential effects on fetal development may be. As one doctor sums it up, "Unquestionably a well balanced diet during pregnancy remains the best source of most of the vitamins. . . . Large doses of certain minerals and fat-soluble vitamins may be harmful and should be avoided during pregnancy. Despite some contrary reports, a definitive case can be made that additional supplies of iron, calcium, and folic acid above that gotten in the average diet should be taken during pregnancy and there is also evidence that increased intake of vitamin B-1 and B-6 might be beneficial to pregnant women."[13]

Calcium and Toxemia of Pregnancy

The complications of pregnancy toxemia, including elevated blood pressure, the spill of protein in the urine, and fluid retention, increases the risk to the fetus and the mother. The process by which this condition develops in women during the third term of gestation is not well understood. Recently, however, it has been found that not only does a high-quality, unrefined diet using the basic food groups help reduce the risk of toxemia, the increased dietary calcium intake also has a beneficial effect.[14]

Supplementation with 440 milligrams of calcium per day reduced the incidence of toxemia in one population from 14.6 to 4.8 percent. The toxemia of pregnancy may or may not accompany a condition called gestational diabetes in which in the last trimester of pregnancy the woman has elevated blood pressure and the symptoms of diabetes. Gestational diabetes may be the result of a vitamin B-6 deficiency. In a recent study it was found that administration of vitamin B-6 at the level of about 50 milligrams per day to women with this condition led to normalization of blood glucose and an elimination of the symptoms of diabetes.[15]

Vitamins and calcium work along with the trace elements in controlling the metabolism and development of the fetus. One of the most exciting recent areas of understanding in the nutrition and growth of the fetus is the role that the elements zinc, manganese, and chromium play in establishing the proper sequence of events during pregnancy.

Trace Elements and Pregnancy

Deficiencies of zinc, manganese, and chromium have been shown to lead to increased risk to birth defects in animals studied.[16] And it has been recently reported that when animals were fed a diet moderately deficient in zinc from the seventh day after conception until delivery, the offspring of these animals showed depressed immune function, and that, in addition, the second and third generations, all of which were fed diets that contained normal levels of zinc, continued to manifest reduced immunity, although not to the same degree as in the first generation. The authors go on to suggest, "Dietary supplementation beyond the levels considered adequate might allow for more rapid or complete restoration of immunity [in zinc deprived infants]."[17]

What other effects does zinc have in proper fetal development? It was found that the zinc content of the blood of mothers giving birth to babies who were small was significantly lower than that of mothers giving birth to normal-weight babies, and the authors of this study conclude that maternal tissue zinc depletion is associated with fetal growth retardation.[18] It has also been found that mothers who give birth to infants who have a condition where the spine does not close correctly, called spina bifida cystica, may have an abnormality in zinc availability or metabolism during pregnancy.[19]

Reduced fertility in the woman, fetal growth retardation, abnormal fetal development, and prolonged labor are all consequences of zinc deprivation.[20] A zinc deficiency may also be associated with calcium deficiency in the elevated blood pressure and toxemia of pregnancy.[21] It was also found that infants who had higher incidences of congenital defects at birth (undescended testes and changes in the fingers and hands) were delivered from adolescent mothers whose blood zinc levels were well below the mean for their group. These same women were also found to generally have higher levels of blood pressure and be at greater risk to pregnancy toxemia.

The level of zinc intake considered sufficient during pregnancy is

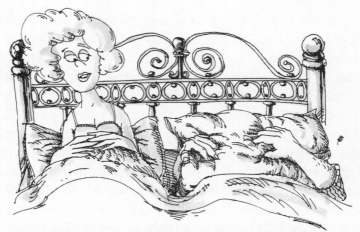

WAKE UP, JOHN, I HAVE THIS TREMENDOUS CRAVING FOR AUTOMOBILE BUMPERS.

in the range of 20 to 30 milligrams per day (total amount in diet plus any supplement). Zinc absorption is aided by the presence of adequate levels of iron, vitamin B-6, and picolinic acid which comes from trypto-phan, an amino acid found in high-quality protein such as lean meat, fish, eggs, and milk products. Supplementation with zinc, vitamin B-6, iron, and dietary tryptophan in one study led to fetal growth accelera-tion and improved zinc status.[22]

Another trace element linked with proper fetal development dur-ing pregnancy is chromium. Chromium is known to be very important in stabilizing the body's ability to properly metabolize blood sugar, which is the major source of energy for the developing fetus. When chromium is deficient, there may be an interruption in the proper breakdown of blood sugar, thereby leading to complications in the development of the fetus. The level of chromium in the mother's hair may be an important indicator of her overall chromium status and reveal what risk the fetus may have in relation to chromium defi-ciency.[23]

An intake level of chromium of 100 micrograms per day is considered desirable for pregnant women, particularly in the last trimester. The best food sources for chromium include liver, brewer's yeast (particularly chromium-enriched brewer's yeast), whole-grain products, and yeast breads.

Essential Fats and Pregnancy

Essential fatty acids, found in high content in unsaturated vegetable oils, are extremely important for the proper stimulation of the developing nervous system and the regulation of a class of hormones called prostaglandins. If a mother's diet is excessively high in saturated animal fats (which are low in these essential fatty acids) or if the mother is on a weight loss diet during pregnancy where she is not taking in adequate levels of fatty acids, there may be an adverse impact on the development of the nervous system of the fetus.

Most nutritionists suggest that at least 1 percent of a person's total calories should come as essential fatty acids, a level that may need to be slightly higher during pregnancy. This higher need and the possibility that elevated blood cholesterol levels of the mother are associated with increased risk to heart disease in later life of her child make it urgent for the mother during pregnancy to try to keep her total animal fat intake down and replace it with unsaturated vegetable oils. The total fat intake during pregnancy should not be more than 20 to 25 percent of the calories, the majority of which should come from vegetable oils. Use of oils in salad dressings, homemade mayonnaise, or in stir-frying of vegetables are alternatives.

Protein and Pregnancy

Protein in the pregnant women's diet should be of high quality and balanced with proper vitamin and mineral intake. The babies and placentas taken from 462 deliveries showed that those women who had a balanced protein and calorie intake during pregnancy had slightly larger birth-weight babies than women who utilized high-protein sup-

Table 7

Range of Nutrients Required by Pregnant Women

Protein		80–120 g
Calories		1,800–2,600 cal.
Fluids		3–5 pts
Salt		6–8 g
Essential Fats		3–10 g
Vitamins:		
	A	5,000–20,000 IU
	D	400–800 IU
	E	100–400 IU
	C	200–1,000 mg
	B-1	5–100 mg
	B-2	5–100 mg
	B-3	10–200 mg
	B-6	5–100 mg
	B-12	5–200 mcg
	folic acid	800–2,000 mcg
	pantothenic acid	50–200 mg
	biotin	50–100 mcg
Minerals:		
	phosphorus	1,400–1,800 mg
	calcium	1,000–1,200 mg
	magnesium	300–600 mg
	iron	20–60 mg
	copper	2–5 mg
	zinc	20–40 mg
	manganese	5–10 mg
	chromium	50–100 mcg
	selenium	100–200 mcg
	iodine	200–500 mg

plements during pregnancy; this latter diet showed some adverse effects on fetal growth, ability to reach full term, and newborn survival.[24] This strongly suggests that pregnant women should *not* be on protein-enriched weight loss diets during pregnancy, and that dietary protein during pregnancy be at the level of 80 to 120 grams per day, which is equivalent to a total of 10 to 16 ounces (¾ to 1 pound) of lean meats, fish, poultry, or cheese daily.

Starting the Living
Life Insurance Program

So what have we really said about protecting the unborn? We have tried to establish that the Nutraerobics Living Life Insurance Program starts ideally before conception and continues throughout fetal development. From day zero on, optimal function is dependent upon the optimal environment for the fetus. Since the fetus cannot protect itself, it is exclusively dependent upon what its mother and father provide for it. (Ranges of nutritional intake are summarized in Table 7.) Giving the child an optimal state of nutrition and protecting it from exposure to known harmful materials such as alcohol, toxic chemicals, certain medications, or cigarette smoking just make good sense in providing a full opportunity to that new life.

Many unfortunate health conditions of unknown origin that occur in the child's early or later life may have actually started during the period of fetal development. There is no better gift parents can give to their child than the gift of the optimal environment during pregnancy. Not only does this help the child throughout his or her whole life, the physical and emotional health of the parents benefit as well.

Remember, it was not too long ago that we felt that the fetus was always protected against nutritional deficiency because it drew from the reserves of the mother. Now we know that this is not always the case. There are examples in which the development of the fetus may be compromised so that the mother's status is maintained. Such seems to be the case, for example, with calcium. If a mother is on a lower than optimal calcium intake, it's not her bone calcium that suffers but the bone density of the infant. What is optimal for the mother, however, is going to be optimal for the fetus as they live during these first nine months of the fetus's new life.

The story doesn't end, however, with the arrival of the healthy newborn. From birth on, children need their own Nutraerobics Programs based upon their own individual needs. During infancy and childhood it will be the parents who can recognize these specific needs. Let's direct our attention next to patterning a specific Nutraerobics Program for your child.

Notes

1. F. Pottenger, "The Effect of Heat-Processed Foods on the Dentofacial Structures of Experimental Animals," *American Journal of Orthodontics and Oral Surgery, 32,* 467(1946).

2. L. Hurley, *Developmental Nutrition* (Englewood Cliffs, NJ: Prentice-Hall, 1980).

3. H. J. Evan et al., "Sperm Abnormalities and Cigarette Smoking," *Lancet* (21 March 1981):627–630.

4. T. F. X. Collins and E. V. Collins, "A Comprehensive Study of the Teratogenic Potential of Caffeine in Rats," pp. 1–24, Data Acquisition and Monitoring Division, National Oceanic and Atmospheric Administration, Washington, D.C., 1980; P. E. Palm, E. P. Arnold, and C. J. Kensler, "Evaluation of the Teratogenic Potential of Fresh-Brewed Coffee," *Toxicology and Applied Pharmacology, 44,* 1(1978).

5. M. E. Jacobson, A. S. Goldman, and R. H. Syme, "Coffee and Birth Defects," *Lancet* (27 June 1981):1415–1416.

6. B. S. Burke et al., "Nutrition Studies During Pregnancy," *American Journal of Obstetrics and Gynecology, 46,* 35(1943).

7. J. S. Vobecky and C. Fisch, "Biochemical Indices of Nutritional Status in Maternal, Cord, and Early Neonatal Blood," *American Journal of Clinical Nutrition, 36,* 630(1982).

8. T. Brewer, *Metabolic Toxemia of Late Pregnancy* (New Canaan, CT: Keats, 1982).

9. R. W. Smithells, S. Sheppard, and M. J. Seller, "Possible Prevention of Neural-Tube Defects by Periconceptional Vitamin Supplementation," *Lancet* (16 February 1980):339–342.

10. P. A. Long and N. A. Beischer, "Importance of Abnormal Glucose Tolerance

(Hypoglycemia) in the Etiology of Pre-eclampsia," *Lancet* (30 April 1977):923.

11. L. B. Greentree, "Dangers of Vitamin B-6 in Nursing Mothers," *New England Journal of Medicine, 300,* 141(1979).

12. B. Wilcken, "Maternal Vitamin B-6 Deficiency and Infant Atherosclerosis," *Nutrition Reports International, 1976,* p. 12.

13. K. S. Moghissi, "Risks and Benefits of Nutritional Supplements During Pregnancy," *Obstetrics and Gynecology, 58,* 694(1981).

14. "Toxemia of Pregnancy: The Dietary Calcium Hypothesis," *Nutrition Reviews, 39,* 124(1981).

15. H. J. J. Coelingh Bennink and W. H. P. Schreurs, "Improvement of Oral Glucose Tolerance in Gestational Diabetes by Pyridoxine," *British Medical Journal 3,* 13(1975).

16. C. C. Pfeiffer and B. Barnes, "Role of Zinc, Manganese, and Chromium Deficiencies in Birth Defects," *International Journal of Environmental Studies, 17,* 43(1981).

17. R. S. Beach, M. E. Gershwin, and L. S. Hurley, "Gestational Zinc Deprivation in Mice: Persistance of Immunodeficiency for Three Generations," *Science, 218,* 469(1982).

18. N. J. Meadows and D. L. Bloxam, "Zinc and Small Babies," *Lancet* (21 November 1981):1135–37.

19. K. E. Bergmann and K. H. Tews, "Abnormalities of Hair Zinc Concentration in Mothers of Newborn Infants with Spinabifida," *American Journal of Clinical Nutrition, 3,* 2145(1980).

20. C. A. Swanson and J. G. King, "Zinc Utilization in Pregnant and Nonpregnant Women," *Journal of Nutrition, 112,* 697(1982).

21. F. Cherry and H. K. Batson, "Plasma Zinc in Hypertension/Toxemia in Adolescent Pregnancy," *American Journal of Clinical Nutrition, 34,* 2367(1981).

22. G. W. Evans and E. C. Johnson, "Effect of Iron, Vitamin B-6, Picolinic Acid on Zinc Absorption," *Journal of Nutrition, 111,* 68(1981).

23. G. Saner, "The Effect of Parity on Maternal Hair Chromium Concentration and the Changes During Pregnancy," *American Journal of Clinical Nutrition, 34,* 853(1981).

24. M. Pereira, M. Winick and M. Susser, "Effects of Prenatal Nutritional Supplementation on the Placenta," *American Journal of Clinical Nutrition, 36,* 229(1982).

13

Children and Their Behaviors

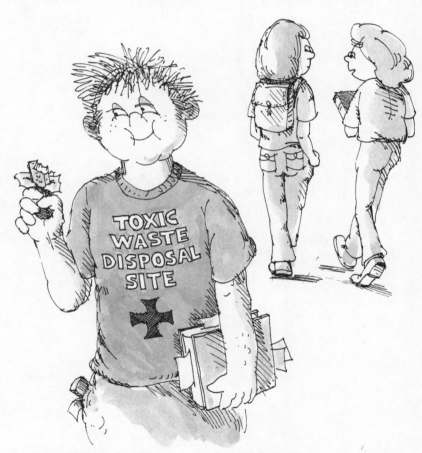

RALPH EATS SO MUCH JUNK FOOD, HIS MOTHER
MADE HIM A SPECIAL T-SHIRT.

Does your child have:

1. Abdominal or chest pain?

1	2	3	4
No	Sometimes	Frequently	All the time

2. Sleep disturbances, restlessness, recurring bad dreams?

1	2	3	4
No	Sometimes	Frequently	All the time

3. Personality changes, depression, aggression?

1	2	3	4
No	Sometimes	Frequently	All the time

4. Nasal congestion, cough, sore throat, or earache?

1	2	3	4
No	Sometimes	Frequently	All the time

5. Fatigue, headaches, or recurring fever?

1	2	3	4
No	Sometimes	Frequently	All the time

If your score exceeds twelve, you may find some important answers to these problems in Chapter 13.

Some of our greatest joys—and sources of exasperation—are our children. Their successes make us proud and exuberant, their failures and difficulties leave us concerned and sometimes frustrated. What can the Nutraerobics Program contribute to maximize your child's success by the improvement of both physical and emotional health? By starting to recognize your child's biotype, you may be on the road to improving his or her health in ways you didn't dream possible.

The symptoms listed at the beginning of the chapter were all found to be associated with undernutrition in children. Patients who had one or more of these listed symptoms, but who could not be found upon medical evaluation to have any known disease, were by more thorough nutritional analysis found to be suffering from a deficiency of one of the B vitamins, vitamin B-1.

The cause of this particular deficiency appeared to be associated closely with the children's heavy consumption of empty-calorie foods: carbonated sweet beverages, candy, snack foods, and other nutritionally marginal foods. The symptoms found in these patients could all be correlated with the preclinical signs of vitamin deficiency but most doctors are not used to recognizing them as such.

Supplementation of these youngsters' diets with vitamins led to improvement although the recovery was slow, generally taking two to three months for marked results. In over half the patients, though, supplementation and dietary improvement led to a significant reduction in symptoms and health-related problems.[1]

Earlier, these children might have been thought to have been suffering from behavioral or physiological problems of unknown origin and been treated with psychological therapy or medications such as sedatives, muscle relaxants, or antihyperactivity drugs. Their symptoms, however, were actually caused by their diets, which were vitamin deficient due to their high consumption of empty- or naked-calorie foods.

Such states of marginal deficiency may be very common, even in our modern affluent society, because of our high dependence on empty-calorie foods. These conditions may possibly even be more dangerous than frank vitamin deficiency symptoms such as those associated with beriberi and scurvy, since the personality changes seen with these conditions in children were frequently aggressive in nature and it took quite a while for the metabolic abnormalities to improve after dietary intervention.

The "Junk Food Syndrome"

Obviously, not all human personality and behavioral problems are explained by faulty diet; however it does appear that some abnormal behaviors, particularly in children, may depend on eating habits that upset delicate biochemical balances in the brain. Such seems to be the case with children who consume upward of 50 percent or more of their calories as empty calories, a problem loosely termed the "junk food syndrome."[2]

The case history of Tracy is illustrative. Tracy was a 12-year-old boy described as highly excitable and failing in school. He displayed little self-control, had recurring bad dreams, and complained of constant stomach pains and fatigue. Since the age of 10, Tracy had become increasingly combative. He constantly started arguments at home and at school. After giving Tracy a comprehensive physical, the pediatrician found nothing medically wrong with him. Although the boy displayed some symptoms of hyperactivity, the doctor doubted this was the problem. His constipation, muscle pain, and lethargy were not typical of hyperactivity; neither was his aggressive behavior. Further evaluation led to the suggestion that Tracy might be suffering from "overconsumptive undernutrition," the "junk food syndrome."

The brain depends upon proper levels of calories, vitamins, and minerals for its manufacture of energy to control mood, mind, memory, and behavior. If the brain is getting adequate calories in the form of blood sugar but not getting adequate levels of vitamins and minerals, it may result in symptoms of behavioral disturbance. This is particularly seen in the most biologically sensitive individuals in our society, our children.

Tracy's parents were advised to eliminate candy, doughnuts, and ice cream from his diet, to add more vitamin- and mineral-rich foods such as fruit, hard-boiled eggs, and whole-grain products, and to supplement with a high-potency B-complex vitamin daily. Within three weeks Tracy had improved remarkably in several ways. His new biochemical tests showed he no longer suffered from the chronic nutritional inadequacies found earlier. His schoolwork improved, and his random aggressiveness virtually disappeared within two months.

Behavior and Biochemical Individuality

There is a very significant individual genetic need for various vitamins for optimal function. In one study it was found that the children who suffered from a variety of B-1 deficiency symptoms did not have low blood levels of vitamin B-1 by standard testing methods. Presumably they were getting adequate levels of vitamins in their diets; however, when the actual ability of these vitamins to operate effectively in cells was examined, it was found deficient in the majority of these children.

Many investigators have identified the unique biochemical needs of certain individuals for levels of vitamins greater than those the average person may require in order to promote optimal function. Apparently healthy normal individuals may differ significantly in the rates at which their cells utilize various vitamins and vitamin metabolism is undoubtedly under genetic control.[3] In a study of "normal, healthy individuals," 7 percent were found to be poor utilizers of vitamin B-6 who may require significantly greater quantities in their diets for optimal function, even though they were not suffering from the classic signs of a vitamin B-6 deficiency. The restoration of proper function could only be established when giving B vitamins at ten to fifteen times the Recommended Dietary Allowance level, which would be difficult to get from diet alone without supplementation.[4]

In a recent attempt to identify those individuals who may need high levels of B vitamins to optimize function, the minimum effective dose of B vitamins to compensate for metabolic sluggishness was studied. It was observed after administering vitamin B-2 and other vitamins of the B family at four times the Recommended Dietary Allowance for one month, that 50 percent of the children had biochemical evidence of B-vitamin deficiency before supplementation as judged by the degree of improved enzyme function that occurred after supplementation. The question is, to what extent did genetic predisposition contribute to this persistent B-vitamin deficiency state which may have been related to chronic clinical manifestations? It's only recently that nutritionists have begun looking at this question of chronic vitamin deficiency based upon biochemical uniqueness.

Vitamins and Brain Function

Some individuals' requirements for members of the B vitamin family and vitamin C may far exceed what are considered to be the normal dietary levels, and intake at normal levels may lead to idiosyncratic symptoms such as headache, irritability, insomnia, and weakness.

A most interesting and highly controversial application of this concept of biochemical individuality and vitamin need in children was work done with a severely retarded child who at the age of 7 was in diapers, could not speak, and had an estimated IQ of between 25 and 30. Analysis of blood and other tissues of this patient indicated nutritional deficiency even though the child was getting what would appear to be nutritionally adequate diet. Utilizing a supplement containing very high levels of nutrients far in excess of what would be considered reasonable, the child began to improve. In a few days he was talking a little and in a few weeks he was learning to read and write and beginning to act like a normal child. By the time he was 9 years of age, he read and wrote at the elementary school level, was moderately advanced in arithmetic, and according to his teacher was mischievous and active. He was able to ride a bicycle, use a skateboard, play ball and the flute, and had an IQ of about 90.[5]

It appeared that even after seven years of suboptimal nutrition relative to *his* need, this child could respond to a meganutrient program in a remarkable fashion, which seems to support the concept that his genetic need for vitamins in order to optimize his function was far in excess of what would be considered adequate for average individuals.

A genetotrophic disease is one in which the genetic pattern of the individual requires a higher supply of one or more nutrients, such that when these nutrients are supplied at the higher level, the disease is prevented or treated. To explore this hypothesis under more controlled conditions, an elegant double-blind, crossover study was devised. In this experiment, sixteen retarded (Down's syndrome), school-age children with initial IQs of 17 to 70 were given nutritional supplements or placebos during a period of eight months. The supplement contained eight minerals in moderate amounts and eleven vitamins, mostly in relatively large amounts as indicated in Table 8.

The amounts of vitamins found in this formulation would be considered wasteful by most medical investigators and nutritionists because it would be assumed that at this level the nutrients could not be used and might even be toxic. During the first four-month period, the five children who received supplements increased their average IQ by 5 to 10 points, while the eleven subjects given the placebo showed negligible change. During the second period the subjects who had been given placebos in the first period received supplements and showed an average increase in IQ of at least 10. Three of the five subjects who were given supplements for both periods, thereby getting supplements for eight months, showed additional IQ gains during the second four months.

Three of four children with Down's syndrome gained between 10 and 25 units in IQ and showed physical changes in the direction of normal. Vision and facial structure improved and growth rates increased.[6]

These are remarkable results, for it is generally thought that a congenital condition such as Down's syndrome is irreversible and that

Table 8

**Daily Doses of Supplemental Vitamins and Minerals
Used in Mental Retardation Study**

Vitamin A (palmitate)	15,000 IU
Vitamin D (cholecalciferol)	300 IU
Thiamin mononitrate	300 mg
Riboflavin	200 mg
Niacinamide	750 mg
Calcium (pantothenate)	490 mg
Pyridoxine hydrochloride	350 mg
Cobalamin	1,000 mg
Folic acid	400 mg
Vitamin C (ascorbic acid)	1,500 mg
Vitamin E (d-α-tocopheryl succinate)	600 IU
Magnesium (oxide)	300 mg
Calcium (carbonate)	400 mg
Zinc (oxide)	30 mg
Manganese (gluconate)	3 mg
Copper (gluconate)	1.75 mg
Iron (ferrous fumarate)	7.5 mg
Calcium phosphate (CaHPO)	37.5 mg
Iodine (KI)	0.15 mg

The daily dose was 6 tablets. The tablets also contained microcrystalline cellulose, povidone, stearic acid, sodium silicoaluminate, hydroxypropyl-methylcellulose, propylene glycol, silica gel, polyethylene glycol, titanium dioxide, oleic acid, and tribasic sodium phosphate as excipients. The placebo tablets contained lactose, microcrystalline cellulose, stearic acid, povidone, propylene glycol, hydroxypropylmethylcellulose, titanium dioxide, and oleic acid.

the best we can do for children with it is to provide them comfort and social support. But have we in fact accepted certain diseases as irreversible, rather than recognizing them as indications of incredibly wide variations in the genetic need for specific nutrients?

Conditional Lethal Mutations

It is possible that all of us carry with us one or more messages in our genes that code for specific need for nutrients above and beyond what would be considered average for most individuals. Fortunately, most of us do not carry the genetic messages that code for such extremely high needs that we cannot even come close to fulfilling them from our diet; therefore, most of us do not experience such serious health problems as Down's syndrome. It is possible, however, that these less significant genetic alterations, if not attended to, can lead to increased risk to degenerative disease and may represent conditional lethal mutations.

The term *conditional lethal mutations* means that these genetic changes, if unattended, may prove lethal to us in mid to late life as degenerative diseases such as heart disease, cancer, or diabetes, but are conditional upon the way we treat our genetic nature through our lifestyle. This represents the whole thrust of the Nutraerobics Program, and its attempt is to identify those biochemically unique features of your and your child's genetic disposition and then to manage those uniquenesses correctly, so as to prevent their lethal expression in mid to late life.

Intelligence and Vitamins

That mental functioning can improve with vitamin supplementation is not a completely new observation. One study reported the average IQ score to be 4.5 units higher in seventy-two students with higher vitamin-C levels in their blood than in seventy-two students matched by socioeconomic criteria who had lower vitamin-C levels, but who were not suffering from scurvy.[7] Most of this difference in IQ was abolished after both groups were given supplemental orange juice for six months, and the authors conclude that intelligence test performances are determined by the "temporary nutritional state of the individual, at least with regard to . . . ascorbic acid."

Another study looked at the effects of an improved diet and an improved diet with vitamins on the IQs, school achievement, and other measurements in twenty learning-disabled children. For six months, large amounts of vitamin C, vitamin B-3, pantothenic acid, and vitamin B-6 were given to ten of the children on a double-blind basis. The improved diet seemed to produce beneficial results; however, there were suggestive greater improvements in IQ and in reading tests that occurred in the group given the supplement.[8]

It should be pointed out that there is as yet no definitive way for absolutely determining optimal vitamin needs for individuals with particular sensitivities. Even in the study on the sixteen retarded children, the researchers point out, "It seems certain that better supplements can be found than the particular combination we tested. . . . Ultimately it should be possible to tailor supplements to meet individual needs; at which time, perhaps, several of the nutrients we included could be reduced or eliminated in individual cases, and possibly even greater amounts of specific nutrients might be called for on an individual basis."

We cannot advocate—on the basis of their study alone—the consumption of such large levels of nutrients by the population-at-large for improved mental functioning, but the study does indicate that the range of nutritional needs may be much farther divergent than we have previously suspected in standard nutrition and medicine. If this is correct, then we may have been missing many people who would be responsive to nutritional therapy by assuming that they are consuming the average diet and by definition must be adequately nourished.

As is so many times the case in making observations, the initial assumption we make may dictate the final conclusion. If we assume that disease is not related to nutrition because we see no signs that we or our children are suffering nutrient deficiency, then it is obvious that we will not look for the potential chronic health effects of suboptimal nutrition. As Louis Pasteur once said, "The chance of making an observation favors the mind that's prepared to make that observation."

The Nutraerobics Program, which is based on the genetotrophic theory of disease, tries to identify those factors that may indicate specific nutritional need above and beyond the "average" and deliver to the individual nutrition that will optimize his or her function based upon biochemical need.

Nutrient Excesses

We must repeat that any substance may be toxic in large quantities and, therefore, one should not consume large doses of nutrients without some knowledge of their need. The desirability of taking a high dose of any nutrient must be based on an analysis of benefits versus potential risks. One should try to maximize benefits while minimizing risks, remembering that a zero level of risk is never possible. The levels discussed in the Nutraerobics Program for supplemental nutrients have been found by clinical studies to be in the safe range to maximize benefits and minimize risks for humans with biochemical need.

Do not use the philosophy "If a little is good, a whole lot more ought to be better"; try to tailor the intake specifically to your own biochemical requirements. Close analysis of your biotype (by going back and reevaluating your responses to the various questionnaires in Chapter 2) after being on an altered nutritional program is useful for improving your understanding of either your own or your child's specific requirements.

Sugar and Its Influence on Behavior

Let's examine what other specific factors of the Nutraerobics Program may influence the health and the behavior of children. A five-year study under the Children's Achievement Program for Educational Readiness evaluated children's achievement in school in relationship to their diets. In this long-term study the participants received diet education and nutritional support, in which highly refined foods and sugars were sharply reduced in their diets and replaced by fresh fruits and juices and whole-wheat flour; chocolate milk, sugar-coated breakfast cereals, and sugared doughnuts were eliminated in preference to French toast and hot oatmeal and raisins for breakfast. Those who had reached the fifth or sixth grade were found to have an accelerated performance in school and were either at or above their regular designated grade levels at the completion of the program.[9]

A similar positive effect was observed in lowering the sugar content in the diets of juveniles who, due to behavior problems of a severe nature, had been placed in juvenile homes or treatment centers. The children and the staffs, with the exception of the chefs, were not informed of the change. Three months after the removal of white sugar, products containing white sugar, and highly sugared beverages from the menu, the children on the modified diet had a 45 percent lower incidence of formal disciplinary action than the control group. This particular improvement continued throughout the remainder of the incarceration of these children and is another illustration of impact on sensitive individuals that the empty-calorie diet may have.[10]

Toxic Elements and Behavior

Exposure to toxic minerals in the environment and their accumulation in the body also contribute to altered behavior and performance in children. One report showed that children who were, by standard testing in their school system, evaluated as learning disabled had much higher hair lead and cadmium levels than did children in a matched group who were not learning disabled. Analysis of levels of heavy metals in the hair has been used as a technique to assess body burden of these potentially toxic minerals and results indicate that there may be a causal relationship between functional problems of the brain and excessive accumulation of toxic minerals in children with learning disabilities.[11]

This observation seems to be corroborated by other studies in which the levels of lead in the teeth of children in the elementary school grades were examined and correlated with their performance and learning abilities in school. Children with higher levels of lead in their teeth had lower performances in school and the greater learning problems. Of the 2,146 children tested, only two really had what would be considered diagnosable lead toxicity by standard medical evaluation, but many more of the children were nonetheless impaired by excess accumulation of lead through exposure in their environments.[12]

In estimating the changes in blood lead levels in the United States over the past four years, it is found that there is still evidence of elevated blood lead in black, Chicano, and Caucasian children.[13] Many investigators feel that blood lead is not a very reliable tool for assessing lead body burden in that most of the lead accumulated in the body is deposited within bone and tissue and is not available in the blood; therefore, this report may actually be a low estimate of the true spectrum of problems associated with excessive lead in our children.[14]

There have been recent suggestions in medical literature that screening children, particularly in urban areas, for lead burden may be important as a preventive health tool. Most of the lead these children are getting is not from eating lead-based paints, but from inhaling and ingesting background lead from foods, dust, and air. Foods such as tuna and tomatoes, which come in cans with leaded solder seams, are contaminated with the lead and may be one of the contributors to an increased burden of lead in our environment.[15]

A relationship between lead exposure and accumulation in the child and deficiency in intelligence has also been reported.[16] Lead seems to interrupt the ability to utilize the vitamin folic acid effectively and may have an adverse impact upon cellular development and regeneration.[17] This interruption of folic acid metabolism may result in the observed behavioral and psychological changes that occur in children as the result of exposure to lead.[18]

Excess accumulation of lead has also been found associated with autism in children.[19] The present understanding of lead and its role in the nervous system of children underscores the importance of screening for lead as a necessary part of the medical evaluation of all autistic and similar patients.

Preventing Lead Absorption

Due to these panoramic effects of lead on the behavior and functioning of children, a recent editorial advocated that child health programs consider routine periodic screening of all children from 1 to 5 years of age for lead exposure. The article goes on to point out that the United States has been successful in reducing other preventable childhood illnesses and, with a concentrated effort, the achievable goal of a dramatic reduction in undue lead absorption would improve the psychological functioning of lead-sensitive children.[20]

Sources of exposure are house dust, canned foods, polluted atmospheres, and lead-containing ceramic glazes. Reduction of exposure to these sources is the first step in reducing children's body burden of lead. The second step is decreasing its absorption and increasing its rate of elimination from the body, which is best accomplished when the child is on an iron-and calcium-rich diet with adequate vitamin C and vitamin E. These nutrients are known to both prevent the absorption of lead into the blood and to hasten its elimination from the body. Children should be getting adequate iron at the level of 10 to 20 milligrams a day, calcium at 600 to 800 milligrams a day, vitamin C at 500 to 1000 milligrams a day, and vitamin E at 50 to 100 units a day to prevent a potential excess burden of lead.

Again, not all children are at equal risk to the accumulation of lead at the same level of exposure. Children differ in their abilities to absorb and accumulate lead; therefore, some children may need a greater intake of the nutrients that block lead's absorption or hasten its elimination from the body than other children. Inspection for the subtle signs of lead excess, which include behavioral problems, classroom performance difficulties, and inability to concentrate or stay at tasks for an extended period of time, may all suggest the necessity for screening for excessive lead body burden in your child.

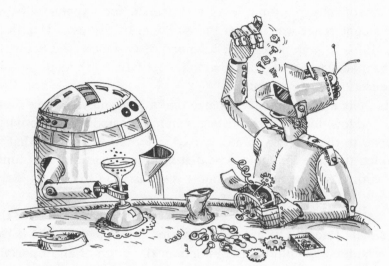

PERSONALLY, I FIND NATURAL FOOD MUCH MORE SATISFYING
THAN SYNTHETIC OILS.

The "Feingold Diet"

The late Dr. Benjamin Feingold, in his best-selling book *Why Your Child Is Hyperactive,*[21] espoused the theory that excessive food additives, food colorings, and natural salicylates (found in berries, cherries, apples, and mint) in children's diets contribute greatly to behavior disorders and hyperactivity. Reactions to Dr. Feingold's hypothesis from the scientific community and from parents were quite different. The scientific-medical community discounted Dr. Feingold's hypothesis because it lacked proof; parents, however, reported success with the diet. The field of behavioral pharmacology became suddenly very popular and better respected as a scientific discipline.

Our environment contains an increasing number of new chemicals, some of them to be found in foods. Most of the clinical trials done on food additives before they are allowed to be used do not measure any possible effects of these substances on behavior.

There still exists considerable debate as to whether the Feingold diet is scientifically reinforcible as a treatment for hyperactivity. A consensus conference was held at the National Institutes of Health in January, 1982, to seek positions on defined diets such as the Feingold diet in the management of childhood hyperactivity. At this symposium several questions were examined.

1. Is there any empirical evidence that a low-salicylate, low–food coloring and low–food additive diet has an impact upon hyperactivity? The answer to this seemed to be a mixed yes. Studies indicate that in a controlled trial the Feingold type diet improved learning and function in children and seemed to be most responsive in the younger-age children.[22]

2. Is there any biological explanation to support the effect of the Feingold diet? Recently it has been reported that one food dye, FDC Red Dye Number 3, inhibits the uptake in the brain of an important neurochemical that has a responsibility for transmitting messages. If true, this observation presents a mechanism by which this food coloring could affect behavior. It's also possible that direct toxic effects and allergic responses to certain food colorings or additives could lead to the observed findings.

3. If defined diets are effective, how and under what circumstances should they be employed? The panel concluded that defined diets may not be useful or possible in all cases of childhood hyperactivity. It may be impossible for some families to implement and manage an additive-free dietary program for a child because this diet is dependent upon the consumption of foods that are not convenience or highly preprocessed items, but necessarily made from fresh, unprocessed, raw materials. The panel, therefore, recommended changes in the law to require labels to list food additives and substances that may migrate to the foods from the wrappers and containers, so that parents could make an informed choice at the supermarket as to what foods to buy in the trial of the low–food additive diet with their child.

Recently, a pediatric allergist has commented that one of the problems with previous studies that did not demonstrate the success of the Feingold diet may have been that too low a level of food additives were used in the study group of children, compared to what children normally consume in their diets. The level of food additives now consumed by children may be 100 to 400 milligrams a day on the average, which is four to eight times higher than the level used in many of the studies.[23] When asked how you can recognize children who might respond to a Feingold diet, she replied, "Look at them. If they have dark circles under their eyes, bright red ears, and a glassy look when the Jekyll and Hyde behavior develops, the answer may be a food. These children often have associated classical hay fever or asthma symptoms, headaches, abdominal complaints, leg aches, and behavior problems. The symptoms are often triggered by the very foods they crave. Sugar, peanut butter, popcorn, orange juice, apple juice are the foods they love. Suspect the child who will not drink milk but craves dairy products. These are the patients who might respond to an attempt at dietary management."

Children as Indicators of Health

So what can we conclude from this discussion of children's behavior and physical function and their relationship to the diet and environment? First, children may be one of the most sensitive biological indicators in a population of the impact of diet on behavior. If, in fact, a variety of behavioral problems are developing in our children due to the consumption of calorie-rich, nutrient-poor diets, it may be a signal to the adult population that they are equally at risk to health-related effects of consuming this diet for a long period of time. Improving dietary quality by reducing empty calories and increasing the relative level of vitamins and minerals in the diet can help improve such subtle indicators as psychological functioning.

The second important conclusion is that the statistical average level of adequacy of nutrients may not be the optimal level for specific children. Biochemical individuality may dictate a need above and beyond that which is considered average by ten or more fold.

Table 9

Additives and Foods to Be Eliminated in the Feingold Diet

All instant breakfast drinks
or protein powders that are colored

All luncheon meats

Colored butter or margarine

All candies

BHT

BHA

Aspirin

Oil of Wintergreen

All cough drops

Synthetic ice creams

Benzoic acid

Methyl benzoate

All powdered desserts

Flavored yogurt

All soft drinks

Antacid tablets

Natural Salicylate-Containing Foods:
    berries
    apples
    cherries
    green pepper
    mint-flavored items
    cider vinegar
    cloves
    catsup
    colored cheeses
    grapes
    oranges
    peaches
    plums
    apricots

Source: B. F. Feingold, *Why Your Child Is Hyperactive* (New York: Random House, 1975).

Lastly, we have seen that exposure to environmental agents such as lead may contribute to certain psychological and behavioral problems in children. Again, increasing the quality of the diet so that a greater intake of iron, calcium, vitamin E, and vitamin C are routinely consumed will reduce the risk of lead absorption and accumulation.

Other environmental agents such as food colorings and food additives may have adverse behavioral effects in some sensitive children. The message and treatment is again the same: utilize highly unprocessed foods as much as possible, foods with few or no coloring or additive agents, and be a label reader and beware of the ingredients listed in Table 9. These approaches may not cure all behavioral or learning disability problems, but at least they will provide you with attractive alternatives toward their management, alternatives that are under your control, reasonably inexpensive, and at worst will do no harm.

Now that we have looked at the whole family of vertical disease problems from pregnancy to old age, it's time to put your Nutraerobics Program into a package that can be implemented. The final chapter is your guide to the implementation of your personalized Nutraerobics Program.

Notes

1. D. Lonsdale and R. J. Shamberger, "Red Cell Transketalase as an Indicator of Nutritional Deficiency," *American Journal of Clinical Nutrition, 33,* 205(1980).

2. J. Bland, "The Junk Food Syndrome," *Psychology Today* (January, 1982):92.

3. B. B. Anderson and D. L. Mollin, "Abnormal Red-cell Metabolism of Pyridoxine Associated with Thalassemia," *British Journal of Haematology, 41,* 497(1979).

4. M. S. Bamji and G. Radhaiah, "Relationship Between Biochemical and Clinical Indices of B-vitamin Deficiency," *British Journal of Nutrition, 41,* 431(1979).

5. H. Turkel, *New Hope for the Mentally Retarded* (New York: Vantage Press, 1972).

6. R. F. Harrell et al., "Can Nutritional Supplements Help Mentally Retarded Children?" *Proceedings of the National Academy of Sciences U.S.A., 78,* 574(1981).

7. A. L. Kubala and M. M. Katz, "Intellectual Performance and Plasma Ascorbic Acid of School Children," *Journal of Genetics and Psychology, 96,* 343 (1060).

8. J. Kershner and W. Hawke, "Diet Influences on Learning Disability," *Journal of Nutrition, 109,* 819(1979).

9. N. Warden, M. Duncan, and E. Sommars, "Nutritional Changes Heighten Children's Achievement," *International Journal for Biosocial Research, 3,* 72(1982).

10. S. J. Schoenthaler, "The Effect of Sugar on the Treatment and Control of Antisocial Behavior," *International Journal for Biosocial Res., 3,* 1(1982).

11. R. O. Phil and M. Parkes, "Hair Element Content of Learning Disabled Children," *Science, 1981,* 204(1977).

12. H. L. Needleman and P. Barrett, "Deficits in Psychologic and Classroom Performance of Children with Elevated Dentine Lead Levels," *New England Journal of Medicine, 300,* 689(1979).

13. K. Mahaffey and R. S. Murphy, "National Estimates of Blood Lead Levels: United States 1976–1980," *New England Journal of Medicine, 307,* 573(1982).

14. M. Laker, "On Determining Trace Element Levels in Man: The Uses of Blood and Hair," *Lancet* (31 July 1982):260.

15. C. Patterson and D. M. Settle, "Lead in Albacore: Guide to Lead Pollution in Americans," *Science, 207,* 1167(1980).

16. H. L. Needleman and D. Bellinger, "Lead Associated Intellectual Deficit," *New England Journal of Medicine, 306,* 367(1981).

17. J. A. Blair and M. A. Moore, "Lead and Tetrahydrobiopterin Metabolism: Possible Effects on IQ," *Lancet* (24 April 1982):964.

18. G. Winneke, "Neurobehavioral and Neuropsychological Effects of Lead," *Lancet* (4 September 1982):550.

19. D. J. Cohen and D. F. Harcherik, "Blood Lead in Autistic Children," *Lancet* (10 July 1982):94.

20. J. S. Lin-Fu, "Children and Lead," *New England Journal of Medicine, 307,* 615 (1982).

21. B. F. Feingold, *Why Your Child Is Hyperactive* (New York: Random House, 1975).

22. J. M. Swanson and M. Kinsbourne, "Food Dyes Impair Performance of Hyperactive Children on a Laboratory Screening Test," *Science, 207,* 1485(1980).

23. D. Rapp, "Food Additives and Hyperactivity," *Lancet* (15 May 1982):1128.

14

Implementing Your Nutraerobics Program

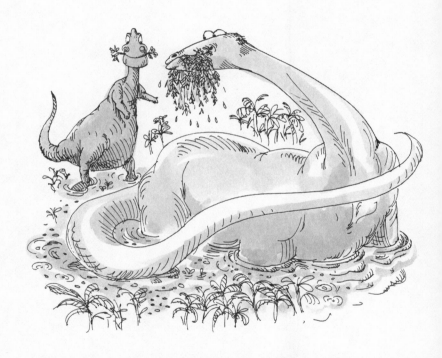

CHANGE ? WHY SHOULD WE CHANGE ? HAVEN'T WE ALREADY
GOT EVERYTHING WE COULD EVER POSSIBLY WANT ?

1. Do you have bad skin?

1	2	3	4
No	Sometimes	Commonly	Very bad

2. Do you have vision problems including glaucoma, myopia, or cataracts?

1	4
No	Yes

3. Does your skin age and wrinkle too quickly?

1	2	4
No	Somewhat	Yes

4. Is your hair thin and lacking luster?

1	2	4
No	Somewhat	Yes

5. Do you tend toward scarring when cut, or have skin rashes?

1	2	4
No	Somewhat	Yes

6. Do you heal poorly?

1	2	4
No	Somewhat	Yes

7. Do you suffer from an irritable bowel condition?

1	2	3	4
No	Occasionally	Frequently	All the time

If your score exceeds 18, the specific examples used in this chapter should be helpful for you.

If the Nutraerobics Program can be so successful in preventing and possibly even treating many of the common diseases, why has it not been more generally accepted by the medical community in the United States?

There are many reasons why a valuable new health improvement concept is not readily accepted by the medical community. One is that doctors are trained to deliver disease treatment, not preventive medicine. Therefore, they are less likely to utilize new knowledge about health enhancement until interest on the part of health-care consumers is great enough to force them to become proficient in this field.

Also, for full application and acceptance, a new concept in health care must show benefit to corporate entities within the health-care delivery sector. There is no way to patent vitamins, minerals, and exercise and lifestyle modification, so there is little economic motivation for health-care corporations to be involved. Until it can be demonstrated to these corporate entities that there is a business in health enhancement, there will be little support from the health-care industries and insurance providers.

There has always been a lag between the development of a new concept in health care and its final acceptance by the medical community. Of one hundred and eleven significant breakthroughs in medicine, the medical community accepted only 8 percent in less than one year, 26 percent within ten years, 43 percent within twenty years, and 82 percent within fifty years.[1] It was twenty-one years from the time Rous and Turner prolonged the life of blood cells until the final development of the blood bank, and sixty-four years from Tyndall's observation that penicillin mold inhibited bacterial growth until the drug penicillin was discovered. As two doctors themselves point out, "Health-care practitioners often see the health-care system of the United States as immutable to change."[2]

No standard medical textbook outlines a low-technology health-care program oriented toward the consumer like the Nutraerobics Program. Modern medicine moves to greater and greater degrees of heroic high-technology intervention with procedures such as dialysis, nuclear medicine, artifical organs, and coronary bypass surgery; the direction is toward specialization and away from the generalist concept of preventive medicine.

And we see new problems arising from these specialized approaches. For example, "preventive" chemotherapy after breast cancer surgery has only a 4 percent benefit; its mortality rate is 4.4 percent, and some remaining number suffer serious side effects.[3] Who decides when and how to use an available high-technology therapy like this and what its specific risk/benefit relationship is? How about the marvelous medical breakthroughs like coronary bypass surgery? A recent investigation of patients who had had successful bypass operations indicates that the disease progressed in the absence of lifestyle changes in the treated patients.[4]

Modern medicine must realize it does not have to give up what it does well—that is, treat disease—it must only recognize that by concentrating some energy on a program such as the Nutraerobics Program to help people keep healthy, it can better use its financial and human resources in the treatment of disease. The Nutraerobics Program works. It saves money, prevents disease, and enhances the quality of life.

In a very interesting recent study in which executives of telephone companies in Japan and the United States were compared as to their incidence of heart disease, it was found that American executives who had a higher animal-fat diet and a more sedentary lifestyle were fatter and had higher blood cholesterol levels with higher blood pressures, and were at much higher risk to coronary heart disease, than were the Japanese executives under similar occupational stress but with differing diets and lifestyles.[5] An interesting secondary observation of this study was that first-generation Japanese who were living in the United States and working as telephone company executives had the high risk to heart disease of their fellow Americans rather than of their counterparts in Japan, indicating that lifestyle and not just genetics plays a major role in determining risk to heart disease and the other major killer diseases.

The Health-Care Consumer

Consumer interest in lifestyle enhancement is here. Pressure to improve the delivery of preventive medicine is now being placed upon all sectors of the health-care delivery system including doctors, hospitals, out-patient clinics, insurance agencies, and public service and health facilities. Consumer interest in nutrition became evident in a recent study of routine patients seeking out the care of medical doctors —67 percent of the patients used nutritional supplements on a regular daily basis, although they had very little understanding of why they used them or what they were good for. Eighty percent of the supplement users believed that the supplements were effective, somehow increasing energy vitality or strength. Sadly, 62 percent of the supplement users had never discussed their use with their physicians, obviously as a result of either their fear of what the physicians would say or their belief that the doctors knew very little about nutritional supplements so they needn't bother asking.[6] As the authors of the study point out, "Viewed in this context, supplement taking may be interpreted as an expression of a health-care need." The time is right for the implementation of a successful health enhancement program such as the Nutraerobics Program.

When to Implement the Program

When should the Nutraerobics Program be implemented? From infancy on. In a study of 250 infants who had eczemic-like skin problems and asthma, 50 percent had allergies to various foods and breast-feeding was in no way protective against the problem.[7] Designing the diet to minimize exposure to the food allergen and making sure that the infant is properly nourished with zinc, vitamin B-6, and essential fatty acids and has adequate stomach acid secretion can all lead to alleviation of such symptoms.

The early development of arteriosclerosis might even start at the fetal stage if the mother is not properly nourished with vitamin B-6 during pregnancy.[8] Supplementation of the pregnant woman's diet with adequate vitamin B-6 is suggested and the level should be tailored to meet her needs based upon her biotype.

Studies also have indicated that the level of dietary calorie intake for infants may have a great impact upon their predisposition to obesity and other weight-related health problems in later life. It is reported that in animals restriction of calories to prevent the condition of overweight led to increased lifespan and reduced cancer rate.[9]

The conclusion drawn from this work is that the Nutraerobics Program can be implemented anytime throughout the lifespan, but the earlier you start to recognize your biotype and design your environment and nutrition to meet your needs, the better will be your probability of leading a long, healthy life.

The Environment and Nutraerobics

Remember, the Nutraerobics Program goes beyond just diet. It encompasses your total lifestyle and environment. Even things like excessive noise can be hazardous to your health. As a former U.S. Surgeon General points out, "Calling noise a nuisance is like calling smog an inconvenience. Noise must be considered a hazard to the health of people everywhere."[10]

Different people respond to noise in different ways; identical noise exposures produce different blood pressure, heart rhythm, and hormone levels in different individuals. A recent study offers a very troubling picture of noise effects. One doctor studied his patients' visits to him over the course of a week and related the home noise exposure to the presence of health problems. He found that there were three times as many psychological problems and twice as many heart and blood pressure problems in those people who lived in the higher-noise regions than in those who lived in the lower-noise regions. Traffic sounds, rock bands, aircraft noise, and noisy industrial jobs increase neurologic and intestinal disturbances and the Environmental Protection Agency suggests that "cases of ulcers in certain noisy industries have been found

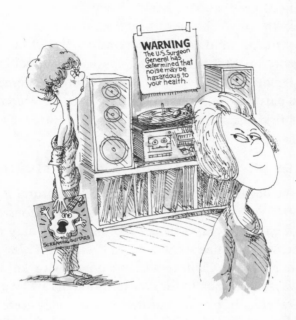

to be up to five times as numerous as what normally would be expected."

Is noise the only occupational exposure of concern in the Nutra-erobics Program? No, the program is also interested in exposure to chemicals and physical agents within the occupational environment that can lead to increased risk to many diseases. One of the most notable examples is asbestos exposure, which was virtually unheard of as a health risk twenty years ago.[11] Asbestos has been shown to increase the risk of mesentheliomal cancer (an unusual cancer of the lower stomach). Over 3000 contemporary manufactured products contain asbestos. At present, several million Americans are employed in industries that make or use asbestos products and countless millions of American citizens are exposed to asbestos in the course of their daily lives. It was not until Dr. Irving Selikoff continued to point to the association between asbestos exposure and cancer in the face of considerable criticism from his colleagues that it was finally accepted as another potential occupational health hazard.[12]

Exposure to vinyl chloride, benzene, particulate air pollution, arsenic, heavy metals, and cold-tar derivatives are all known occupational and environmental hazards that can have a direct impact upon health. The workingplace environment, including the home, should be looked at as part of your total health picture in a comprehensive evaluation of risk association.

Natural or New Is Not Always Healthy

Not all the hazardous things are synthetic. Natural is not always healthy, either. We have already discussed in a previous chapter the cancer risk of eating moldy grains or peanuts that may contain the powerful carcinogen called aflatoxin. In October, 1978, a group of individuals in northern California came down with an acute blood disease that was traced back to the consumption of raw goat's milk (the goats were presumably free of disease but obviously were not).[13]

Pasteurization has led to a much lower incidence of milk-borne diseases, but to think that pasteurization, just because it is a commercial process, must damage the nutritional quality of the milk is to miss the other side of the question. What is the cost-benefit tradeoff with regard to the increasing risk in nonpasteurized dairy products of bacterial diseases?

Even natural products like alfalfa sprouts may have an adverse health effect when consumed in excess. A recent report indicates that monkeys who were fed 40 percent of their calories as alfalfa sprouts and seeds developed a symptom related to systemic lupus erythmatosus.[14] It was found that this was the result of a toxic substance called canavanine in the alfalfa seeds and sprouts. Obviously, consumption of modest amounts of alfalfa sprouts will cause no problem, but in the extreme case, where a considerable portion of the calories come from even this natural product, there may be some adverse effects.

The message is clear: extreme diets can be as hazardous as extreme lifestyles. There will always be one or two individuals who seem to flourish with the most bizarre lifestyle, but for the majority of individuals, bizarre diets or lifestyles may have long-term adverse health effects.

Also, just because a thing is new, does not necessarily mean it is better. The early excitement for the surgical treatment of morbid obesity by removing part of the intestine is now tempered by the understanding that many individuals who undergo this surgery not only develop severe nutritional problems but may also develop arthritis as an immune hypersensitive reaction caused by the delivery of bacterial debris from the intestinal tract into the bloodstream.[15]

Once dimethyl sulfoxide (DMSO) was hailed as the panacea for all arthritis and muscle pain. It has now been shown to have potential adverse side effects when taken internally in large quantities.[16] Topical application of DMSO in small amounts may prove safe and useful in the management of some pains of osteoarthritis and muscle trauma, but extrapolating that safety to the use of large quantities internally without supervision is unwarranted.[17]

The Importance of Exercise in Nutraerobics

In putting your Nutraerobics Program together, exercise is of utmost importance, but what kind and how much is advisable? Aerobic exercise, the type of exercise that provides adequate levels of oxygen to each cell, is capable of contributing to the following health improvements if done regularly: improved heart and lung function, decreased body fatness, decreased appetite, increased alertness, better sleep, decreased blood fats, decreased resting pulse, improved circulation, increased bone density, and improved intestinal regularity.

Aerobic exercise is achieved when your pulse rate during your exercise is 180 beats per minute minus your age in years. (For example, if you are 60 years old, a good target exercise pulse, or your training zone, is 180 minus 60, or 120.) It is most important to keep the level of activity constant for at least fifteen minutes. You don't have to be a jogger. Any form of exercise that can sustain your pulse at a constant rate within your training zone for fifteen minutes is acceptable. Examples include swimming, dancercise or jazzercise, stationary bicycle or rowing machine, exercise classes, dance, vigorous walking, raquetball (if done for exercise, not competition), and skipping rope.

As you exercise aerobically, you actually increase the number of "furnaces," called mitochondria, in your cells that burn food to produce energy. Your ability to efficiently produce energy for muscle contraction, immune function, cell reparation, and brain function all depend upon your state of aerobic competency, which in turn depends upon your nutrition, exercise, and lifestyle program.

On the other hand, heavy exercise can be a stressor. Studies now indicate that women involved in very heavy exercise programs may lose calcium from their bones and possibly be at greater risk to osteoporosis in later life. It is also recognized that many women who train as competitive athletes are found to have irregular or no menstrual periods. The long-term implications for health are as yet unclear, but it does suggest that heavy training is a stressor on the body and may require greater or different nutritional support than lighter exercise.

Moderate aerobic exercise is not optional in the Nutraerobics Program—it is essential. If your response is "I don't have time to exercise," then the question is "Do you find time to eat?" If you can find time to eat, then you can also find time to exercise. The total time per day allotted to exercise may be no more than fifteen to twenty minutes, but even if it's one hour from start to shower and finish, that's **less than 4 percent of your whole day.** If you don't have that amount of time, then your priorities need reviewing. Get involved with an exercise support group such as your local Y, exercise class, health club, or spa and stick with it.

Balancing the Midline

The Nutraerobics Program utilizes approaches that have been tried and proven both safe and effective in promoting health and reducing the risk of disease. The focus is on trying to define your optimum level of health rather than just keeping you free of obvious disease. The most interesting thing about optimum levels is that they generally exist between two extremes that may both be related to ill health. Generally, deficient substances or adequate substances in deficient quantities can produce deficiency symptoms, whereas the same substance in excess can produce toxicity symptoms and the symptoms of both deficiency and toxicity may be very similar. The optimum level is the midline in between, which is based upon your own specific biological requirements. For example, low blood cholesterol and high blood cholesterol have both been associated with increased risk to disease; a midline blood cholesterol between 170 and 180 is ideal for most individuals.[18]

The time to start implementing your Nutraerobics Program is now. Let's now define your optimum as best we can, based upon the information that you have read through and thought about in the first thirteen chapters of this book. On the following pages you will find your Nutraerobics Program Summary Checksheet, on which you can design your program in summary. Read the instructions and then start filling it out. By using your biotype, we hope to be able to chart your path towards optimal health.

How to Use
Your Nutraerobics Program Summary Checksheet

1.   Review your biotype as determined in Chapters 2 and 3.

2.   Review all 27 variables on the checksheet.

3.   Write in the levels you have determined you need for each of these factors based on your biotype.

4.   For those factors you are not sure about, review the suggested chapters to see how they relate to your biotype.

5.   When two or more levels of the same factor are suggested from different chapters, select the largest amount.

6.   From your diet and present lifestyle make a list of those factors you have to change or supplement to be within your determined optimal range.

7.   If you have indicated the need for a large number of food supplements (pills), it may mean you need to concentrate more on dietary improvement to reduce dependency on supplements. Depending upon your lifestyle and genetic requirements, there may be need for selected supplementation of specific nutrients, but good nutrition **starts** with a good diet.

Nutraerobics Program Summary Checksheet

	Suggested range per day	Optimal amount for your biotype	Chapters to find information
1. Protein			
vegetable	25–70 g	_____	7, 8, 9
animal	25–70 g		10
2. Fat			
saturated	15–30 g	_____	3, 4, 6
unsaturated	20–40 g		7, 8, 9
3. Carbohydrate			
starches	190–380 g	_____	5, 7, 13
sugars	40–80 g		
4. Fiber supplement	15–35 g	_____	8, 9, 12, 13
5. Gums (pectin, guar, glucomannan)	0–5 tsps	_____	5, 7
6. Calories (based upon metabolic rate)	1,200–3,500	_____	6, 8
7. Body weight-to-height ratio:			
increase	*See body mass*	_____	6, 7, 9
decrease	*index*		
8. Blood pressure:			
increase	110–140	_____	7
decrease	70–85		
9. Digestive function improvement (enzymes, acid, fiber)		_____	8, 11
10. Smoking reduction	0–as little as possible	_____	8
11. Alcohol reduction	0–2 drinks/day	_____	7, 8
12. Exercise tolerance improvement	Check resting pulse and recovery time	_____	6, 7, 10

Nutraerobics Program Summary Checksheet

	Suggested range per day	Optimal amount for your biotype	Chapters to find information
13. Occupation and/or environment change		_____	4, 14
14. Lighting change (natural sunlight, naked eye)	0.5–2.0 hrs. exposure/day	_____	11, 13
15. Relaxation therapy	0.5–2.0 hrs./day	_____	4, 14
16. Essential oils (MaxEPA) or fatty acids	0–50 grams/day	_____	7, 11
17. Fat-soluble vitamins			
A (retinol)	2,500–25,000 IU	_____	8
D (cholecalciferol)	200–1,000 IU	_____	10
E (tocopherol)	100–800 IU	_____	7, 8
18. Water-soluble vitamins			
B-1 (thiamin)	5–50 mg	_____	5, 13, 14
B-2 (riboflavin)	5–50 mg	_____	5, 13
B-3 (niacin)	10–3,000 mg	_____	3, 5, 13
B-6 (pyridoxine)	10–300 mg	_____	3, 12, 13
B-12 (cobalamine)	10–1,000 mcg	_____	3, 9
biotin	50–400 mcg	_____	6, 14
pantothenic acid	20–1,000 mg	_____	11
folic acid	400–3,000 mcg	_____	9, 12
choline	10–100 mg	_____	4, 5
inositol	100–2,000 mg	_____	7
C (ascorbic acid)	500–6,000 mg	_____	5, 7, 10, 12
19. Major minerals			
calcium	800–1,400 mg	_____	7, 10
magnesium	400–600 mg	_____	5, 7, 10
sodium	3,000–5,000 mg	_____	7, 10
potassium	4,000–6,000 mg	_____	6, 7
phosphorus	1,200–1,500 mg	_____	10

	Suggested range per day	Optimal amount for your biotype	Chapters to find information
20. Trace minerals			
iron	10–30 mg	_____	5, 9, 13
zinc	10–30 mg	_____	9, 11, 12, 13
copper	2–10 mg	_____	6, 8, 10, 11, 13
chromium	50–300 mcg	_____	5, 7, 12
manganese	2–20 mg	_____	7, 8
iodine	100–1,000 mcg	_____	9
fluorine	50–100 mcg	_____	10
21. Accessory nutrients (not for everyone)			
carnitine	500–2,000 mg	_____	7, 9
beta-carotene	5,000–20,000 I.U.	_____	8
tyrosine	500–3,000 mg	_____	5, 7
lecithin (phosphatidyl choline)	20–100 g	_____	4
tryptophan	500–2,000 mg	_____	5, 7
bioflavonoids	100–2,000 mg	_____	5
22. Reduce toxic mineral burden: lead, mercury, cadmium, aluminum		_____	13
23. Increase fluid intake	2–5 pints	_____	6
24. Decrease allergy-producing foods and environmental substances	determined from testing	_____	11
25. Decrease exposure to ultraviolet light or X-rays		_____	8
26. Hobbies and leisure time activities		_____	4, 14
27. Intellectual stimulation or pursuits		_____	4, 14

Going On to the Next Step

From the completion of your Nutraerobics Program Summary Checksheet, you now should know what level of animal and vegetable protein per day is optimal for you, what type of fat and carbohydrate intake is best for you, and how much sugar in your diet would be considered acceptable. Remember, some people are extremely sugar-sensitive and sugar may have to be limited very carefully if you are one of them.

In reviewing body weight-to-height ratio, blood pressure, digestive function, and lifestyle habits such as smoking, alcohol consumption, exercise, and occupational exposure, you should now have a good idea as to where to concentrate your energies in the design of your new modified lifestyle for improved health.

From the information that you have pored through in the first thirteen chapters of this book, you have undoubtedly learned a considerable amount about your specific needs for various vitamins and minerals. The optimal place to get these would be by revising your diet to include foods that contain them; however, as has been pointed out, you may have a certain genetic need that exceeds your ability to get that level in optimal amounts from your diet alone. Start by dietary revision and then, if necessary, use selected supplementation to reinforce your requirements.

In each case you may need to go back and reread through the chapters that discuss allocation of the levels of need to your biotype for each of those specific agents. If you've taken good notes in your reading to this point, you should not have to do much review, but remember that the time you spend now in reflecting will pay the later dividends of a Nutraerobics Program better tailored to your specific needs.

Vision, Hair, and Skin

Individuals who have properly put together their Nutraerobics Program have experienced health improvements in areas they did not initially expect. Three areas where improvements in function have been seen, although these were not areas of primary concentration, are vision, hair, and skin.

Strong evidence suggests that the risk to cataract is increased in nutritional inadequacy, particularly with regard to vitamin B-2,[19] and other evidence suggests that cataracts are in part related to the poor management of blood sugar through what are called the insulin-insensitive pathways.[20] Nearsightedness may be in part related to a chromium deficiency.[21] By designing your Nutraerobics Program for optimal health, you may have already started on the road toward preventing cataracts and improving your vision.

Hair, an actively growing protein, is extremely dependent upon the overall tissue repair and protein manufacturing machinery in your body. As your health improves, your ability to manufacture new protein and promote better hair growth may also result. Zinc, biotin, the essential amino acid methionine, and proper protein digestion and assimilation have all been identified as being important in the stimulation of proper hair growth and texture. A pantothenic acid deficiency has been implicated in the premature graying of the hair. As an added bonus to the other benefits of your program, you may start to see improvements in hair texture and density.

Many skin problems are a secondary manifestation of overall chronic ill health. Proper levels of zinc, the essential fatty acids, vitamin B-6, vitamin A, reduction of exposure to food or environmental allergens, and improved digestion and elimination have all been shown to be useful in the treatment of skin problems such as eczema and seborrhea.[22]

The program pays dividends. Not only are you going to realize directly an improvement in your overall health by reducing your risk to the major killer diseases, but you will also see improvement in many of the other things that we associate with aging, some of which may be cosmetic.

I-Centered Versus We-Centered

So far we have concentrated on the I-centered needs, those specific problems relating to improvement of your individual health; now let's address the broader issue of community health. You may perfectly design your Nutraerobics Program to your individualized biotype, eat right, exercise, relax, and have the most stimulating and rewarding of occupations, but still be exposed to contaminants such as dioxin from herbicides, or polychlorinated biphenyls, or residues of DDT, or formaldehyde, or photochemical oxidants, or chlorinated hydrocarbons in your water supply.[23] In Michigan, 1231 adults were examined for body tissue levels of polychlorinated biphenyls and exposure was identified in 97 percent of these individuals. Recently a syndrome called "Kawasaki syndrome," an acute illness of unknown cause seen in children under 5, was associated in eastern Colorado with the use of a commercial rug shampoo.[24]

What we have here is a "suprapersonal" health concern, that is, one that exceeds the I-centered concern in that it has to do with the health of the whole community. As individuals start to feel better from the implementation of their own personalized health improvement programs, it is hoped they will have enough energy to redress some of the problems we have at the community level with regard to pollution and despoilment of our environment.

The quality of life and mental and physical health may relate to problems that are beyond our own immediate control and require societal action. One individual cannot clean up his or her own air, water, noise, waste, and chemical contamination or alter the commercial food supply system; however, many working together can. It is important that people first feel well enough, that they have the resources available to direct toward the solution of these major problems, and then, second, that they have the motivation and concern to do so.

Often the comment is made, "What can one person do? That is

a government problem." Solutions to these problems start with the individual just as alteration of our health-care system started with the individual and grew to the large numbers who are now striving for new forms of preventive health-care. You can start by making pertinent decisions in your own local environment concerning the quality of life and health.

Start your environmental cleanup program by reducing, as much as you can, your dependency upon petrochemically derived cleaners and other agents, especially those of unknown biological impact. Be concerned about what happens in your own neighborhood. Make it important in your life to know what role the quality of your environment plays in determining your and your family's health. It is very difficult to quantify the health effects of a clean environment and sometimes in the face of economic pressures, environmental quality can be compromised; however, studies indicate that long-term exposure to environmental toxins can be one of the major contributors to community risk to disease.

Putting It into Perspective

At this point you may be feeling that your life has to be very intense and you have to think about everything you do, and that this in itself will be a psychological stress you have to deal with. The aim of this book is to confront you with various aspects of your lifestyle that may contribute to your disease and ill-health patterns but not to exclude the importance of living life for what it is. Life should be filled with humor and joy and be something worth living just for the enterprise. When your mind is at ease, then you are smiling with the world, your food is better digested and assimilated, and your body has a better opportunity to utilize oxygen in the way that it should.

Think, for a moment, about plucking a shiny, yellow lemon off a sun-kissed lemon tree and smelling that fragrant aroma. Then cut the lemon with a knife and watch the juice spurt out in every direction. Smell that beautiful, fragrant aroma of a ripe and succulent, but tart, fruit. Then think about holding the lemon over your mouth and squeezing the juice and feeling it hit your tongue with that bracing, astringent effect of making you want to pucker; all of your salivary glands at the back of your mouth are recoiling in response to the astringent effect of the lemon. Can you now taste the lemon, feel the flow of saliva or the tightness in your salivary glands from just this brief visualization exercise? If so, you've demonstrated to yourself exactly the importance of the relationship between your mind and your body. When you've prepared your body correctly, it can work in harmony with the environment. Your food is better digested, assimilated, and utilized. Most of the major degenerative diseases and problems associated with older age have strong relationships to the way people perceive themselves in the world and whether they are in harmony or disharmony with the music of the environment. If your biotype indicates that your health is controlled by stress, then concentrate on relaxation. Practice slowing down. Plan ahead for leisure time and keep to your schedule. Have time for yourself each day, and a vacation away from it all each year of significant enough duration to "put it all into perspective." If you are still too "stressed," you may need planned stress-reduction techniques such as biofeedback, meditation, or other relaxation techniques.

A Case Study for Nutraerobics

Good examples of that relationship between mind and body are conditions such as ulcerative colitis and Crohn's disease (a nonspecific inflammatory bowel disease), both of which have increased worldwide and have emerged as two of the most important health problems of our time. Ulcerative colitis and Crohn's disease are characterized by bleeding, diarrhea, cramping and abdominal pain, weight loss, and ulceration of the intestine with need for surgery. The prognosis is not good. The condition is inflammatory and progressive and complications can lead to generalized malnutrition.[25]

No analogs of these diseases have been found in animals; nor has it been possible to reproduce them experimentally. These conditions are more common in countries that are highly developed and Western-ized, such as the United States, England, and Scandinavia. Evidence now suggests that excessive intake of refined sugar and low-fiber diets are preliminary to the development of these inflammatory bowel dis-orders. Low zinc and pantothenic acid intakes and certain food addi-tives are also suggested to be possible contributors to the development of inflammatory bowel disorders.[26]

Food allergy is also suspected in a number of cases to be a con-tributing cause of these conditions, and environmental stress or distress syndrome is also implicated. The story reads almost like a chapter out of this Nutraerobics book. A genetic predisposition to a particular prob-lem is compounded by a suboptimal diet, exposure to environmental assaulting agents, and a distressful lifestyle, which shows itself first at the first boundary line of the body's defense, which is the intestinal mucosa.

Oriental medicine over 2000 years ago correlated psychological problems with intestinal diseases. Diet, a genetic predisposition, and lifestyle all play a role in determining risk to a disease such as inflam-matory bowel disease. Yes, you can give a zinc supplement or calcium pantothenate to individuals with this condition, but if their minds are not ready, and they are not smiling with the world, then the benefit of the supplementation approaches zero.[27]

Taking Responsibility for Your Health

So it starts by taking the first step toward gaining responsibility for your own health. It starts with as simple a step as joining a health club, or deciding that maybe exercise isn't too difficult for you. If you could sell a drug that would help people lose weight, slow the aging process, prevent a heart attack, and increase self-esteem, you would make a fortune, but if you try to convince people to change their lifestyles, exercise, eat right, and learn how to enjoy the world without killing themselves through the Nutraerobics Program, many people initially might think you were crazy.

Just starting with exercise might be a great beginning. Nerve impulses traveling from the eyes to the brain move 5 to 10 percent faster in runners than in nonrunners when both subjects are at rest. Men who participated in one aerobic exercise program did not experience the expected 9 to 15 percent decline in physical work capacity that ordinarily occurs between the ages of 45 and 55.[28]

Once again, we're talking about reducing the rate of biological aging. If you don't like to start with exercise, then how about starting with nutritional improvement? If not that, how about an evaluation of your workingplace environment or your level of intellectual stimulation or better yet, how about looking at it all in a comprehensive Nutraerobics Program? Review your checksheet to see where you are going to get started in the integrated program. The key at this point is obvious: you can intellectualize the subject to death, but if you don't put yourself into it and become a participant, you will never reap the rewards of your vertical disease prevention program.

If you can't yet deal with problems like lack of exercise, smoking, excessive weight, and excessive alcohol use, then you may not be psychologically ready to implement the program. Some investigators say that people do not change their lifestyles unless they are adequately educated to the alternatives.[29] No longer can this be an excuse for you. You've read and studied the Nutraerobics Program, you know about alternatives, and you have explored your biotype. So we have come down to personality factors and belief systems. Even constipation has recently been related to psychological and personality factors.[30] Constipated individuals benefit from higher dietary fiber intake and may be at greater risk to cancer of the colon, diverticulitis, diabetes, and atherosclerotic diseases.

If you are ready to grab hold of the responsibility for a portion of your health and are willing to make some changes in the basic way that you lead your life, then improved health by application of the Nutraerobics Program is for you. If, however, you already feel that you have adequate health, or that you cannot make compromises in your lifestyle, or that you just enjoy being involved in a personal experiment to see if you have "designer" genes that will stand the wear and tear of an abusive lifestyle—then just consider the time you spent reading this book as an intellectually stimulating and provocative experience.

If, however, you are ready to apply the Nutraerobics Program, using your biotype, then you are ready to break out of what Hans Selye talks about as a "general adaptation syndrome," which is a pattern of reactions that individuals develop to compensate for obnoxious or stressful qualities of their environment or lifestyle.[31] Once you have decided that the way to approach health is not adaptation but rather reconstruction, you have truly taken the big step forward in implementing a Living Life Insurance Program. The prospect of having a population of older individuals who are healthy enough to bring the wealth of wisdom and experience that they have from living on this planet sixty or more years to addressing many of the social problems that we have today is an exciting opportunity. This may be within the grasp of our culture if we can adopt a program like the Nutraerobics Program and move in later years toward not only life with wisdom, but also life with health. Remember: health is not a mystery. You have the keys in your head, heart, and hands.

Notes

1. J. H. Comroe and R. D. Dripps, "The Top Ten Advances in Cardiovascular-Pulmonary Medicine 1945–1975," Dept. Health and Human Services Publ. No. 78-1521, Washington, D.C., 1977.

2. J. W. Salmon and H. S. Berliner, "Why Contemporary Medicine Is Failing," *American Journal of Acupuncture, 8,* 191(1980).

3. H. Vorherr, "Adjuvant Chemotherapy of Breast Cancer: Reality, Hope, Hazard?" *Lancet* (19 December 1981):1413.

4. S. F. Seides and S. E. Epstein, "Long-term Anatomic Fate of Coronary-Artery Bypass Grafts and Functional Status of Patients Five Years After Operation," *New England Journal of Medicine, 298,* 1213(1978).

5. Y. Sakai and R. W. Stone, "Cardiovascular Risk Factors Among Japanese and American Telephone Executives," *International Journal of Epidemiology, 6,* 7(1977).

6. E. C. English and J. W. Carl, "Use of Nutritional Supplements by Family Practice Patients," *Journal of the American Medical Association, 246,* 2719(1981).

7. R. R. Gordon and R. Allen, "Immunoglobulin E and the Eczema-Asthma Syndrome in Early Childhood," *Lancet* (9 January 1982):72.

8. C. I. Levene and J. C. Murray, "The Aetiological Role of Maternal Vitamin B-6 Deficiency in the Development of Atherosclerosis," *Lancet* (19 March 1977): 628.

9. R. Weindruch and R. L. Walford, "Dietary Restriction in Mice Beginning at 1 Year of Age: Effect on Life-span and Cancer Incidence," *Science, 215,* 1415(1982).

10. J. Raloff, "Noise Can Be Hazardous to Our Health," *Science News, 121,* 377(1982).

11. M. R. Becklake, "Exposure to Asbestos and Human Disease," *New England Journal of Medicine, 306,* 1480(1982).

12. J. E. Craighead and B. T. Mossman, "The Pathogenesis of Asbestos-Associated Diseases," *New England Journal of Medicine, 306,* 1446(1982).

13. J. J. Sacks and N. F. Brooks, "Toxoplasmosis Infection Associated with Raw Goat's Milk," *Journal of the American Medical Association, 248,* 1728(1982).

14. M. R. Malinow and P. McLaughlin, "Systemic Lupus Erythematosus-like Syndrome in Monkeys Fed Alfalfa Sprouts: Role of a Nonprotein Amino Acid," *Science, 216,* 415(1982).

15. J. Kangilaski, "Arthritis May Follow Jejunoileal Surgery," *Journal of the American Medical Association, 246,* 933(1981).

16. R. S. Muther and W. M. Bennett, "Effects of Dimethyl Sulfoxide on Renal Function in Man," *Journal of the American Medical Association, 244,* 2081(1980).

17. J. R. Beljan et al., "Dimethyl Sulfoxide —Controversy and Current Status," *Journal of the American Medical Association, 248,* 1369(1982).

18. E. Cheraskin and W. M. Ringsdorf, "The Biologic Parabola: A Look at Serum Cholesterol," *Journal of the American Medical Association, 247,* 302(1982).

19. H. W. Skalka and J. T. Prochal, "Cataracts and Riboflavin Deficiency," *American Journal of Clinical Nutrition, 34,* 861(1981).

20. G. E. Bunce, "Nutrition and Cataract," *Nutrition Reviews, 38,* 322(1980).

21. B. Lane, "Myopia and Accommodation Problems in Chromium Deficiency," *Journal of Vision Research, 12,* 435(1980).

22. S. Wright and J. L. Burton, "Oral Evening Primrose Oil Improves Atopic Eczema," *Lancet* (22 November 1982):1120.

23. J. R. Beljan et al., "Health Effects of Agent Orange and Dioxin Contaminants," *Journal of the American Medical Association, 248,* 1895(1982); M. S. Wolf and I. J. Selikoff, "Human Tissue Burdens of Halogenated Aromatic Hydrocarbons," *Journal of the American Medical Association, 247,* 2112(1982).

24. P. A. Patriarca and M. P. Glode, "Kawasaki Syndrome: Association with the Application of Rug Shampoo," *Lancet* (11 September 1982):578.

25. J. B. Kirsner and R. G. Shorter, "Recent Developments in 'Non-specific' Inflammatory Bowel Disease," *New England Journal of Medicine, 306,* 775(1982).

26.   J. B. Kirsner and R. G. Shorter, "Second of Two Parts on Inflammatory Bowel Disease," *New England Journal of Medicine, 306,* 837(1982).

27.   "Zinc Deficiency in Crohn's Disease," *Nutrition Reviews, 40,* 109(1982).

28.   B. Liebman, "A Look at the Benefits of Exercise," *Nutrition Action,* (November 1981):9.

29.   C. A. Lambert and S. J. Spaight, "Risk Factors and Lifestyle: A Statewide Health-Interview Survey," *New England Journal of Medicine, 306,* 1048(1982).

30.   D. M. Tucker and G. E. Inglett, "Dietary Fiber and Personality Factors as Determinants of Stool Output," *Gastroenterology, 81,* 879(1981).

31.   H. Selye, *The Stress of Life* (New York: McGraw-Hill, 1956).

Index

Abortions, spontaneous, 291
Acarbose, 152
Accessory nutrients, 73
Acetaldehyde, 16
Acetylcholine, 108
Acne, cystic, 174
Acquired Immunodeficiency Syndrome, 283–284
Additives. See Food additives
Adenosine, 150 ·
Adolescence, 230, 232, 237
Adrenal glands: and blood pressure, 26, 29; and brain function, 118, 119, 120; and weight management, 29, 137, 145
Adrenaline, 26, 106, 108, 148, 216
Adriamycin, 213
Aerobic exercise, 147, 150, 157, 335–336, 347
Aerobics, 6
Affluence, 198
Aflatoxin, 210–211, 334
Age. See Biological age; Life expectancy
Aggression, 118, 121, 233, 310, 311
Aging, 4–5, 7–8, 77–101, 344, 347–348; and bone status, 251, 252–253, 256; and brain function, 95–96, 108, 127; and immune system, 98, 211
AIDS. See Acquired Immunodeficiency Syndrome
Alcoholic beverages, 16, 35, 41, 59, 63, 87; and bone status, 251, 258, 259; and cancer, 173, 198, 201, 207–208, 214; and heart disease, 173, 176; liver function and, 16, 173, 207–208, 214; male physiology and, 243; during pregnancy, 292, 303; and sodium-potassium ATPase, 136
Alcoholism, 44, 113
Alertness, mental, 120, 121, 335. See also Intelligence
Alfalfa sprouts and seeds, 334
Allergies, 18–19, 28, 29, 43, 119, 347; and arthritis/arthralgia, 266, 277, 280–281, 282; and behavior disorders, 116–117, 278, 322, 323; and bone status, 261, 266; of children, 322, 323, 331; immune system and, 98, 273, 277–281, 282; and skin problems, 18, 117, 278, 331, 343
Aluminum, 98–99, 126–127, 261, 262
Aluminum cookware, 99, 127, 262
Alzheimer's disease, 95, 108
Amenorrhea, 233
American Heart Association, 175–176, 191
Amino acids, 73, 154, 155, 180; and blood pressure, 99, 108; and brain function, 106, 107–108, 110, 113, 114, 127–129,

150; for hair, 41, 343; and heartbeat, 154, 155; and heart disease, 188, 189–191; and immune system, 276; and male infertility, 242–243; for osteoarthritis, 244; and thyroid, 17, 28; and weight management, 147, 150, 155
Amygdalin, 204–205
Amylase inhibitor, 152
Amyotrophic lateral sclerosis (ALS), 98, 99, 126–127
Anaerobic metabolism, 254
Analgesics, 116
Anderson, Robert, 23
Anemias, 45, 46, 70, 94, 110, 228–229; and healing time, 44; pernicious, 70, 110
Ankle swelling, 29
Anorexia nervosa, 159, 232–233
Antacids, 99, 127, 262
Antibiotics, 44
Antibodies, 272
Antimetabolites, 203
Anxiety, 68; and appetite, 148; blood sugar and, 19, 120, 121; oral contraceptives and, 235; with premenstrual tension, 233
Apgar scores, 295
Appestat, 148
Appetite, 148–150; compulsive, 135, 148–149, 230, 295; exercise decreasing, 147, 150, 157, 335; loss of, 68, 160, 232; and ovulation, 238
Apple juice, 323
Apple pectin, 123
Apples, 321
Apricot pits, 205
Arachidonic acid, 189
Arginine, 180, 283–284
Aromatic hydrocarbons, 199, 207, 208
Arsenic, 207, 217, 334
Arteriosclerosis, 44, 189, 331–332. See also Atherosclerosis
Arthralgia, 244, 266
Arthritis, 266; and immune system, 98, 273, 275, 277, 280–283; iron and, 230, 283; sunlight and, 244; after weight loss surgery, 335. See also Osteoarthritis
Asbestos, 199, 207, 333–334
Aspirin, 230, 282
Asthma, 323, 331
Asymptomatic preliminary stage, of nutrient depletion, 68
Atherosclerosis, 69, 172–179 passim, 188, 191, 297, 348
Attention span. See Concentration ability
Australia, 297
Autism, 319–320

Autoimmunity, 273, 275
Automobile exhaust, 262

Back pain, 42, 236
Bacon, 34, 201, 216
Baked goods, 34–35, 121, 149, 177, 311. *See also* Breads
Balance disturbances, 120, 126, 152, 243
Bananas, 280
B-complex vitamins, 20, 33, 60, 70–71, 158, 311–312; and aging, 95, 96–98, 108; and alcohol consumption, 16, 63; and brain function, 95, 108, 311–312; and bulimia, 233; and cancer, 202, 215, 217; eye condition and, 27; for hair, 41; and hand/feet discomforts, 42, 296; during pregnancy, 296–297, 298, 300, 331–332; and skin problems, 17, 18, 27, 217; and sleeping problems, 20–21; with smoking, 63; and stress, 17; for tongue condition, 28, 41. *See also individual B vitamins*
Beans, 34, 123, 146, 183
Beef, 34, 116, 180, 278
Beer, 214
Beets, 229
Behavioral problems, 105–129 passim; with allergies, 116–117, 278, 322, 323; blood sugar and, 19, 105, 106, 119–126 passim; bulimia and, 232; of children, 113–121 passim, 309–325 passim; with empty-calorie foods, 35, 309–311; iron and, 113, 230, 325; sex-related hormones and, 227–228, 233. *See also* Lifestyle
Belgium, 171
Bellevue-Redmond Medical Facility, 84–85
Benzene, 207, 334
Beriberi, 61, 67
Berries, 65, 321
Beta-carotene, 17, 73, 201, 209–210, 274–275
Betaine hydrochloride, 229–230
Beverages, 59, 64, 121, 293, 309. *See also* Alcoholic beverages; Coffee; Juices; Milk; Soft drinks; Tea
Beverly Hills Diet, 151–152
Bicycling, stationary, 157, 336
Bile, 29
Biofeedback, 283
Bioflavonoids, 41, 44, 73
Biological age, 4–5, 79, 86–87, 347–348
Biotin, 41, 158, 343
Biotype, 12, 13
Birth control, 63, 214–215, 234–235, 237
Birth defects, 290, 291–292, 296, 299
Birth weights, 294
Bladder cancer, 216–217

Bleeding, 27, 41, 44, 346
Blood acidity, 254
Blood bank, 329
Blood-brain barrier, 106, 108
Blood cells. *See* Red blood cells; White blood cells
Blood cholesterol. *See* Cholesterol
Blood disease, 334
Blood lead, 319
Blood pressure, 26, 99, 330; brain function and, 107, 108; coffee and, 216; fasting and, 151; noise and, 332; personality traits and, 24; salt/sodium and, 29, 35, 99, 136, 185–186; vitamin E and, 70. *See also* High blood pressure
Bloodstream, 271
Blood sugar, 19; and brain function, 19, 105, 106, 119–126; chromium and, 94, 123–125, 300; fiber and, 182, 183; and PMT, 234; during pregnancy, 294–295, 298, 300; and vision, 343; with weight-reducing efforts, 151, 152, 154, 156
Blood triglycerides, 183, 189
B-lymphocytes, 271, 272, 273, 274, 284
Body mass index, 26–27, 141, 142. *See also* Weight-to-height ratio
Bone meal, 257
Bone status, 19, 34, 42–43, 69, 241, 249–268; aluminum and, 99, 261, 262; calcium and, 19, 28, 35, 42, 43, 99, 249–268, 336; chemotherapy and, 203, 204; copper and, 94, 260, 261, 282; estrogen and, 239, 241, 253, 264; exercise and, 238, 265, 335, 336; fetal, 291
Bowels. *See* Intestines
Brain function, 20, 67, 105–130, 227; and aging, 95–96, 108, 127; and allergy, 116–117, 119, 278, 280, 322, 323; and appetite, 148, 150; blood sugar and, 19, 105, 106, 119–126; of children, 113–121 passim, 230, 309–325 passim; exercise and, 117, 119, 126, 336; fetal, 117–118, 292. *See also* Psychological disturbances
Bran, oat, 182, 281
Breads, 34, 57, 122, 178; fiber in, 35; during pregnancy, 293, 301; vegetable gums in, 122, 123
Breakfast, 33, 64, 123
Breastfeeding, 240, 258, 297, 331
Breasts: cancer of, 138, 198, 200, 204, 214–215, 239, 330; fibrocystic disease of, 215, 239–240
Breathing difficulty, 28
Breath shortness, 45, 160, 278
Breath smell, 30

Brewer's yeast: chromium-enriched, 94–95, 124–125; during pregnancy, 301; selenium-rich, 242, 276; for tongue sensitivity, 41; vitamin B-3 in, 42
Brown fat metabolism, 18, 137, 143–145, 146–147, 157
Bruising, easy, 41, 44
Brussels sprouts, 212
Bulimia, 159, 232–233
Burkitt, Denis, 181
Burkitt's lymphoma, 204
Bursitis, 98
Butter, 35, 57, 58, 59; and cholesterol, 34, 58, 178, 184; heart disease and, 177, 178, 184
Buttermilk, 256, 261
B vitamins. *See* B-complex vitamins; *individual B vitamins*

Cabbage, 136, 201, 212
Cadmium, 45; and bone loss, 261, 262; and brain function, 115, 318; and heart disease, 187; and high blood pressure, 187; in water, 187, 217
Caffeine, 147, 215, 240, 291–292
Cakes, 35, 121, 149
Calcitonin, 252, 255, 262
Calcium, 33, 35, 39, 60, 63, 241; aluminum and, 99, 127, 262; and back pain, 42; and blood pressure, 45–46, 186–187, 299; bone/tooth status and, 19, 28, 35, 42, 43, 99, 249–268, 336; and dysmenorrhea, 236; fingernail problems and, 43; growth spurts and, 19; heartbeat irregularities and, 43; and lead, 262, 320, 325; leg/muscle cramping and, 45–46, 252, 256; during pregnancy, 256, 258, 294, 296, 298, 299, 304; weight loss diets and, 137, 156
Calcium gluconate, 257
Calcium lactate, 257
Calcium pantothenate, 274
Calculus formation, 28, 252, 258
Canada, 184
Canavanine, 334
Cancer, 61, 93, 195–223, 283, 334; and alcohol consumption, 173, 198, 201, 207–208, 214; asbestos and, 199, 207, 333–334; chemotherapy and, 202–204, 205, 213, 214, 330; constipation and, 215, 281, 348; fiber and, 181, 201, 215, 216; fibrocystic disease and, 239; genetic disposition for, 18; and selenium, 201, 202, 211, 212, 215, 242, 276; and weight management, 137–138, 211, 332

Candies, 35, 64, 121, 149, 309, 311
Canned foods, 58, 262, 319, 320
Capillary fragility, 41, 44
Caramel snacks, 121
Carbohydrates, 28, 33, 34, 55–57; and brain function, 108; and dysmenorrhea, 237; and weight management, 146, 150, 152, 154, 155, 156, 159. *See also* Starch; Sugars
Carbon monoxide, in blood, 174
Carbon tetrachloride, in water, 217–218
Carnitine, 73, 189–191, 242–243
Carpal tunnel syndrome, 29–30, 97–98
Casein, 155
Cataracts, 343
Cell reparation, 336. *See also* Healing time
Cellulose, 201
Ceramic glazes, lead-containing, 320
Cereals: and bone status, 260–261; and cancer, 201; for children, 64, 121; chromium in, 124; fortified, 64; and heart disease, 178, 183
Cerebral allergy, 116–117, 278
Ceroid pigments, 96
Cervical dysplasia, 235–236
Cheeses, 57–58; and calcium, 35; and cholesterol, 34; and heart disease, 177, 178; protein from, 34, 156, 303; tyramine in, 280
Chemotherapy, 112, 202–204, 205, 213, 214, 330
Cherries, 321
Chicken, 34, 178. *See also* Eggs
Children, 307–326, 331, 332; bone/tooth status of, 256, 260; brain function of, 113–121 passim, 230, 309–325 passim; and fluorides, 264; fortified foods for, 64; growth retardation in, 276
Children's Achievement Program for Educational Readiness, 317–318
Chlorinated hydrocarbons, 199, 218, 344
Chlorination, water, 199, 218
Chlorine, 60
Chloroform, 217
Chocolate, 116, 136, 240, 278, 280
Cholesterol, 34, 57, 58, 228, 335, 337; and cancer, 210; chromium and, 94, 188; and heart disease, 29, 30, 44, 160, 169–189 passim, 301, 330; weight management and, 135, 156
Choline, 95–96, 108, 110
Chondroitin sulfate, 191
Choriocarcinoma, 203, 204
Chromium, 60; aging and, 94–95; and blood sugar, 94, 123–125, 300; and cancer,

202; and cholesterol, 94, 188; and
  healing time, 44; during pregnancy, 298,
  299, 300–301; toxicity with, 71; and
  vision, 343; for xanthomas, 44
Chronic degenerative disease family, 4
Circulation, 27, 44, 45, 335
Citrus fruits, 33, 41, 61, 201, 251, 278
Citrus products, 116, 216, 316, 323
Cleaning materials, 292, 344, 345
Cleft palate, 291
Cocoa, 136
Coenzyme Q, 212
Coffee, 116, 216, 240, 278, 280, 292
Cola, 240. *See also* Soft drinks
Cold-tar derivatives, 334
Colitis, 29, 274, 283, 346–347
Collagen, 153, 155, 259, 260
Colon: cancer of, 198, 200, 201, 204, 213,
  215–216, 281, 348; spastic, 256;
  ulcerative, 274, 283, 346–347
Coloring agents, 207
Coma patients, 129
Community health, 344–345
Concentration ability, 67, 114; allergy and,
  278; blood sugar and, 19, 126; iron and,
  230; lead and, 320
Condiments, 177, 181
Conditional lethal mutations, 315
Confectionary goods, 121, 254. *See also*
  Candies
Confusion, mental: with allergies, 278; blood
  sugar and, 19, 120, 121, 295; with
  premenstrual tension, 233; with
  Wernicke-Korsakoff syndrome, 243
Connor, William, 91
Constipation, 18–19, 348; and brain function,
  118, 310; and colon cancer, 215, 281,
  348; fiber and, 18, 156, 182–183, 215,
  281, 348; immune system and, 281;
  weight loss diet and, 156
Contraceptives, oral, 63, 214–215, 234–235
Cookies, 34–35, 121, 149
Cooking methods, 37–38, 57, 177, 178, 184,
  301
Cookware, aluminum, 99, 127, 262
Copper, 19, 43, 44, 45, 60, 94; anemias and,
  45, 94, 229; and bone status, 94, 260,
  261, 282; and brain function, 113; and
  cancer, 211, 215; and heart disease, 94,
  187; and immune system, 19, 211,
  281–283; and suntanning, 17, 94;
  thyroid and, 17, 28, 146; toxicity
  possible with, 71; and weight
  management, 146, 154, 155
Copper aspirinate, 282

Copper salicyclate, 282
Corn, 65; allergy-producing, 116, 278; and
  blood acidity, 254; blood sugar and,
  120, 123, 125; and cholesterol, 181
Corn chips, 149
Corn oil, 147, 184
Corn sweeteners, 59, 178
Coronary bypass surgery, 330
Cough, recurring, 28
Cream, 177
Crohn's disease, 274, 346–347
Cucumber, 136
Cured foods, 58, 201, 216
Cyanide, 205
Cyanogenic glycoside, 205
Cyclamate, 59
Cysteine, 41
Cystic mastitis, 215, 239–240
Cystine, 41, 155
Cytochrome P-450, 207–208
Cytochromes, 144, 207–208

Dairy products, 36, 58, 61, 177, 323; and
  bone status, 35, 251, 254, 256, 257, 261;
  and cancer, 209, 216; during pregnancy,
  293, 296, 300. *See also* Butter; Cheese;
  Milk
Dance, 336
Dancercise, 157, 336
Dandruff, 27
Dates, 35
DDT, 217, 344
Decaffeinated coffee, 216
Deep-fried foods, 37, 57, 177, 178
Delaney amendment, 197
Dental-care personnel, toxic exposure of, 126
Dental restoration work, faulty, 258
Depression, 68, 107–126 passim;
  hypoglycemia and, 19, 120, 125, 295;
  medications for, 148; with oral
  contraceptives, 234, 235; with
  premenstrual tension, 233
Dermatitis, 18, 30, 296. *See also* Eczema
Diabetes, 61, 125; and bone status, 254;
  chromium and, 94, 125; constipation
  and, 348; maturity-onset, 18, 27, 94,
  125; and pregnancy, 294–295, 298;
  vegetable gums and, 183; weight
  management and, 27, 125, 137, 138,
  152, 156
Diarrhea, 18–19, 152, 236, 278, 346
Diastolic pressure, 26, 174
Diethylstilbestrol, 207
Digestive cancers, 198, 201, 215–217, 333.
  See also Colon

Digestion problems, 29, 30, 35, 266; with
fatty foods, 21; fiber for, 181; and
immune system, 273, 274; with proteins,
41; with starch blockers, 152;
underweight from, 159, 160. *See also*
Intestines
1,25 Dihydroxivitamin D, 253
Dimethylglycine (DMG), 73, 128–129
Dimethyl sulfoxide (DMSO), 335
Dioxin, 344
Dips, fat-rich, 57
Dismutase, superoxide, 212
Distillation, water, 218
Distress, 16–17, 23, 283, 347
Diuresis, 137
Diuretics, 26
Diverticular disease, 281, 348
Dizziness, 120, 152
D,L-phenylalanine, in treatment of arthritis,
98
DNA, 297
Dolomite, 257
Dopamines, 106, 112, 148
Doughnuts, 149, 311
Down's syndrome, 313–315
Dreams, 20–21, 43, 114
Driving, reckless, 87
Drugs, 87, 282; aluminum in, 99, 127, 262;
behavior-modifying, 108, 110, 112; birth
control, 63, 214–215, 234–235;
caffeine-containing, 240;
cholesterol-reducing, 170; for heart
disease management, 171;
hunger-producing, 148; nutrient
antagonisms to, 30–31, 63, 230;
pain-killing, 116; during pregnancy,
117–118, 303; vitamin K and, 44;
weight-affecting, 139, 148. *See also*
Chemotherapy
Dust, lead in, 262, 319, 320
Dysmenorrhea, 236–237, 238

Earlobe crease, 17–18
Early warning risk factor intervention, 8–10,
89, 91
Ear wax, 30
Eclampsia, 293
Eczema, 18, 30; allergy-causing, 18, 278,
331, 343; zinc and, 18, 30, 232, 276,
331, 343
Eggs, 33, 36, 58, 59, 209, 216; allergies to,
116, 278; for children, 311; and heart
disease, 179–180, 181; during pregnancy,
293, 300
Eicosapentaenoic acid (EPA), 185, 236

Electroshock, 112
Emaciation, 232
Emotions, 105, 107, 110, 112, 115; and blood
sugar, 19, 105, 295; thyroid and, 119.
See also Anxiety; Distress; Mood;
Psychological disturbances
Empty-calorie foods, 35, 37, 61, 62–63, 66;
and bone loss, 251; for children,
309–311; during pregnancy, 293; and
weight management, 61, 148–149, 150
Endocrine system, 118–119, 120, 123,
145–146, 147, 148, 150. *See also*
Adrenal glands; Thyroid
Endorphins, 116, 117, 150, 151, 157
Energy level, 19, 140–141, 264. *See also*
Hyperactivity; Lethargy; Tiredness
England, 152, 171
Environmental hazards, 332–334, 344–345,
347; and brain function, 126–127,
318–320, 325; and cancer, 198–200, 207,
208, 212, 217–218, 333–334; in drinking
water, 99, 127, 187, 199, 217–218, 344;
fetal development and, 291, 292. *See
also* Toxic elements
Environmental Protection Agency, 217,
332–333
Enzymes: chemotherapy inhibiting, 203; and
cancer, 208, 212; digestive, 152, 160,
281; and weight problems, 136
Epidemiology, 197–198
Epilepsy, 127, 128
Equilibrium loss, 120, 126, 152, 243
Eskimos, 184–185
Esophagus, cancer of, 198, 201
Essential fatty acids: cholesterol and, 30,
301; in eggs, 33; and immune system,
98, 277; for infants, 331; during
pregnancy, 301; and skin problems, 18,
30, 331, 343
Essential nutrients, 73
Estradiol, 214
Estrogens, 227; and bone status, 239, 241,
253, 264; and cancer, 214–215, 239; and
cholesterol, 228; and fibrocystic disease,
239; melatonin and, 215, 244; smoking
and, 239
Estrone, 214
Ethylene dichloride, 216
Ewing's tumor, 204
Exercise, 87, 335–336, 347; and bone status,
238, 265, 335, 336; and brain function,
117, 119, 126, 336; for circulation, 44,
45, 335; for digestion, 30; and heart
disease, 44, 176–177; for menopausal
women, 238; and menstruation,

237–238, 336; for stress reduction, 117, 283; vitamin B-6 and, 240; and weight management, 147, 150, 155, 156–157, 159, 160, 238, 335
Exorphins, 116–117, 280
Eyes: condition of, 27, 41, 230, 243, 278, 343; fetal development of, 290; sunlight exposure of, 119, 215, 244–245

Family history. *See* Genetic disposition
Fasting, 151, 254
Fatigue. *See* Tiredness
Fats, 21, 34, 37, 55–56, 57, 59–60, 62; and bone status, 254; and cancer, 197, 200–201, 215; and cholesterol, 34, 172–184 passim, 330; and female hormones, 215, 236, 237, 301; and heart disease, 34, 172–189 passim, 301, 330; and immune system, 276–277; and weight management, 146, 147, 148–149, 154, 160. *See also* Essential fatty acids; Oils
FDA. *See* Food and Drug Administration
FDC Red Dye Number 3, 322
Feet, problems with, 42, 296
Feingold (Benjamin) diet, 321–323, 324
Female physiology. *See* Women
Ferrous fumarate, 230
Ferrous sulphate, 230
Fetal alcohol syndrome, 292
Fetal development, 117–118, 227–228, 229, 287–305, 331–332
Fever, 139
Fibers, dietary, 33, 35, 64, 73; and cancer, 181, 201, 215, 216; and cholesterol, 174, 178, 181–183; and intestinal function, 18, 30, 156, 182–183, 201, 215–216, 281, 346, 348; and weight management, 149, 150, 156
Fibrocystic disease, 215, 239–240
Fibronectin, 151
Figs, 35
Finger bending abilities, 29–30, 97–98
Fingernail problems, 43, 229
Fish, 58, 156, 177, 178, 180–181, 278; canned, 319; oils in, 34, 98, 184–185, 236, 277; during pregnancy, 300, 303; smoked, 201
Flax seed oil, 244
Flour, 63, 124
Flufenamic acid, 236
Fluid balance, 158
Fluid consumption, 30, 35. *See also* Beverages; Water, drinking
Fluid loss, 137, 158

Fluid retention, 29, 136, 298
Fluorescent lights, 119
Fluoride, 262–264
Fluorine, 60
Fluorosis, 264
Flushing, 16, 70–71, 111, 296
Folic acid, 30, 33, 41, 42, 63, 235–236; anemia and, 45, 229; and bone/tooth status, 28, 260, 264–265; and brain function, 110, 113, 114, 319; and cancer, 203, 214; and healing time, 45; and immune system, 28, 273, 277; during pregnancy, 294, 297, 298
Food additives, 58; and behavior disorders, 321, 322–323, 324, 325; and bone loss, 255; and intestinal problems, 323, 346; and cancer, 197, 202
Food and Drug Administration (FDA), 152–153, 186, 197, 235
Formaldehyde, 344
Fortified foods, 59, 63–64
Framingham Study, 169
Fried foods, 37, 57, 177, 178, 301
Frozen food, 38
Fructose, 59, 147, 156, 178
Fruit juice, 155, 156, 215, 316, 323
Fruits, 34, 57, 59, 61, 183, 274; allergies to, 280; and bone status, 254, 256; and cancer, 201, 209, 212; for children, 311; in historical diets, 65; for night vision, 41; during pregnancy, 293; in weight loss diets, 152, 156. *See also individual fruits*

Gall bladder function, 21
Gallstones, 29
Gamma-aminobutyric acid (GABA), 107, 127
Garlic concentrate, 73
Garlic oil, 183
General adaptation syndrome, 23, 348
General Mills, 64
Genetic disposition, 290, 347; toward B-vitamin deficiency, 312; toward cancer, 18; conditional lethal mutations in, 315; toward depression, 117; toward diabetes, 18; toward heart disease, 18, 44, 169, 172–173; toward high blood pressure, 18; toward obesity, 17, 135–136, 137. *See also* Birth defects
Genetotrophic theory of disease, 12, 313, 317
Gestation. *See* Pregnancy
Glucomannan, 123, 183
Glucose tolerance factor (GTF), 124
Glycine, 127

Glycoproteins, 211
Glycosaminoglycans, 191
Gonorrhea, 243
Gori, Gio, 90
Grains, 33, 57, 59, 61, 242; and bone status,
    254, 256, 260–261; and brain function,
    124, 125, 311; and cancer, 201, 211,
    242, 334; and heart disease, 178, 180,
    183, 242; in historical diets, 65; during
    pregnancy, 301; for tongue sensitivity,
    41; for weight management, 146, 159.
    *See also individual grains and grain
    products*
Gravies, 37
Graying, premature, 343
Growth: rapid spurt of, 19; retardation in,
    276, 291, 299
Guam, 126
Guanosine, 150
Guar gum, 123, 183
Gum, chewing, 148
Gum condition (in mouth), 28, 41, 252,
    256–260 passim
Gums, vegetable, 73, 122, 123, 156, 183, 201

Hair, 343; chemotherapy and, 203;
    chromium in, 300; copper and, 94, 343;
    lead in, 318; protein and, 20, 27, 41,
    152, 343; vitamin A toxicity and, 69,
    210, 274; zinc and, 41, 276, 282, 343
Haldol, 110
Ham, 34, 201
Hands: B vitamins and, 42, 296;
    neurotransmitters and, 107
Hay fever, 323
HDL, *see* High-density lipoprotein
Headaches, 266; with allergies, 43, 117, 278,
    279–280, 323; with dysmenorrhea, 236;
    from vitamin deficiency, 312; with
    vitamin overages, 69, 70, 210, 274; with
    weight loss drugs, 139
Healing time, 44–45, 118, 125, 191, 276, 282
Health-care industry, 88, 329
Heart attack, 24, 160, 167, 185, 189
Heartbeat, 43, 153, 154, 155, 160, 278. *See
    also* Pulse rate
Heartburn, 21, 99
Heart disease, 26, 61, 93, 165–194, 330;
    blood pressure and, 26, 137, 160, 169,
    174, 185–186, 187, 330; and cholesterol,
    29, 30, 44, 160, 169–189 passim, 301,
    330; constipation and, 182–183, 348;
    with copper deficiency, 94, 187; earlobe
    crease and, 17–18; ear wax and, 30;
    fetal development and, 297, 301,
    331–332; and fish oil, 34, 184–185; leg

coloring and, 44; and life expectancy,
    93; noise and, 332; personality related
    to, 24, 169; selenium and, 242; surgery
    for, 175, 330; vitamin D toxicity and,
    69; vitamin E and, 189, 213; weight
    problems and, 137, 160
Height. *See* Weight-to-height ratio
"Helper" cells, 283
Helplessness feelings, 7
Herbicides, 199, 344
Herpes, 180
High blood pressure, 330; cadmium and,
    187; calcium and, 45–46, 186–187, 299;
    genetic disposition toward, 18; and heart
    disease, 137, 160, 169, 174, 185–186,
    187; obesity and, 136–137, 160; during
    pregnancy, 298, 299; PSMF and, 156;
    sodium/salt and, 29, 35, 99, 136,
    185–186; tyrosine and, 108
High-density lipoprotein (HDL), 172–174,
    176, 177, 185, 188, 189
Historical diets, 65
Hodgkins disease, 204
Hoffer, Abram, 20, 111
Homocysteine, 114, 188
Horizontal disease, 4
Hormones: adrenal, 26, 29, 106, 108,
    118–119, 148, 216; blood sugar
    regulation by, 120, 123, 124, 125, 343;
    and bone status, 239, 241, 252, 253–254,
    258, 262, 264; and brain function, 106,
    108, 116–126 passim, 148, 150, 151,
    157; and cancer, 202, 215, 216, 219; for
    lactation, 240, 297; parathyroid, 252,
    255, 262; sex-related, 215, 219, 227–228,
    231, 236–245 passim, 277, 301. *See also*
    Estrogens
Hot dogs, 201
Huntington's disease, 95, 108
Hydrogen peroxide, 271
Hydroxyapatite, 252, 259
Hydroxylase, 208
Hyperactivity, 310, 321–322
Hypercarotenemia, 209
Hyperexcitable personalities, 42, 113, 119
Hyperglycemia, 120, 124, 125
Hypersensitive immune system, 272–283
    passim, 335
Hypertension. *See* High blood pressure
Hypoglycemia, 19, 120, 124, 125, 294–295
Hypothalamus, 118, 146, 148, 150
Hypothyroidism, 17, 151, 231–232, 240

Ice craving, 230
Ice cream, 34–35, 121, 149, 178, 311
Imagery, for stress reduction, 283

Immune system, 19, 26, 67, 68, 271–285;
and Acquired Immunodeficiency
Syndrome, 283; aging and, 98, 211; and
cancer, 199–213 passim, 219, 276, 283;
empty-calorie foods and, 61; exercise
and, 283, 336; stress and, 23, 284–285;
and tooth/gum status, 28, 258, 260; and
weight management, 151, 211, 335; zinc
and, 19, 98, 202, 211, 260, 275–276,
277, 281–283, 299
Immunotherapy, 202, 206, 283
Incomplete protein breakdown products
(IPBs), 116–117
Infants, 264, 297, 331, 332
Infection susceptibility, 137, 229–230, 232,
276
Infertility, 231, 242–243, 293
Inosine, 150
Inositol, 42, 73
Insecticides, 292
Insomnia, 67, 68, 114; prostaglandins and,
236; tryptophan and, 107–108; vitamins
and, 20–21, 312
Institutional foods, 37, 58
Insulin, 120, 123, 124, 125, 343
Intelligence, 7, 115, 312, 313, 315–317,
318
Interferon, 211
Intestines, 29, 30, 172, 256, 266, 346–347;
allergies and, 18–19, 29, 117, 266, 278,
281, 347; cancer of, 138, 198, 200, 201,
204, 213, 215–216, 281, 348;
chemotherapy and, 203, 204, 213;
diverticular disease in, 281, 348; fiber
and, 18, 30, 156, 182–183, 201,
215–216, 281, 346, 348; and food
additives, 323, 346; and immune system,
273, 274, 278, 281, 283, 335; iron and,
229, 230; mineral toxicity and, 71;
personality traits and, 24; starch
blockers and, 152; ulceration of, 274,
283, 346–347; vitamin K and, 44;
vitamin toxicity and, 69, 274; weight
loss surgery on, 138, 335. See also
Constipation; Diarrhea
Iodide, 202
Iodine, 60, 63; in soil, 124; thyroid and, 17,
28, 63, 146, 231
Iowa farmers, 176
Iron, 19, 39, 41, 46, 60, 63; anemia and, 44,
45, 228–229; behavioral problems and,
113, 320, 325; and healing time, 44, 45;
and immune system, 19, 275, 283;
female physiology and, 228–230, 294,
298, 300; and lead, 320, 325
Irritability, 67, 68, 312

Itai-itai disease, 262
Italy, 171

Japan, 173–174, 330
Jaw alignment, 258. See also Periodontal
disease
Jazzercise, 336
Jogging, 157, 336
Joints, 98, 256, 259, 266. See also Arthritis
Juices, 155, 156, 215, 316, 323
Junk food syndrome, 310–311. See also
Empty-calorie foods
Justification theory, 74

Kaposi's sarcoma, 283
Kawasaki syndrome, 344
Kefir, 216, 256
Kidney problems, 19, 30; blood pressure
and, 26, 174; bone status and, 252;
obesity and, 137; vitamin C and, 30, 70
Kwashiorkor, 67

Labor, in childbirth, 299
Lactalbumin, 155
Lactation, 240, 258, 297
Lactic acid buildup, 296
Lactobacillus acidophilus, 216
Lactobacillus bulgaricus, 216
Lactose intolerance (milk allergy), 16, 116,
261–262, 278, 280, 323
Laetrile, 204–205
Lamb, 34
Lard, 59
L-dopa, 148
Lead, 45, 126; and bone status, 257, 261,
262; children and, 318–320, 325; in
drinking water, 217; male fertility and,
243
Lean body mass, 26–27, 141–142, 237
Learning ability, 107, 115–116, 121,
318–319, 320. See also Intelligence
Lecithin, 73, 95, 108
Lectins, 260–261
Leg discoloration, 44
Leg pain, 43, 45–46, 160, 252, 256, 323
Legumes, 34, 35; and blood sugar, 123, 125;
and brown fat metabolism, 146–147;
and cholesterol, 180, 183
Leisure-time activity, 117
Lente diet, 183
Lethargy, 67, 232, 310. See also Tiredness
Leukemia, 203, 204
Leukotrienes, 277
Levy, R. I., 169, 170
L-glutamine, 110, 244
Lhermitte's syndrome, 45

Life expectancy, 79, 92–93
Lifestyle, 331, 332, 334–335, 345–346,
    347–348; and aging, 81–93, 99, 251,
    252–253, 347–348; and bone/tooth
    status, 251, 252–253, 258–259, 266; and
    cancer, 93, 173, 197–219 passim; and
    conditional lethal mutations, 315; and
    depression, 117; and heart disease, 93,
    169–171, 330; and immune system,
    205–206, 211, 213, 219, 284; sex-related
    hormones and, 227–228, 237, 244, 253.
    See also Sedentary lifestyle
Light, 119. See also Sunlight exposure
Lignin, 201
Lincoln University, Missouri, 94
Linseed oil, 98
Lip condition, 27, 42, 296
Lipectomy, 138–139
Lipofuscin pigments, 96
Liquid protein diets, 153, 154
Liver (meat), 41, 242, 301
Liver function, 71, 111; alcohol and, 16, 173,
    207–208, 214; and cancer, 207–208, 210,
    211, 214, 215; and cholesterol, 172, 180,
    228; in immune system, 272, 274;
    vitamin A and, 69, 209, 210, 274; and
    weight management, 146, 149, 151
Lungs, 45, 83–84, 335; cancer of, 198, 201,
    204, 207, 208, 209–210, 274–275
Lymphatic system, 271
Lymph glands, 271
Lymphocytes, 211, 271–276 passim, 282, 284
Lymphoma, 203, 204
Lysine, 180, 243

Macro elements, 60
Macronutrients, 55–56
Magnesium, 19, 60, 63, 99, 127; and alcohol
    consumption, 16, 243; bone/tooth status
    and, 28, 42, 43, 99, 256, 257, 259, 261,
    262, 264; and cancer, 202; and
    dysmenorrhea, 236; heart disorders and,
    43, 187; and hyperexcitability, 42; and
    immune system, 202, 276; leg/muscle
    cramping and, 45, 46, 187; weight loss
    diets and, 137, 154, 156; and
    premenstrual tension, 233–234; and
    stress, 17; and Wernicke-Korsakoff
    syndrome, 243
Maize, 65
Malabsorption, 27, 159, 229–230
Maldigestion, 29, 41, 159, 160, 266
Male physiology, 159, 173–174, 227, 228,
    233, 239–245 passim, 291
Malnutrition of too much of too little, 61

Manganese, 19, 60, 71, 113; and cancer, 211,
    212, 215; during pregnancy, 298, 299
Manic depression, 113, 116
Marasmus, 67
Margarine, 34, 35, 57–58, 59, 177, 178, 184
Marginal deficiency, 66–68
Marijuana, 243
Mast cells, 277, 278, 280–281
MaxEPA, 98, 185, 236
Mayonnaise, 181, 301
Meat products, 177, 201
Meats, 37, 42, 57, 58, 59, 61, 156; and bone
    condition, 241, 251, 254, 255, 256; and
    cancer, 200, 209, 215; and heart disease,
    177, 178, 180–181; in historical diets,
    65; during pregnancy, 300, 303; and
    tongue condition, 41. See also individual
    meats
Medications. See Drugs
Melancholic genes, 117
Melanin, 17
Melatonin, 119, 215, 244
Memory, 105, 107; aging loss of, 95–96, 108,
    127; children's problems with, 115;
    Wernicke-Korsakoff syndrome and, 243
Men, 159, 173–174, 227, 228, 233, 239–245
    passim, 291
Menopausal and postmenopausal women,
    238, 240–241, 253, 261
Menstrual cycle, 230, 231, 233–234,
    236–239, 336
Mental functions. See Alertness, mental;
    Brain function; Concentration ability;
    Confusion, mental; Learning ability;
    Memory
Mental illness. See Psychological
    disturbances
Mental outlook, 7, 87, 283–284
Mental retardation, 312–315
Mercury, 126, 217
Mescaline, 112
Mesentheliomal cancer, 333
Metabolic poisoning, 264
Metabolic switching, 140–141, 159
Metabolic weight equation, 139–141
Metabolism, 18, 20, 21; anaerobic, 254; and
    brain function, 105; brown fat, 18, 137,
    143–145, 146–147, 157; chemotherapy
    and, 203
Methionine, 41, 154, 155, 243, 343
Methylxanthines, 240
Michigan, 344
Micro elements. See Trace elements
Microhemorrhages, 27
Micronutrients, 60

Migraine headaches, 279–280
Milk, 33, 35, 58, 61, 63, 156, 334; allergies
    to, 16, 116, 261–262, 278, 280, 323; and
    bone status, 35, 251, 252, 261–262; and
    heart disease, 177, 178; during
    pregnancy, 296
Milk products. *See* Dairy products
Millet, 254
Minerals, 60–62, 71, 72, 179; and aging,
    92–95; and brain function, 105, 314; and
    cancer, 61, 212–213, 276; and heart
    disease, 61, 174, 185–188; and immune
    system, 61, 273, 275–276; during
    pregnancy, 294, 295, 297–298, 299–301;
    with weight management, 61, 150,
    158–159. *See also individual minerals*
Mint, 321
Mitochondria, 134, 157, 336
Molybdenum, 60
Monosodium glutamate (MSG), 16
Montreal Olympics, 237
Mood, 105, 114, 119–123, 125, 126. *See also*
    Depression
Morbid obesity, 136–137, 335. *See also*
    Obesity
Morphine, 116
Mouth corners, cracks/redness at, 27, 229,
    296. *See also* Teeth; Tongue condition
Mucopolysaccharides, 191
Mucous membrane dryness, 69, 274
Multiple Risk Factor Intervention Trial
    (MRFIT), 170–171
Mumps, 243
Muscle exercise, 240, 336
Muscle loss, 126, 152, 154
Muscle tissue, 146, 240, 251
Muscle weakness/pain, 278; and allergy, 43,
    278; blood sugar and, 295; and brain
    function, 114, 129, 310; calcium and,
    45–46, 252, 256; dimethyl sulfoxide and,
    335; with fluoride, 264; iron and, 229;
    magnesium and, 45–46, 187; vitamin
    B-1 for, 43, 296; weight-loss efforts and,
    139, 152
Mutations, conditional lethal, 315
Myesthesia gravis, 275
Myristanol, 129

National Cancer Chemotherapy Program,
    203
National Cancer Institute, 199, 212
National Institutes of Health, 322
National Research Council, 197, 200
Nausea, 139, 203, 264, 296–297
Nearsightedness, 343

Neck tenderness, 28
Nervous system, 106, 116, 129, 283–284;
    calcium and, 35; copper and, 71, 94;
    fetal, 118, 292, 301; folic acid and, 236;
    lecithin and, 95, 108; mineral toxicity
    and, 71, 126–127, 319–320; vitamin
    toxicity and, 69; vitamin B-1 and, 110
Neural-tube defect, 294
Neuroendocrinology, of immune system,
    283–284
Neurotransmitters, 105–130, 148, 150, 280.
    See also Brain function
Niacin. *See* Vitamin B-3
Niacinamide, 71, 98, 111, 244
Night vision, 41
Nitrates, 216
Nitrosamines, 216
N,N-dimethylglycine, 73, 128–129
Noise, 119, 332–333
Nose bleeding, 44
Nose cracks/redness, 27, 229
Nucleic acids, 150, 297
Nutritional pharmacology, 71
Noradrenaline, 106, 108
Nutrition and Physical Degeneration, 266
Nutrition scan, 33
Nuts, 34, 65, 116, 201, 334

Oat bran fiber, 182, 281
Oat-cell cancer, 209
Oats, 181
Obesity, 61, 136–157 passim;
    anorexic/bulimic and, 233; genetic
    disposition toward, 17, 135–136, 137;
    infant nutrition and, 332; surgery for,
    138–139, 335. *See also* Weight
    management
Occupational health hazards, 126, 198, 207,
    332–334
Octacosanol, 129
Oil concentrates, 73, 129
Oils, 37, 59–60; and cancer, 200–201; for
    dysmenorrhea, 236; heart disease and,
    34, 177, 181, 183–185; and immune
    system, 98, 277; weight management
    and, 148. *See also* Vegetable oils
Olive oil, 184
Olympics, Montreal, 237
Omega-3-eicosapentaenoic acid, 185, 236
Oral health problems, 27, 61, 229, 296. *See
    also* Gum condition; Teeth; Tongue
    condition
Oral hygiene, 258, 259
Orange juice, 216, 316, 323
Organ meats, 34. *See also* Liver

Organ reserve, 79
Orthomolecular psychiatry, 20, 109–114, 115
Oslo, 171
Osmond, Humphrey, 20
Osteoarthritis, 244, 252, 253, 259, 265;
    dimethyl sulfoxide for, 335; obesity and,
    137
Osteogenic sarcoma, 204
Osteoporosis, 19, 34, 251, 253, 259, 261, 265;
    exercise and, 336; fluoride for, 264;
    smoking and, 239, 259; vitamin D for,
    69, 261, 264
Ovaries, 227; cancer of, 138, 198, 214,
    234–235; chemotherapy and, 203–204;
    cysts in, 230, 235; phagophagia and, 230
Overconsumptive undernutrition, 61, 310
Overcooking, 37
Oxalate stone formation, 19, 30, 70, 252
Oxygen, 106, 157, 174, 271

Pain killers, 116, 150
Paint fumes, and fetal development, 292
Pancakes, 33
Pancreas function, 21, 120, 124, 152
Pancreatic cancer, 198, 216
Pancreatic enzyme supplements, 281
Pancreatin tablets, 281
Pantothenic acid, 17, 274, 316, 343, 346
Para-aminobenzoic acid (PABA), 17, 217
Parathyroid gland, 252
Parathyroid hormone, 252, 255, 262
Parkinsonism, 98, 99, 126, 148
Pasta, 35, 57
Pasteur, Louis, 317
Pasteurization, 334
Pauling, Linus, 110, 213
Peach pits, 205
Peanut butter, 323
Peanut oil, 147, 184
Peanuts, 116, 334
Peas, 183
Pectins, 123, 201
Pellagra, 54, 67, 111
Penicillin, 329
Periodontal disease, 19, 251, 253, 257–258,
    259, 260, 265
Pernicious anemia, 70, 110
Personality disorders, 42, 107–121 passim,
    233, 310. See also Psychological
    disturbances
Personality traits: of anorexics/bulimics, 159,
    233; heart-disease-related, 24, 169;
    time-urgency-related, 24
Pesticides, 199, 292
Peyronies disease, 242

Phagophagia, 230
Phagocytosis, 271
Phenylalanine, 106, 108
Phenylpropanolamine, 139
Phosophatidyl choline, 95
Phosphorus, 60, 156; and bone/tooth/gum
    status, 19, 28, 252–264 passim; and iron
    absorption, 229; during pregnancy, 294
Photochemical oxidants, 344
Physiological stage, of nutrient depletion, 68
Pickled foods, 201, 216
Picolinic acid, 300
Pies, 121
Pigments: aging, 96; tanning, 17, 94, 217
Pineal gland, 119
Pituitary, 118, 120, 145–146
Plaque: in arteries, 175, 177, 188, 191; on
    teeth, 28, 252, 258
Plateaus, weight, 158
Platinum, 203
Poisoning. See Toxic elements
Poland, 171
Pollution: air, 262, 320, 334; and cancer,
    198, 199, 218; water, 199, 218
Polychlorinated biphenyls (PCBs), 217, 344
Popcorn, 323
Pork, 34, 201, 216
Postural hypotension, 26
Potassium, 33, 60; and blood pressure, 186;
    heartbeat and, 43, 154, 155; weight
    management and, 136, 137, 154, 155,
    156
Potato chips, 149
Potatoes, 34, 35, 37, 59; allergies to, 278;
    and blood sugar, 120, 123
Poultry, 34, 57, 59, 177, 178, 303. See also
    Eggs
Pregnancy, 287–305; calcium during, 256,
    258, 294, 296, 298, 299, 304; hormone
    medications during, 117–118; and
    immune system, 274, 283, 299; iron
    during, 229, 230, 294, 298, 300; stress
    with, 118, 227–228, 258, 283; vitamin
    B-6 during, 296–297, 298, 300, 331–332
Premenstrual tension (PMT), 233–234
Preventive medicine, 88–91, 329, 330, 331
Price, Weston, 265–266
Pritikin diet, 146
Processed foods, 38, 58, 59, 66; and
    bone/tooth status, 251, 253, 254, 262,
    264, 266; fortified, 59, 63–64; heart
    disease and, 178; and iron absorption,
    229; lead in, 262, 319, 320. See also
    Empty-calorie foods; Food additives
Progesterone, 227, 228

Prohibition, 59
Prolactin, 240, 297
Prometol. *See* Wheat germ oil concentrate
Prostacyclin, 185
Prostaglandin F-2 alpha, 236
Prostaglandins, 236, 277, 301
Prostate cancer, 138, 198, 200, 204
Prostate gland, enlargement of. *See* Prostatic hypertrophy
Prostatic hypertrophy, 244
Protein, 33, 34, 55–57, 243; and bone/tooth status, 34, 241, 252, 256, 259, 261; and brain function, 106, 116–117, 280; and hair, 20, 27, 41, 152, 343; and healing time, 44; and heart disease, 172, 178, 179–180, 211; and immune system, 151, 273, 276–277, 280, 281; during pregnancy, 300, 301–303; and weight management, 41, 146–160 passim, 211, 276, 303
Protein efficiency ratio (PER), 155
Protein powder replacement diets, 153, 156
Protein-sparing modified fast (PSMF), 153–157
Psychiatry, orthomolecular, 20, 109–114, 115
Psychological disturbances, 20, 105–126 passim; of children, 113–121 passim, 310, 319, 320, 325; with dysmenorrhea, 236; noise and, 332; weight-affecting, 137, 148, 159, 233. *See also* Anxiety; Behavioral problems; Depression
Psychosis, 107–116 passim
Psychotherapy, 112
Pulse rate, 26, 151, 157, 335
Purification, water, 199, 218
Purines, 150
Pyorrhea, 257. *See also* Periodontal disease
Pyruvic acid buildup, 296

Radiation therapy, 202, 203, 204, 205
Radioactive elements, 217
Raisins, 35
Raquetball, 336
Recommended Dietary Allowances (RDAs), 39, 54–55, 74, 211; in breakfast cereals, 64; of B vitamins (general), 70–71, 311, 312; of folic acid, 114, 297; during pregnancy, 294, 295, 296, 297; sex differences in, 228, 229; of vitamin B-1, 42; of vitamin B-3, 111; of vitamin B-6, 39, 98, 114; of vitamin C, 39, 260, 274
Rectum, cancer of, 201
Red blood cells, 271, 297
Redundancy, 14
Relaxation, 117

Reproductive function, 94, 203–204, 227–245 passim, 291, 293; cancer and, 138, 198, 204, 214, 234–235; hormones related to, 215, 219, 227–228, 231, 236–245 passim, 277, 301. *See also* Estrogen; Pregnancy
Respiratory function, 28, 83–84, 323, 331. *See also* Breath shortness; Lungs
Retardation: growth, 276, 291, 299; mental, 312–315
Reverse osmosis units, 218
Rhabdomyosarcoma, embryonal, 204
Rhubarb, 30
Riboflavin. *See* Vitamin B-2
Rice, 120, 122, 123, 125, 181, 254
Rickets, 67
Risk factor intervention, early warning, 8–10, 89, 91
Rowing machine, 336
Rye, 181

Saccharin, 216–217
Safflower oil, 147, 184, 277
Salad dressings and oils, 34, 59, 177, 181, 301. *See also* Oils
Salicylates, 321
Salt, 29, 35, 36–37, 57, 58, 121; and blood pressure, 29, 35, 99, 186; and cancer, 201; iodine with, 63
Saponins, 73
Sauces, 37, 181
Sausages, 34, 201
Scheroderma, 275
Schizophrenia, 107, 109, 111, 113, 116
Sclerosis, 251
Scurvy, 54, 61, 67, 315
Seborrhea, 18, 343
Sedentary lifestyle, 66, 93; and appetite, 150; and bone status, 251, 252, 265; and heart disease, 169, 330
Seeds, 201, 334
Seizure disorders, 106, 127–129
Selenate, 276
Selenite, 276
Selenium, 60, 201; and cancer, 201, 202, 211, 212, 215, 242, 276; and hair condition, 41; and healing time, 45; and immune system, 202, 211, 212, 276; and male infertility, 242; and prostatic hypertrophy, 244; toxicity with, 71
Selikoff, Irving, 333–334
Selye, Hans, 348
Senate, U.S., 55–57, 186
Serotonin, 106, 108, 148
Sesame oil, 147, 184
Set-point theory, 137, 143, 144

Sex-related physiology. *See* Men; Reproductive function; Women
Sharks, 210–211
Shellfish, 180–181, 278
Silicon, 60
Singlet oxygen, 271
Sinus drip, 28
Skin problems, 44, 174, 276, 343; with allergies, 18, 117, 278, 331, 343; cancer, 217; with tanning, 17, 94, 217; vitamin A and, 28, 209, 210, 274, 343. *See also* Dermatitis
Skipping rope, 336
Sleep, 20–21, 43, 114, 335. *See also* Insomnia
Smell sense, 45
Smoked foods, 58, 201, 216
Smoking, 63, 87, 93; and bone status, 239, 251, 258, 259; and cancer, 198, 201, 207, 208, 213, 214, 274–275; and fetal development, 291–292, 303; and heart disease, 169, 171, 174, 175, 187; and menstruation, 238–239
Snacks, 34–35, 58, 64, 121, 293, 309
Sodium, 57, 58, 60, 136, 185–186. *See also* Salt
Sodium-potassium ATPase, 136
Soft drinks, 34–35, 59, 121, 309; and appetite, 148; behavioral problems and, 35, 121, 309; and bone status, 255, 256; and fibrocystic disease, 240
Soils, food-bearing, 124, 127, 212
Solvents, and fetal development, 292
Soy, 155, 278
Soy beans, 181
Soy oil, 147
Speech loss, 126
Sperm, 204, 242–243, 291
Spiller, Gerald, 71–73
Spina bifida cystica, 299
Spinach, 30
Spreads, fat-rich, 57, 59, 181, 301
Starch, 34; and blood sugar, 120, 121, 125; in weight management, 146–147, 152–153, 156, 159
Starch blockers, 152–153
State-by-state incidence, of heart disease, 167–168
Steroid hormones, 227
Steroids, anabolic, 207
Sterols, plant, 180, 181
Stir-frying, 301
Stomach acid, 99, 229–230, 262, 331
Stomach cancer, 201, 216, 333
Stools, 21, 29

Stress, 16–17, 22–24, 26, 79, 227–228, 346; allergy and, 347; appetite-stimulating, 148; and bone status, 251, 258, 336; and brain function, 117, 118, 121, 126, 148; from exercise, 336; and immune system, 23, 284–285
Stress Power, 23
Stroke, 24, 26, 160, 167, 174, 185
Sudden infant death syndrome, 297
Sugars, 20, 33–37 passim, 57, 59, 62, 323; and brain function, 115, 120, 121, 125, 317–318; in fortified foods, 64; and heart disease, 172, 178; and intestinal diseases, 323, 346; during pregnancy, 293; and tooth/gum status, 28, 260, 261; and weight management, 147, 148–149, 152, 156, 160
Sunflower seed oil, 147, 184, 277
Sunlight exposure, 244–245; and bone status, 42, 252, 253, 254; burn from, 17, 217; cancer from, 217; melatonin released by, 119, 215, 244
Superoxide, 212, 271
"Suppressor" cells, 283
Surgery: for cancer, 202, 203, 204, 205; for cholesterol reduction, 175; coronary bypass, 330; for intestinal problems, 274; for weight loss, 138–139, 335
Surveillance system, immune, 199–200, 271–272. *See also* Immune system
Sweden, 228
Sweet potatoes, 59
Swimming, 157, 336
Switched metabolism, 140–141, 159
Systemic lupus erythematosus (SLE), 275, 334
Systemic therapy, for cancer, 202

Tannenbaum, Albert, 197
Tannin, 229
Tanning, 17, 94, 217
Tardive dyskinesia, 108
Taste sense, 45, 93–94, 148, 232, 282
Taurine, 73, 110, 127–129, 155
Tea: allergy-producing, 116, 278, 280; and cancer, 212; and fibrocystic disease, 240; and iron absorption, 229; and sodium-potassium ATPase, 136
Teeth, 19, 28, 233, 251–266 passim, 319
Temperature: bodily reactions to, 17, 118; cooking, 37, 184
Testes, 204, 227, 242, 243
Testosterone, 227, 228, 239, 242
Thiamin. *See* Vitamin B-1
Thirst, 125

Thorazine, 110
Throat tenderness, 28
Thrombosis, coronary, 185
Thymosin, 283, 284
Thymus gland, 211, 276
Thyroid, 17, 28, 118–119, 230, 252; and
    blood sugar, 120; iodine and, 17, 28, 63,
    146, 231; and weight management, 137,
    145–146, 151, 159
Tics, 107
Time urgency stress, 24
Tiredness, 46, 112, 117, 264, 278, 295. *See
    also* Weakness
T-lymphocytes, 211, 271–272, 273, 274, 276,
    282, 283, 284
Tobacco products, 176, 207. *See also* Smoking
Tomatoes, 319
Tongue condition, 28, 41, 42, 229
Torula yeast, 124
Total (cereal), 64
Toxemia, 293, 298, 299
Toxic elements, 303, 332–334; and aging,
    98–99, 127; amydalin and, 205; and
    bone loss, 261, 262; and brain function,
    126–127, 318–320, 325; and cancer,
    198–200, 207, 208, 212, 217–218,
    333–334; in chemotherapy, 203–204,
    213; in drinking water, 99, 127, 187,
    199, 217–218, 344; fetal development
    and, 291, 292; in food additives, 322.
    See also Cadmium; Lead
Toxic levels, of nutrients, 68–71, 317, 337; of
    fluoride, 264; of iron, 230; of vanadium,
    116; of vitamin A, 38, 69, 209, 210, 274;
    of vitamin D, 38, 69, 254
Trace elements, 60, 71, 187–188, 298,
    299–301. *See also individual elements*
Transmethylation theory, 112
Trampolining, 157
Triacantanol, 129
Triglycerides, blood, 183, 189
Tryptophan, 300; and brain function, 106,
    107–108, 113, 150; and dysmenorrhea,
    236; and PMT, 234; and weight
    management, 150, 155
Tuna, 319
Turnip greens, 136
Turkey, 34
Type A personality, 24
Type B personality, 24
Tyramine, 280
Tyrosine, 17, 28, 99, 108, 147, 150

Ulcerative colitis, 274, 283, 346–347
Ulcers, 283, 332–333

Ultratrace elements, 64
Underweight problems, 159–160, 232–233
United States Department of Agriculture
    (USDA), 58–59, 229, 275
United States Dietary Goals, 57, 186
United States Environmental Protection
    Agency, 217, 332–333
United States General Accounting Office,
    217
United States heart disease incidence,
    167–168
United States Senate, 55–57, 186
University of Alabama Medical School, 175
University of Illinois, 129
University of Minnesota, 175
University of Southern California Medical
    School, 175
Uric acid problems, 30
Urination problems, 30, 46, 125, 229, 298;
    and prostatic hypertrophy, 244
Uterine cancer, 198, 214, 215
Uterine cysts, 235–236

Vaccination, 272
Vanadium, 60, 116
Vegetable gums, 73, 122, 123, 156, 183, 201
Vegetable juices, 155, 156
Vegetable oils, 34, 35, 57, 59; and cancer,
    201; and heart disease, 177, 183–184;
    and immune system, 276; during
    pregnancy, 301; and weight
    management, 147, 160
Vegetable proteins, 180, 181, 276
Vegetables, 34, 35, 41–44 passim, 57–61
    passim; beta-carotene in, 201, 209, 274;
    and bone status, 254, 256; cooking
    methods for, 37; and dysmenorrhea,
    237; during pregnancy, 293, 301; in
    weight loss diets, 156. *See also
    individual vegetables*
Vegetarian diets, 36, 41, 180, 230, 276
Ventricular arrhythmia, 153
Vertical disease, 3–4, 130, 160, 266
Vinblastine, 203
Vincristine, 203
Vinyl chloride, 207, 334
Vision. *See* Eyes
Vitamin A, 39, 60, 63, 92; and cancer, 209,
    210, 274–275; during pregnancy, 294,
    295–296; and skin problems, 28, 209,
    210, 274, 343; toxicity of, 38, 69, 209,
    210, 274; and vision, 41
Vitamin B (general). *See* B-complex vitamins
Vitamin B-1, 27, 42, 61, 96–97; and brain
    function, 110; children and, 309, 311;

Vitamin B-1 (cont.)
and heartbeat irregularities, 43; and
muscle condition, 43, 296; during
pregnancy, 296, 298; and weight
management, 160; and
Wernicke-Korsakoff syndrome, 243
Vitamin B-2, 27, 42; and aging, 96–97; and
brain function, 113; for children, 312;
during pregnancy, 294, 296; and skin
problems, 44; and tongue condition, 28,
41; and vision, 343; and weight
management, 160
Vitamin B-3 (niacin), 27, 42, 54; and brain
function, 110–111, 112, 113, 316; and
osteoarthritis, 244; during pregnancy,
296; sunburning and, 17; and tongue
condition, 28, 41; toxicity margin with,
70–71
Vitamin B-6, 16, 39, 63, 240; and aging,
96–98; and bone/tooth/gum status, 28,
260, 264–265; and brain function, 110,
111, 113, 114, 119, 316; and carpal
tunnel syndrome, 29–30, 97–98; for
children, 311, 331; and dream recall, 43;
with dysmenorrhea, 236; and heart
disease, 188; and immune system, 273;
with oral contraceptives, 63, 235; during
pregnancy, 296–297, 298, 300, 331–332;
and premenstrual tension, 234; for skin
problems, 17, 30, 44, 343
Vitamin B-12, 36, 45, 235–236; and anemias,
45, 70, 229; and back pain, 42; and
bone/tooth/gum status, 28; and brain
function, 110, 113; and immune system,
273, 277; during pregnancy, 297
Vitamin C, 27–45 passim, 54, 60, 61, 63,
243; and Acquired Immunodeficiency
Syndrome, 283–284; and aging, 92, 98,
99; and bone/tooth/gum status, 19, 28,
41, 258, 259–260, 261; and brain
function, 110, 111, 113, 116, 119, 312,
315–316; and cancer, 201, 210, 211, 213,
215, 216; for children, 312, 315–316,
320, 325; and heart disease, 188–189;
and immune system, 19, 28, 98, 210,
211, 213, 260, 273–274, 277; and iron,
229, 230; and lead, 320, 325; during
pregnancy, 294, 297; for stress, 17;
toxicity margin with, 70; and weight
management, 158
Vitamin D, 60, 63, 99; and bone/tooth/gum
status, 42, 43, 69, 252, 253–254, 261,
262, 264; during pregnancy, 296;
toxicity of, 38, 69, 254
Vitamin E, 46, 54–55, 60, 63; aging pigments
and, 96; and bone status, 260; and

breast fibrocystic disease, 215, 240; and
cancer, 201, 202, 210, 211, 213; for
children, 325; and eye condition, 27;
and heart disease, 189, 213; and
immune system, 275, 276, 277; and lead,
320; and life expectancy, 93; and male
physiology, 242, 244; during pregnancy,
296; toxicity with, 69–70
Vitamin K, 27, 44, 60
Vitamins, 60–62, 68–71, 72, 179; and aging,
92–95; and brain function, 105,
309–310, 311, 312–317; and cancer, 61,
212–214; children and, 309–310, 311,
312–317; and cholesterol, 174; and
immune system, 61, 273–275; during
pregnancy, 293–294, 295–298; and
weight management, 61, 150, 158–159.
See also individual vitamins
Vomiting, 139, 203, 233

Waffles, 33
Waist-to-hip ratio, 27
Walking, 336
Water, drinking: aluminum in, 99, 127;
cadmium in, 187, 217; and cancer, 199,
217–218; chlorinated hydrocarbons in,
199, 218, 344; chromium in, 124; for
fluid balance, 35; fluoride in, 263–264;
purification of, 199, 218; softeners for,
99, 127
Weakness, 112, 139, 312. *See also* Muscle
weakness/pain
Weight, birth, 294
Weight gain diet, 159–160
Weight loss diets, 38, 63, 137, 139, 146–147,
149–159; during pregnancy, 301, 303;
protein deficiency in, 41, 151, 152, 153,
154, 155, 276
Weight management, 18, 29, 38, 130,
133–163; anorexic/bulimic and, 159,
232–233; brain function and, 118, 125,
126, 148, 150; and cancer, 137–138, 211,
332; chromium and, 94; empty-calorie
foods and, 61, 148–149, 150; exercise
and, 147, 150, 155, 156–157, 159, 160,
238, 335; and genetic disposition, 17,
135–136, 137; infant nutrition and, 332;
of menopausal women, 238; and protein,
41, 146–160 passim, 211, 276, 303;
surgery for, 138–139, 335
Weight-to-height ratio, 26–27, 57, 141–142,
160; and arthritis, 98; and cancer,
137–138, 215; and estrogen, 215; and
heart disease, 137, 169; and high blood
pressure, 137; and obesity, 136,
137–138, 146

Wernicke-Korsakoff syndrome, 243
Wheat, 116, 120, 123, 181, 278, 280
Wheat germ, 201
Wheat germ oil concentrate, 129
Wheaties, 64
White blood cells, 211, 271, 274, 277, 278, 280–281; beta-carotene and, 209; chemotherapy and, 203; and heart disease, 174
Why Your Child Is Hyperactive, 321
Williams, Roger, 12
Wilm's tumor, 204
Wine, 136, 214
Women, 63; and anorexia nervosa, 159, 232–233; bone status of, 239, 241, 253, 261, 264; bulimia of, 232–233; and cervical dysplasia, 235–236; exercising by, 237–238, 240, 336; and fibrocystic disease, 215, 239–240; and hypothyroidism, 231–232, 240; and iron, 228–230, 294, 298, 300; lactating, 240, 258, 297; lung cancer in, 207; menopausal/postmenopausal, 238, 240–241, 253, 261; and menstrual cycle, 230, 231, 233–234, 236–239, 336; migraine headaches of, 279; and oral contraceptives, 63, 214–215, 234–235; vitamin B-6 for, 63, 234, 235, 236, 240, 296–297, 298, 300, 331–332. *See also* Estrogens; Ovaries; Pregnancy
World Health Organization, 171
World War II, 59

Xantine compounds, 240
Xanthomas, 44

Yeast, 116, 124, 212, 278. *See also* Brewer's yeast
Yellow fat, 143
Yogurt, 35, 216, 256, 261

Zinc, 19, 20, 41, 43, 60, 63; and bone status, 258, 260–261, 264–265; and brain function, 113, 115, 119; and cadmium, 115, 187; and cancer, 202, 211, 215; and dysmenorrhea, 236; and eye condition, 27, 41; for hair, 41, 276, 282, 343; healing time and, 44, 45, 276, 282; and heart disease, 187–188; and immune system, 19, 98, 202, 211, 260, 275–276, 277, 281–283, 299; for infants, 331; and intestinal disorders, 346; and liver function, 16; and male infertility, 242; with oral contraceptives, 63, 235; during pregnancy, 298, 299–300; and prostatic hypertrophy, 244; and premenstrual tension, 234; and skin problems, 18, 30, 232, 276, 331, 343; smell sense and, 45; taste sense and, 45, 93–94, 232, 282; and thyroid, 17, 28, 146, 159, 231–232; vegetarian deficiency in, 36; and weight management, 146, 159, 160, 211, 232, 233